Population Health

Population Health

Practical Skills for Future Health Professionals

Anne M. Hewitt

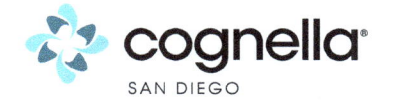

cognella
SAN DIEGO

Bassim Hamadeh, CEO and Publisher
Amanda Martin, Publisher
Amy Smith, Senior Project Editor
Abbey Hastings, Production Editor
Emely Villavicencio, Senior Graphic Designer
Kylie Bartolome, Licensing Coordinator
Ursina Kilburn, Interior Designer
Stephanie Adams, Senior Marketing Program Manager
Natalie Piccotti, Director of Marketing
Kassie Graves, Senior Vice President, Editorial
Jamie Giganti, Director of Academic Publishing

Copyright © 2024 by Cognella, Inc. All rights reserved. No part of this publication may be reprinted, reproduced, transmitted, or utilized in any form or by any electronic, mechanical, or other means, now known or hereafter invented, including photocopying, microfilming, and recording, or in any information retrieval system without the written permission of Cognella, Inc. For inquiries regarding permissions, translations, foreign rights, audio rights, and any other forms of reproduction, please contact the Cognella Licensing Department at rights@cognella.com.

Trademark Notice: Product or corporate names may be trademarks or registered trademarks and are used only for identification and explanation without intent to infringe.

Cover image: Copyright © 2012 iStockphoto LP/porcorex.
Design image: Copyright © 2018 Depositphotos/samart.tiw.

Printed in the United States of America.

This book is designed to provide educational information and motivation to our readers. It is sold with the understanding that the publisher is not engaged to render any type of psychological, legal, diet, health, exercise or any other kind of professional advice. The content of each chapter or reading is the sole expression and opinion of its author, and not necessarily that of the publisher. No warranties or guarantees are expressed or implied by the publisher's choice to include any of the content in this volume. Neither the publisher nor the individual author(s) shall be liable for any physical, psychological, emotional, financial, or commercial damages, including, but not limited to, special, incidental, consequential or other damages. Our views and rights are the same: You are responsible for your own choices, actions, and results and for seeking relevant topical advice from trained professionals.

cognella | ACADEMIC PUBLISHING
320 South Cedros Ave., Ste. 400, Solana Beach, CA 92075

This book is dedicated to all the health management and public health students that I have had the privilege of teaching over the past 30 years. Your enthusiasm, brilliant minds, and friendships have supported me and encouraged the development of a population health text for the next generation of future leaders.

Brief Contents

Preface..xvii
Reviewers xxi

PART I	Populations	1

Chapter 1 Today's Population Health   3

Chapter 2 Focus on Populations: Community, Public, and Global Health Approaches   23

Chapter 3 Public Health Skills for Population Health   51

Chapter 4 Population Health Frameworks   65

PART II	Health	85

Chapter 5 Health Promotion and Wellness for All Populations   87

Chapter 6 Social Determinants of Health: Impact on Population Health   105

Chapter 7 Health for All Populations: Focus on Health Behaviors and Consumerism   129

PART III	Management	147

Chapter 8 Measuring and Assessing Population Health   149

Chapter 9 Risk Management: Population Health's Challenge   165

Chapter 10 Population Health Accountability: Financial and Quality Outcomes   179

Chapter 11 Delivering Population Health Care:
Today's Models   199

| PART IV | Pivoting Toward New Directions | 219 |

Chapter 12 New Population Health Strategies: Patient Engagement and Virtual Care   221

Chapter 13 Today's Challenges and Tomorrow's Opportunities   253

Appendix A: Case Study: The Role of Community Health Needs Assessments for Population Health 281

Glossary 293

Index 307

Detailed Contents

Preface...xvii
Reviewers... xxi

PART I Populations   1

CHAPTER ONE
Today's Population Health   3

Chapter Description   3
Chapter Objectives   4
Key Words   4
What Is Population Health?   4
  Defining Population Health   6
  Discovering Today's Populations   6
  Population Health + Management   8
  Population Health as an Innovation   9
  Why Population Health Management Now?   11
Summary   16
Discussion Questions   17
References   18

CHAPTER TWO
Focus on Populations: Community, Public, and Global Health Approaches   23

Chapter Description   23
Chapter Objectives   24
Key Words   24
Community, Public, and Global Health Approaches   24
Community Health's Population Perspective   28
  Characterizing the Community to Understand the Population   29
  Community Health Workers   30
  Community Health Priorities   31

ix

Community Health Organizations　　32
　　Public Health's Population Perspective　　34
　　　Public Health Achievements　　35
　　　Healthy People 2030　　37
　　　Healthy People 2030: Building a Healthier Future for All　　37
　　　Public Health as a Safety Net　　39
　　Global Health Population Perspective　　41
　　　The World Health Organization　　41
　　　Sustainable Development Goals　　42
　　　Climate Change　　43
　　Summary　　44
　　Discussion Questions　　45
　　References　　45

CHAPTER THREE

Public Health Skills for Population Health　　51

　　Chapter Description　　51
　　Chapter Objectives　　52
　　Key Words　　52
　　Public Health Strategies for Population Health　　52
　　Public Health Tools for Population Health　　53
　　　Exploring Epidemiology　　53
　　　Calculating Disease Rates in Populations　　55
　　Measuring Health Status　　56
　　　Crude and Specific Rates to Characterize Priority Populations　　57
　　Analytical Epidemiology　　58
　　Managerial Epidemiology　　60
　　Summary　　61
　　Discussion Questions　　61
　　References　　62

CHAPTER FOUR

Population Health Frameworks　　65

　　Chapter Description　　65
　　Chapter Objectives　　66
　　Key Words　　66
　　Managing the Health of Populations　　66
　　Key Frameworks for Managing Populations:
　　　The Two Visions　　67

The Triple Aim Vision 67
The Cultural of Health Framework: A Population Health Vision for Communities 69
Collaboration Frameworks for Managing Population Health 70
The Continuum of Collaboration 70
The Collective Impact Framework 71
Implementing Multisectoral Population Health Initiatives 73
Pathways to Population Health Framework 73
Population Health Alliance Framework 74
Summary 79
Discussion Questions 79
References 81

PART II Health 85

CHAPTER FIVE

Health Promotion and Wellness for All Populations 87

Chapter Description 87
Chapter Objectives 88
Key Words 88
Exploring Health Definitions 88
High-Level Wellness and Well-Being 89
Health Assessments for Population Health 92
Healthy Days Measures 92
Health Risk Assessments 93
Population Health Applications of Health Promotion and Disease Prevention 95
Population Health: The Role of Advocacy 96
Expanding the Continuum of Care 98
Health in All Policies 98
Summary 100
Discussion Questions 101
References 101

CHAPTER SIX

Social Determinants of Health: Impact on Population Health 105

Chapter Description 105
Chapter Objectives 106
Key Words 106

Today's American Culture and Population Health   106
Social Determinants of Health   109
The Relationship of SDOH to Population Health Outcomes   112
Population Health Strategies for SDOH   113
The Upstream/Downstream Parable   *113*
Population Health Outcomes and Health Equity   114
Cultural Competence in Population Health   120
Summary   120
Discussion Questions   121
References   122

CHAPTER SEVEN

Health for All Populations: Focus on Health Behaviors and Consumerism   129

Chapter Description   129
Chapter Objectives   130
Key Words   130
Changing Health Behaviors: A Population Health Challenge   130
Health Behavior Population Health Strategies   131
Health Behavior Models   133
  Health Belief Model   *134*
  The Transtheoretical Model   *135*
The Impact of Consumerism   137
Behavior Economics   139
Population Health Strategies to Improve Decision-Making   140
Summary   141
Discussion Questions   142
References   143

PART III Management   147

CHAPTER EIGHT

Measuring and Assessing Population Health   149

Chapter Description   149
Chapter Objectives   150
Key Words   150
The Role of Data and Population Health   150
  Data → Information → Knowledge → Wisdom   *150*
Major Health Informatic Tools for Population Health   152

Health Data Analytics   155
Population Health Data Sources   157
Challenges   158
Summary   160
Discussion Questions   160
References   161

CHAPTER NINE

Risk Management: Population Health's Challenge   165

Chapter Description   165
Chapter Objectives   166
Key Words   166
Introduction to Risk Management   166
  What Is a Health Risk?   166
Risk Management Case Study   168
Risk Management and Personalized Care   174
The Cost and Benefit of Population Health Risk Segmentation   175
Summary   176
Discussion Questions   176
References   177

CHAPTER TEN

Population Health Accountability: Financial and Quality Outcomes   179

Chapter Description   179
Chapter Objectives   180
Key Words   180
Population Health Accountability   180
The Impact of Government Health Plans on Population Health   181
Population Health and Cost of Care   183
New Population Health Payment Models   184
Population Health and Shared Financial Risk   186
Value-Based Payment Options for Health Systems and Providers   186
Population Health's Accountability: Quality, Safety, and Equity of Care   188
  The Relationship Between Quality and Performance   190
  Population Health Practice Example   191
  Population Health: Quality Improvement   192
  Population Health Performance Measures   193
Summary   194
Discussion Questions   195
References   195

CHAPTER ELEVEN

Delivering Population Health Care: Today's Models　　　199

Chapter Description　　199
Chapter Objectives　　200
Key Words　　200
Population Health Strategies to Improve Chronic Care Coordination　　200
　Chronic Care Model　　204
Self-Management of Chronic Disease　　205
Transition-of-Care Model　　206
Implementing Coordinated Care　　207
　Post-Acute Care Strategies of Care　　208
　Back to Walter ...　　208
Frameworks for Integrated Care　　209
　Horizontal and Vertical Integration　　210
Accountable Care Organizations　　211
Patient-Centered Medical Homes　　212
Summary　　213
Discussion Questions　　214
References　　214

PART IV　Pivoting Toward New Directions　　219

CHAPTER TWELVE

New Population Health Strategies: Patient Engagement and Virtual Care　　221

Chapter Description　　221
Chapter Objectives　　222
Key Words　　222
Patient–Health Care Professional Interactions　　222
　Population Health: Reframing the Talk　　224
Patient Engagement and Patient Empowerment　　225
Patient Satisfaction and Patient Experience　　229
　Patient Experience　　230
Virtual Care for Successful "High-Tech" Population Health Outcomes　　231
Aligning Virtual Care With Population Health: Mobile Applications　　233
　Mobile Applications and Patient Engagement　　234
Population Health Virtual Care Decision-Making Strategies　　235
Virtual Care: Population Health Technology Applications　　238

Wearable Technology: Wellness, Monitoring, and PROs   238
Impacting Population Health Management Workflows   242
Virtual Care Challenges   244
Summary   245
Discussion Questions   246
References   246

CHAPTER THIRTEEN

Today's Challenges and Tomorrow's Opportunities   253

Chapter Description   253
Chapter Objectives   254
Key Words   254
Population Health: The Challenges Ahead   254
Introduction to Innovation   259
  A Framework for Innovation: Design Thinking   261
  Step 1: Empathy   262
  Step 2: Define the Problem   263
  Step 3: Ideate   263
  Step 4: Design a Prototype   263
  Step 5: Test the Prototype   264
Reorganizing to Reengineering: New Models for Population Health   264
Transition to Transformation: Collaboration Shifts to the Co-Production of Health   267
Advancing Collaborations to the Co-Production of Health   268
  Population Health and the Co-Production of Health Initiatives   270
Managing Change for Future Population Health Initiatives   271
  Managing Resistance to Change   272
Agile Leadership for Population Health's Future   273
Summary   275
Discussion Questions   275
References   275

Appendix A: Case Study: The Role of Community Health Needs Assessments for Population Health 281

Glossary 293

Index 307

ACTIVE LEARNING

This book has interactive activities available to complement your reading.

Your instructor may have customized the selection of activities available for your unique course. Please check with your professor to verify whether your class will access this content through the Cognella Active Learning portal (http://active.cognella.com) or through your home learning management system.

Preface

For future health professionals, population health stands out as the single most important strategy needed to navigate and excel within today's health sector. Regardless of whether one is serving in a clinical or an administrative role, the knowledge and skills necessary to ensure quality of health for all depend on a thorough understanding of population health. Pre-health students need to enter the field prepared with a strong background *before* they begin their experiential learning. The evident need for an undergraduate textbook propelled me to compile the foundations of population health in a format that would be contemporary, useful, and learner-friendly for all pre-health students.

Divided into four sections, this text answers the following essential questions:

- Why do we focus on "populations"?
- How do we uniquely define *health*?
- Which management strategies ensure the best population health care?
- How will population health change in the future?

Each section carefully addresses relevant topics using chapter introductions and summaries, real-world examples with sample patient scenarios, useful tools and skill applications, quizzes, videos, and personalized self-assessment opportunities to build competencies.

Because population health can be a complex topic, each chapter is designed to present a foundational component followed by easy to understand examples and scenarios. In the first section, students progress through an introduction to population health that clearly identifies the original drivers of change that affected the entire health sector and led to our current strategies for health care delivery. Students also learn to distinguish population health from community, public, and global health as well as how population health is transforming the way care is delivered and why patient outcomes affect today's health payment systems. Within this section, students develop skills for calculating epidemiological rates of disease and death. These skills prepare them to apply key population health "how-to" frameworks for delivering value-based care for all populations.

The second section contains three chapters that deepen the students' understanding of *health* by examining health promotion and wellness strategies and explaining factors such as the social determinants of health and the effect of health disparities on at-risk populations. Students learn population health models including the Health in all Policies and Upstream, Midstream, and

Downstream models. These guidelines and other theories help health professionals encourage positive healthy behaviors in patients and influence consumer decision-making for positive lifestyle choices that can reduce health disparities and create health equity.

The third section challenges students to develop competencies in management as all contemporary health professionals will need to implement population health care and improve patient outcomes. Students will learn to measure and assess population health status by aggregating data from electronic health records and other data sources and using health data analytics to plan and execute population health strategies. A key chapter leads students through the complete health risk management process, beginning with a discussion of risk factor identification and followed by exercises on risk segmentation and stratification strategies and matrices. The final two chapters in the management section emphasize the accountability of population health for improved quality, risk-sharing payment models, and safety mandates. Two contemporary delivery models—accountable care organizations and patient-centered medical homes—are presented as examples of population health care delivery options.

The fourth section, which includes the final two chapters, provides students with important perspectives for meeting the future challenges of the health sector and aligning population health skills. Patient experience skills and the rapid assimilation of virtual care (i.e., telehealth) are two of the emerging areas for population health skill development, and these contemporary concepts, models, and patient strategies are covered in depth to prepare students using the latest technologies. The concluding chapter emphasizes the role of innovation and the three-step process design thinking model. Students discuss the impact of disruptors on the health sector and learn new types of organizational alignments with multisector collaborators as co-producers of health. Skill development includes an introduction to change models and the role of agile leadership to prepare them for the future. This textbook also provides an appendix that contains a case study on the role of community health needs assessments (CHNA) for population health. The case study includes the Association for Community Health Improvement–recommended CHNA process and describes additional concepts and materials, such as community benefit, charity care, the County Health Rankings & Roadmaps tool, and Policy Map, an interactive online mapping tool.

In summary, *Population Health: Practical Skills for Future Health Professionals* covers the complex population health approach in a format that ensures student understanding, skills, and competency development and engages rather than overwhelms the student learner. Instructor resources are available to adopting instructors.

Acknowledgments

I would like to express my gratitude to the gifted and talented individuals at Cognella Publishing, including the following, who, with their continual and collegial support, ensured the success of this text:

- Amanda Martin, Publisher
- Amy Smith, Senior Project Editor
- Abbey Hastings, Production Editor
- Rachel Mann, Instructional Designer
- Haley Brown, Project Editor
- Emely Villavicencio, Senior Graphic Designer
- Tiffany Mok, Senior Content Marketing Specialist

A special thank you to Amanda Martin, whose engagement was truly instrumental in developing all aspects of the manuscript.

Lastly, my appreciation to all my Seton Hall University colleagues who continually provide understanding and empathy, appreciated advice, and unwavering academic humor.

Reviewers

Sharon Bradley, RN, MSN, DNP, CCM, CPHQ, NE-BC
Fairfield University and Sacred Heart University
Fairfield County House and Visiting Nurse & Hospice of Fairfield County-Waveny LifeCare Network

Gloria Ann Browning, PhD, RN
University of Tennessee at Martin

Monica J. Hughes, MSN, RN, NE-BC, CNE
St. David's School of Nursing at Texas State University

Raihan Khan
James Madison University

Jessica Omoregie, PhD
University of Mississippi

Mary Jean Ricci, MSN, RNBC
Drexel University College of Nursing and Health Professions

Pamela Smyth, DNP, RN, CHSE
Ferris State University

Ashley A. White, PhD
Xavier University

ACTIVE LEARNING

This book has interactive activities available to complement your reading.

Your instructor may have customized the selection of activities available for your unique course. Please check with your professor to verify whether your class will access this content through the Cognella Active Learning portal (http://active.cognella.com) or through your home learning management system.

Web-Based Resources: Accessing QR Codes and Links

The author has selected some supporting web-based content for further engagement with the learning material that appears in this text, which can be accessed through QR codes or web links. These codes are intended for use by those who have purchased print copies of the book. You may scan them using a QR code reading app on your cell phone, which will take you to each website. You can also search for the link using a web browser search engine. Readers who have purchased a digital copy of the book can simply click on the hyperlinks beneath each QR code.

Cognella maintains no responsibility for the content nor availability of third-party links. However, Cognella makes every effort to keep its texts current. Broken links may be reported to studentreviews@cognella.com. Please include the book's title, author, and 7-digit SKU reference number (found below the barcode on the back cover of the book) in the body of your message.

Please check with your professor to confirm whether your class will access this content independently or collectively.

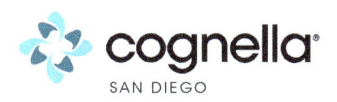

cognella
SAN DIEGO

PART I

Populations

P art I welcomes you to learn about **populations** and why understanding today's health care systems means knowing population health skills and strategies to ensure the well-being and quality of life for all Americans. Population health is an innovative health care delivery approach that differs from community, public, and global health. Chapter 1 starts the learning pathway by defining *population, population health,* and *population health management.* You will learn why unmet population needs such as health disparities helped change the unsustainable medical model (fee-for-service) of health care to a value-based, patient-centered health approach. Chapter 2 provides an overview of the commonalities and differences between the new population health approach and the missions, roles, and activities of community, public, and global health organizations. Topics covered include public health's duty as a safety net provider, the value of community health workers, workplace health, and global health's oversight of climate change. Chapter 3 introduces the basics of descriptive, analytical, and managerial epidemiology that can explain the causes and geographic locations of disease in vulnerable populations. You will learn how data from various epidemiological sources recently helped the health sector identify cases and find at-risk groups during the COVID-19 pandemic. Chapter 4 introduces important population health management frameworks. These how-to guidelines include the Triple Aim®, the American Hospital Association's Pathway to Population Health, and the Population Health Management Framework. For future health professionals, Part I provides a framework for understanding the role of population health.

CHAPTER ONE

Today's Population Health

Chapter Description

This chapter explains the role and purpose of population health and introduces the many events that aligned to form this innovative health care delivery approach. This chapter presents the (1) definitions of populations and population health, (2) important national health events that identified unmet health needs, (3) evolution of population health management as a strategy, (4) five major legislative mandates that served as health sector catalysts, and (5) highlights of the unique characteristics of today's population health. The foundations and development of population health as one of contemporary health care delivery options is covered in this first chapter.

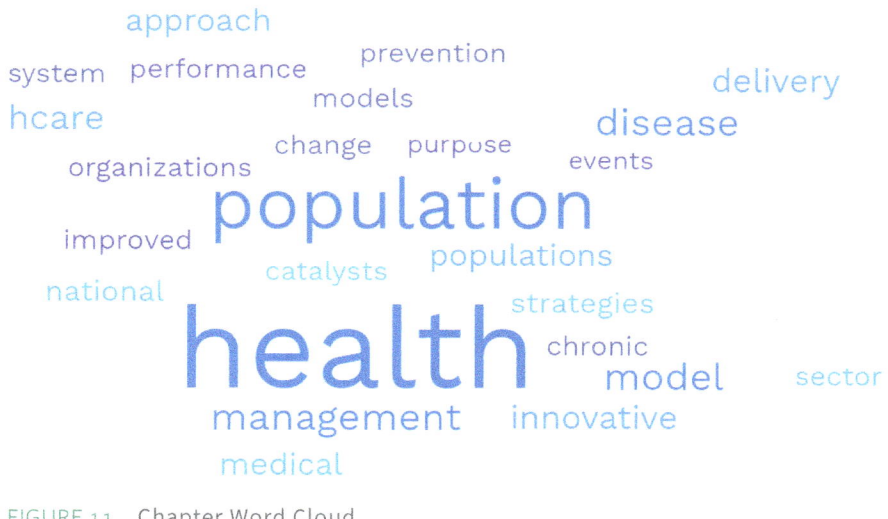

FIGURE 1.1   Chapter Word Cloud

Chapter Objectives

After completing this chapter, students will be able to:

1. Define population health
2. Discuss population health as a strategy for providing health care for all populations
3. Explain three innovative population health strategies that significantly changed the health care delivery system
4. Compare the National Priorities Partnership and the Four Pillars of Population Health Models.
5. Identify the major legislative acts that became catalysts for population health
6. Summarize the major characteristics of population health

Key Words

Accountable care	Health	Morbidity	Population health management
Chronic disease	Health disparities	Mortality	Volume to value
Communicable disease	Health promotion	Pay for performance	
	Hot spotting	Population	
Disease prevention	Medical model	Population health	
Fee-for-service			

Welcome to *Population Health: Practical Skills for Future Health Professionals*!

What Is Population Health?

What is population health? Do not be concerned if you are not yet familiar with a definition for the term. Population health is a relatively new concept for many health professionals, and the definition you learn may depend on who you ask. A survey of hospital and insurance CEOs, payors, consultants, and other health stakeholder leaders revealed that only two out of 37 individuals responded with the same definition for the meaning of *population health* (Pizzi, 2015). What does that suggest for our future population health leaders? Simply, we need to view population health as an emerging field that involves diverse community partners and new types of organizational relationships, which have as a common focus the provision of quality health care for all. One crucial point to remember is that population health is different from public, community, or even global health.

Chapter 2 discusses the commonalities and differences between these various health approaches.

Let's quickly review two basic concepts before exploring not only the various definitions, but also the functions and distinctive characteristics that form the population health approach.

- ***Health*** is one of the very first definitions that preclinical, health administration, and other health profession students' study. The World Health Organization (WHO) defines *health* as the "state of complete physical, mental, and social well-being, and not merely the absence of disease or infirmity" (WHO, 1946). Within this definition is an obvious concern for each person—which is especially important considering this statement was written immediately following the devastation of World War II. The primary emphasis is placed on the individual's right to a healthy life regardless of circumstances.

- ***Population***, a term derived from the late Latin word *populas*, refers to people or multitudes. The unique approach of population health involves not only concentrating on the individual but also considering a population perspective as a health care delivery option as well. We need to understand that populations are not simply composed of single persons, but they also include the context of where people live, work, and play in their local communities (Carlson, 2020).

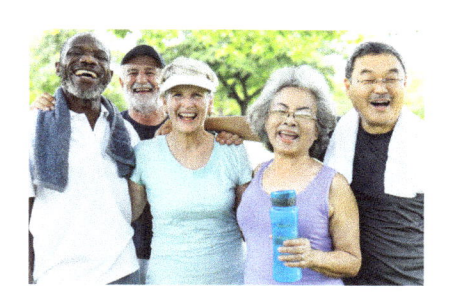

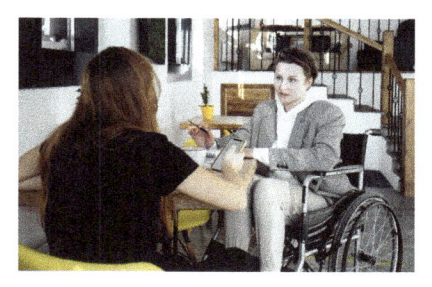

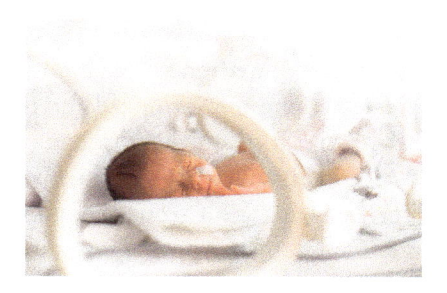

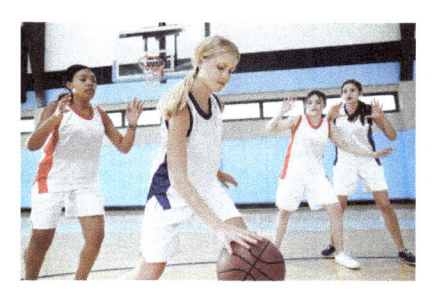

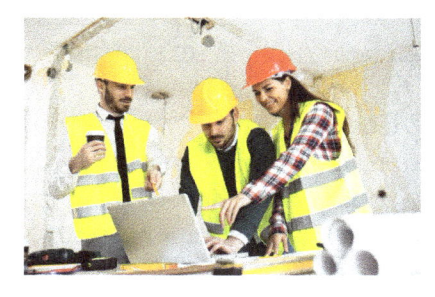

FIGURE 1.2 Today's Populations

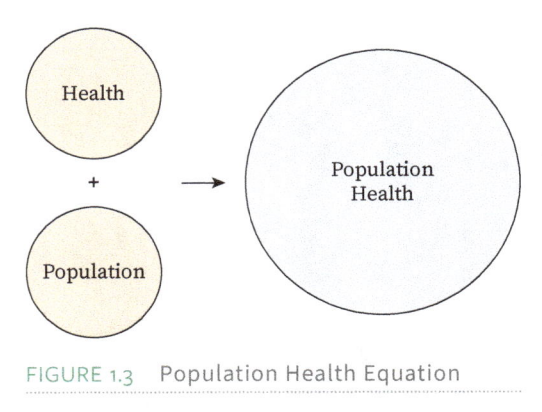

FIGURE 1.3 Population Health Equation

If we combine these two concepts, the resulting health approach is referred to as *population health* (see Figure 1.3).

Although the equation looks simplistic, it has taken many years to encourage America's health system to adopt a population approach. As the WHO's definition of *health* expanded to include the dynamic and changing nature of health over a lifetime and the impact of the external environment on health was recognized, selecting a population health approach slowly became the best option to improve health outcomes.

Defining Population Health

What is a population health approach? What are the outcomes? Who is accountable? Which populations? Who is the payor? Although the idea of population health was introduced in Canada during the 1990s (Coburn et al., 2003), Kindig and Stoddart clearly explained population health's two major contributions as a primary focus on groups (populations) combined with an emphasis on health outcomes (2003). Another commonly cited definition refers to *population health* as a "framework that includes approaches from the social, physical, and biological environments, lifestyle behaviors, and health policy learning domains" (Public Health Agency of Canada, 2001). Population health always uses a group perspective versus focusing on a single individual's health status. Note that population health's twin emphasis on the health and well-being of populations *and* the health outcome provides a critical distinction between population health and public, community, or even global health approaches (Hewitt, 2021). Population health will require partners across many sectors—including public health agencies, health care organizations, community organizations, and local businesses—to integrate investments and policies across all determinants (Kindig, 2015).

Discovering Today's Populations

One of the primary functions of population health entails defining who is the population. Previously, U.S. populations were often described by geographic regions, such as nations, states, municipalities, and communities, or, in the case of local public health agencies, either small mandated, local areas or large metropolitan areas and cities.

Practical Skill: Student Activity

Let's assume the students enrolled in this course will be our population of interest. What do you have in common? What are your differences? Do you have the same level of health? Now imagine that your population is a city such as Buffalo, New York. Wouldn't there be many types of populations in one geographic area? Now read the spotlight below, "The Real World of Hot Spotting," to understand the importance of determining a population's characteristic.

The Real World of Hot Spotting

Most Americans normally seek health care visits with their doctors when they feel ill with unpleasant physical symptoms or require a flu shot or when it is time for a regular checkup. This is a true story of another American subpopulation who, when discovered, caused the health sector to rethink the status quo and helped reinforce the need for population health. In the early 2000s, a young physician practicing in Camden, New Jersey, one of the country's poorest cities, discovered a breakdown in the U.S. health system (Brenner, 2015). Brenner witnessed individuals, often with extreme and multiple medical conditions, continually seek treatment only from local emergency departments because they lacked a primary care provider and/or any type of coordinated care plan. That information led him to start collecting data that linked health care usage and cost by location. In a 6-year time frame, he uncovered evidence that showed that 900 residents living in two specific city blocks, one with a nursing home and another with a housing project, accounted for 4,000 hospital visits and hospital bills totaling $200 million (Gawandi, 2011). Brenner presented a TEDx Talk on health care hot spotting that highlights his personal journey.

Source: Brenner, J. (2015). Healthcare Hot Spotting—Dr. Jeffrey Brenner. YouTube, TEDx Free Library of Philadelphia, February 3, 2015. https://tinyurl.com/mr8nk45k

Brenner's story and amazing findings led to one of the most important aspects of the population health approach: the ability to define and target a population by their needs. The term ***hot spotting*** refers to a strategy designed to identify at-risk subpopulations and lacking a coordinated system of care to manage their chronic illnesses (Caron, 2017). Evidence over the years suggests that just 1% of the American population, or the *super utilizers*, can account for 25% of medical spending, and 5% of the population accounts for nearly half of all annual health care spending in the United States (Cohen, 2009; Ortaliza et al., 2021). Population health will continue to focus on these priority subpopulations to improve health outcomes. Now you know that hot spotting is not just looking for an internet wireless access point!

Let's take the concept of defining a population of interest a little further. Can you identify criteria for defining a population of interest? Find a partner and jot down all the types of populations that you can possibly name! What about athletes, employees, ethnic groups, and disabled persons? Who else?

Population Health + Management

Now that we understand the scope and purpose of population health as system approach, we need to be concerned with strategies to deliver the care. Note that the initial population health approach lacks the third and most critical component: management. In the past, management of institutions, medical practices, state and federal agencies, and public health organizations were separate activities and seen as distinct in many ways with separate missions (Bialek et al., 2020). Therefore, combining the many components of population health requires innovative management. *Management* is simply the process of controlling people and things (Wagner, 2018; Adobe Communications Team, 2019). If population health seeks to provide quality health care for populations, then managing those populations will require business skills to ensure the best health outcomes.

Today's health sector has combined three approaches: **population**-focused care, **health** for all Americans, and innovative **management** strategies to form a stable foundation for the next 20 years of health care. National organizations suggest that population health will require complete structural integration to deliver three major goals: (a) improved health effectiveness, (b) cost-efficiency, and (c) quality of care (Institute for Health Improvement, 2022). These goals, shown in Figure 1.5, emphasize population health's aim to enhance health outcomes for all populations.

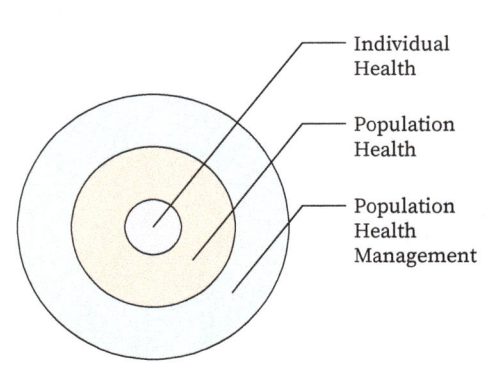

FIGURE 1.4   The Population Health Circle

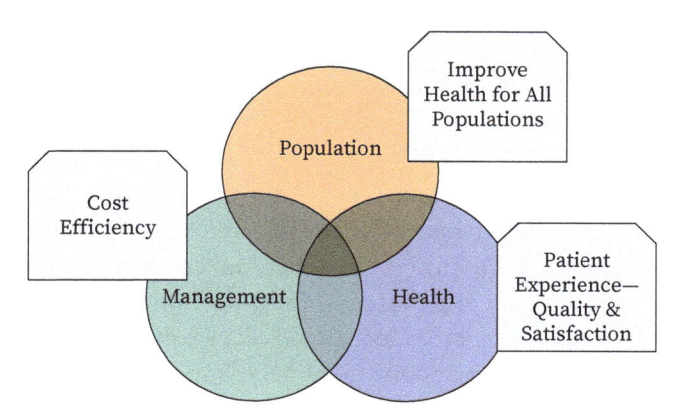

FIGURE 1.5 The Intersection and Functions of Population Health Management

Defining a complex approach such as population health is not an easy task. The American Hospital Association (AHA) recommends a definition that emphasizes clinical health outcomes as a process focused on "improving clinical health outcomes of a defined group of individuals through improved care coordination and patient engagement." The final phrase, "supported by appropriate financial and care models," describes the linkage between management and population health approaches (AHA, n.d.). Another useful definition stresses organizational structure and supervision and refers to *population health* as "healthcare delivery systems to ensure clinically effective, cost effective, and safer health outcomes" (Hewitt, 2021). The population health management strategy depends on an extraordinarily complex set of processes necessary for one of the largest industry sectors in the country to meet the challenges of providing health services for every American.

Population Health as an Innovation

You might be asking yourself, why is this new? Hasn't the health sector always tried to reach these goals? The answer is both yes and no. Of course, optimum health status will always be the goal of our national health system, but the pathways have changed dramatically. The population health approach challenged and continues to transform the standard way of delivering health care in critical areas and distinct ways. Consider the following important examples, which will be discussed in detail in several future chapters.

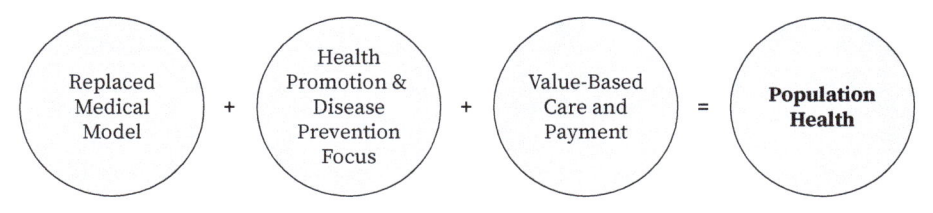

FIGURE 1.6 Population Health Examples of Health Care Changes

- Prior to the emergence of population health, the established medical model framework dominated health care delivery. The **medical model** focuses exclusively on the individual as the organizational center of the entire clinical health care delivery system with an emphasis on treatment as primary and the hospital as the center of healthcare (Medical Model, 2012). Population health integrated the key concept of meeting **populations'** needs and not just focusing on the individual and transformed the health delivery structure by expanding options for how, where, when, and by whom health care was provided. Health care can now be found 24 hours a day and often with no appointment necessary!
- The population health approach also fully integrated two public health strategies, **health promotion** and **disease prevention**, throughout the health system and prioritized their importance as part of holistic health care. Why? In 1900, the major causes of **morbidity** (illness) and **mortality** (death) were pneumonia (influenza), tuberculosis, and gastrointestinal infections, which are all examples of communicable (infectious) diseases (Elflein, 2022). In 2000, national health statistics revealed heart disease, cancer, unintentional injuries, and stroke, all **chronic diseases** or lifestyle related, as the primary reasons for mortality (Ahmad & Anderson, 2021). This dramatic health outcome shift forced the health sector to pivot from an approach that prioritized treating **communicable diseases** to one that stressed lifetime wellness and lifestyle health promotion. Today, one of the busiest buildings on any college campus is the gym and exercise center, and the same can be said for the community senior center.

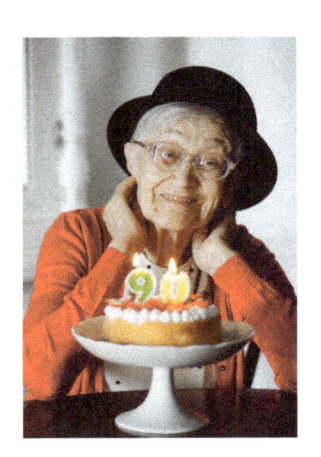

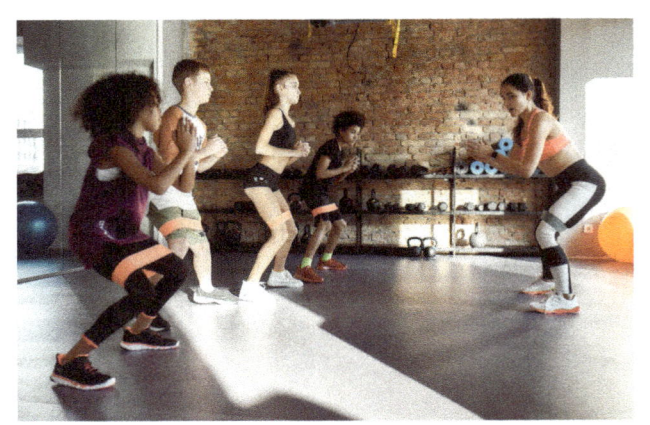

FIGURE 1.7   Health Promotion for All Populations

- The medical model, described above, relied on a traditional **fee-for-service** exchange system. For example, a physician provided a single service, and the health payer then reimbursed the doctor in a fee-for-service exchange system (Healthinsurance.org, n.d.). As you can imagine, the more services that were provided, the greater the income was for both the physician and the sponsoring hospital. The population health approach is to link the payment with the health outcome and not just the provision of treatment. This concept is referred to as ***pay for performance***. Our current health care exchange system continues to make this major transition from a **volume to a value** framework by which health providers are rewarded and incentivized to ensure their patients remain healthy (Buehler et al., 2018). After a visit to a doctor, an urgent care center, or an emergency department, have you ever received a text message asking how well you are doing? That message is linked to a population health–based, cost-effective, value-based approach to health care.

These brief examples highlight a few population health-related changes in health care delivery services, such as integration of lifestyle health promotion and innovative alignment between reimbursement and health outcomes. Why were these transitions in health care delivery required when the United States was known to provide some of the most excellent health care in the world?

Why Population Health Management Now?

In the early 2000s, doubt concerning the quality and sustainability of the entire U.S. health care system became apparent as reports indicated many Americans had unmet health needs in part caused by related social and economic impacts. Health care delivery strategies were fragmented, and various components were siloed and lacked pathways for seamless care (Sperling, 2020). Population health strategies emerged as solutions to alleviate those overwhelming challenges. We can categorize these major health care barriers as either consumer-/patient-oriented or health sector factors as shown in Figure 1.8.

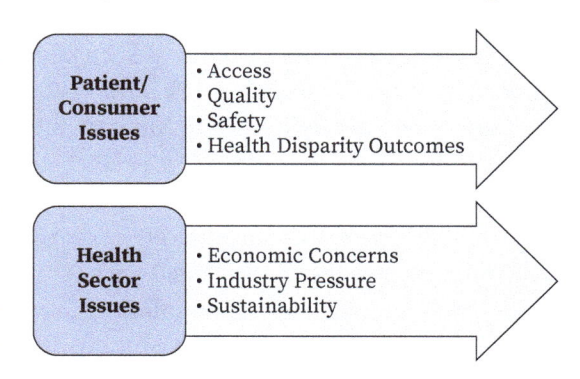

FIGURE 1.8   Patient-/Consumer-Based Unmet Health Needs and Health Sector Concerns

Consumer/Patient Issues

Populations consist of patients who are also consumers, and they may or may not want or have the capability to purchase health insurance. The most pressing and unrelenting unmet health need facing the country for years has been the rising number of uninsured and underinsured in the American population

(Tolbert et al., 2020). Many families within this enormous subpopulation lack access to basic primary care. In 2010, just before population health began its rise as a primary health system delivery model, 48.2 million nonelderly individuals lacked health insurance, and now 10-plus years later, the number has been reduced to 30 million (Finegold et al., 2021). This tremendous decrease has been attributed to legislative initiatives and population health models of care designed for at-risk populations.

In addition to access to care, quality of care emerged as another major concern. An important Institute of Medicine report titled *Crossing the Quality Chasm: A New Health System for the 21st Century* highlighted the enormous variation in health care outcomes (National Academy of Medicine [NAM], 2001). Quality remained an issue when a decade later a study reported that after an inpatient hospitalization, the odds of an individual patient accessing an emergency department within 30 days had increased to one in five, and more than half of these patients were readmitted to the hospital (Brennan et al., 2015). An inherent part of quality care is safety, and in the 1999 Institute of Medicine (IOM) report, *To Err Is Human*, the authors noted that as many as 98,000 patients die from preventable medical errors in U.S. hospitals each year (NAM, 2000). Population health's focus on quality care indicated a clear response to this troubling health sector issue.

The lack of health care access and accountability associated with inadequate quality and safety issues contributed to negative health outcomes across the American population. Of continuing concern are the entrenched **health disparities** among minority groups. Recent statistics show that an African American infant is 14 times more likely to be born premature compared to a White baby's likelihood of nine times (Scommegna, 2021). A 2020 national report from the Office of Minority Health found that 50% of Hispanics develop diabetes in their lifetime and are also 50% more likely to die from the disease than Whites (Hostetter & Klein, 2018). These two dramatic examples illustrate the enormous gap in health care outcomes in our country. The population health approach continues responding to this need with targeted incentives for health systems to improve outcomes for all populations, especially those with special risks.

Major Health Systems and Sector Issues

The nation's health sector also recognized that America's status quo delivery system consisted of sporadic and unconnected care due to health silos. *Health silos* refer to fragmented care in which providers and health organizations do not communicate effectively, and this situation leads to duplication and waste in the system (Sperling, 2019). The economic cost of health care, always a concern, rapidly became a major indicator of an American health system in crisis.

The *gross domestic product (GDP)* is an economic term that refers to the total monetary value of the goods and services produced within the country during a specified time (Business Standard, n.d.). The percentage of GDP attributed to health care escalated from 6.9% in 1970 to 17.7% in 2019 and the percent increase always exceeded that of the general U.S. economy and often by more than a 3% margin (Kurani et al., 2022). Figure 1.9 shows the 2020 GDP percentages spent on education and the military defense (Statista, n.d.; Trading Economics, 2023). Notice the dramatic difference among the total amounts and consider that almost 20% of the economy was spent only on health care, and you can comprehend the concern of health care costs.

GDP Comparisons

Education ■ Military ■ Health ■ Other

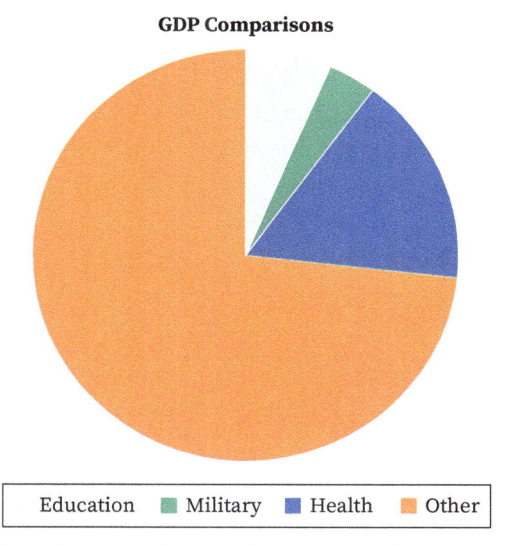

FIGURE 1.9   U.S. 2020 Gross Domestic Product Expenditure Percentage Comparison for Health, Military, and Education Sectors

The second impetus emerged from within the health care industry. Professional health associations, nonprofit health organizations, and health policy experts began to issue reports, recommend calls to action, and develop potential models for population health initiatives. Figure 1.10 presents recommendations from a nationally known group of health care organizations and a recognized health expert in population health.

National Priorities Partnership
- Eliminating Harm
- Eradicating Disparities
- Reducing Illness
- Removing Waste

Four Pillars of Population Health
- Chronic Care Management
- Quality and Safety
- Public Health
- Health Policy

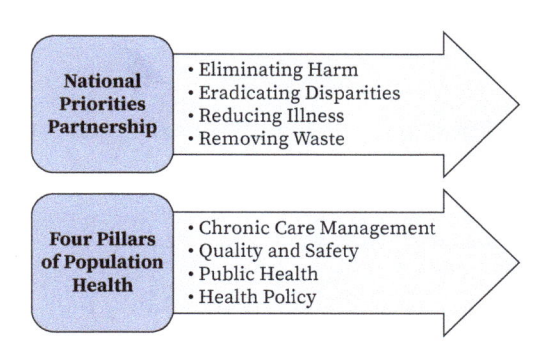

FIGURE 1.10   National Priorities Partnership and Four Pillars of Population Health Models

In 2008, the National Priorities Partnership (NPP), an important group of 50 national health care organizations, proposed four health care challenges. These future aims included strategies that clearly targeted quality, safety, and disparity issues that were already well documented (NPP, 2008). All were designed to encourage movement away from the medical model. Why was this framework so significant? The NPP model represented a consensus among the leading organizations within the health industry and showed an affirmation and approval for moving away from the status quo. A few years later, a recognized population health expert proposed a framework based on four pillars of health that directly aligned key management issues with public health and health policy (Nash, 2012). The innovation within this model was the emphasis on management and the inclusion of legislation (health policy) and public health as a partner. Those pillars reinforced population health's unique strategy of aligning health policy to prioritize public health's emphasis on health promotion and targeting quality and safety of at-risk populations to improve chronic care outcomes.

The combination of patient and consumer unmet needs, increasing industry pressure, and the continuing rise in health care consumption and costs led to thoughtful consideration of the sustainability of the American model of health care. Identification of these challenges was the initial step; the next phase would require support, resources, and guidance to implement change.

Catalysts for Health Care Change

Just as the health experts, policymakers, industry leaders, and nonprofit organizations contributed to the development of a population approach, the federal government produced a series of health policies that both directly and indirectly contributed as change agents for transformation. Figure 1.11, which displays a timeline of the health policy catalysts for change, shows the progression of these important landmark directives and regulations. Notice the brief time frame from 2009 to 2016 when a critical collection of health-related legislation produced tremendous change in the entire industry.

1996—Health Insurance Portability and Accountability Act (HIPAA)

2010—Patient Protection and Affordable Care Affordable Care Act of 2010 (PPACA)

2016—21st Century Cures Act

2009—Health Information Technology for Economic and Clinical Health Act of 2009A (HITECH)

2015—Medicare Access and CHIP Reauthorization Act of 2015 (MACRA)

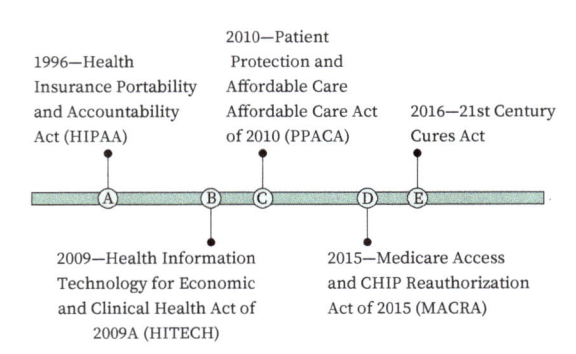

FIGURE 1.11 Five Major Health Policy Catalysts for Change—Timeline

Do you see any similarities in the titles of these federal acts? One apparent theme is access to care as covered in the Health Insurance Portability and Accountability Act of 1996 (HIPAA), the Patient Protection and Affordable Care Act (PPACA), and the Medicare Access and CHIP Reauthorization Act of 2015 (MACRA; Centers for Disease Control and Prevention, 2018; HealthCare.gov, 2010; HIPAA Journal, 2018). Did you guess that the second theme was vulnerable population health issues? Note that MACRA covers Medicare recipients and children (Children's Health Insurance Plan [CHIP]) and the 21st Century Cures Act supports two other subpopulations: those at risk for substance abuse (opioid addiction) and individuals seeking mental health services (American College of Cardiology, 2015; 114th Congress, 2016). Although not obvious by the act's title, the PPACA enabled health care delivery systems' flexibility, the use of health provider incentives, and impetus for major framework change, which allowed population health to become well known and widely adopted. Review Table 1.1 for brief explanations of each of these major legislative works.

TABLE 1.1 The Population Health Alignments With Major Legislation

Federal Legislation Title	Purpose and Impact on Population Health
1996: HIPAA	Expanded in 2000, this law established standards for the electronic exchange, privacy, and security of health information and specifically protected specific data regarding an individual's past, present, or future physical or mental health or condition.
2009: HITECH	One of the first regulations to accelerate the application of health information technology, expectations for quality metrics, and required providers to demonstrate meaningful use from their electronic health records (EHRs).
2010: PPACA	Legislation that generated population health innovations in health promotion policies (community health needs assessments), access and delivery of care initiatives (Medicaid state expansions), new models, and value-based reimbursement frameworks (Medicare Shared Savings Program).
2015: MACRA	Finalized major details on approaches for reimbursing new population health models and is credited with shifting Medicare payments from a fee-for-service to a value-based reimbursement system.
2016: 21st Century Cures Act	Primarily focused on ensuring health information technology delivery related to advancing interoperability, prohibiting information blocking, and enhancing the usability, accessibility, and privacy and security of data.

Practical Skill: PPACA

Given that the health industry in the United States affects the entire population, it is no surprise that it is the most regulated sector by federal, state, and municipal laws (Livni, 2016). Few other health legislation efforts faced political hurdles, scrutiny, and continued legal challenges such as the PPACA (2010). Within the 1,200 pages of the PPACA were both opportunities and innovations that would ensure significant health care delivery transformation (Healthcare.gov, 2010). The three major goals sought to make health insurance more affordable by providing low-income populations with subsidies, increase access by expanding the current Medicaid program to cover more at-risk adults, and provide support and guidance for innovative health care programs and processes (Hewitt, 2021). This legislation hastened the adoption of population health strategies and is considered a major catalyst. Two sections within the PPACA directly affect population health managers and professionals, as they provided mandates and policies that focused on improved patient access and delivery and introduced value-based payment models. See Figure 1.12 for an outline.

Access and Delivery of Care
- Health Insurance Marketplace (Public Exchange)
- Coverage of Preventive Health Services
- Coverage for Annual Medicare Wellness Visit

Value-Based Models
- Accountable Care Organizations Framework
- Medicare Shared Savings Program
- Expanded Medicaid Options for States
- Established the Center for Medicare and Medicaid Innovation

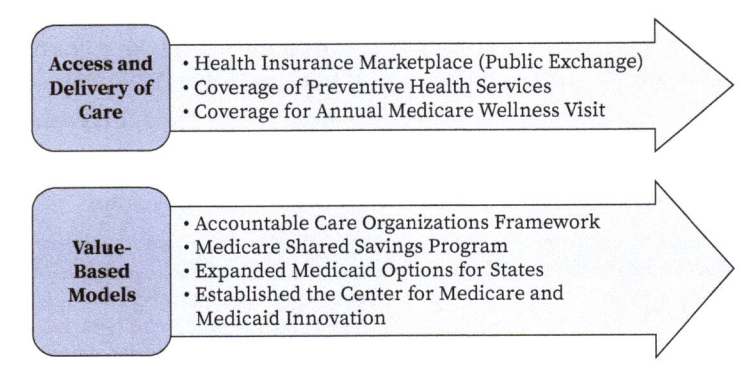

FIGURE 1.12 Access, Delivery of Care, and Value-Based Models From the Patient Protection and Affordable Care Act

Many PPACA-proposed strategies mirrored population health goals that addressed the major unmet health needs of Americans and adopted legislative solutions that built on previous recommendations of health policy experts, health providers and professionals, and major nonprofit organizations. One of the most important aspects of this legislation was the emphasis on **accountable care**. More than a decade later, the concept of accountable care (moving from fee-for-service care to value-based care) continues as the central core of contemporary and future health care delivery systems (Bleser et al., 2023). Another PPACA major accomplishment was the establishment of the Center for Medicare and Medicaid Innovation, which supports development of accountable health communities that assess patients' unmet social needs as well as their clinical health status (Centers for Medicare & Medicaid Services, 2017). The impact and results of the PPACA are still being debated, but its primary role for population health management continues (Jha, 2019).

All five of these major health policies encouraged population health development and adoption by providing targeted initiatives designed to solve both consumer patient issues of access and cost as well as health sector operational and technical challenges for improved health care.

Summary

Although population health as a major health sector approach is recognized today, it requires us to examine the past journey and contemplate the pathway for the future of the 21st century's most recognized health care delivery model to date. Population health emerged as an innovative solution to the American health system in crisis because it focused on integrating three distinct strategies of health, populations, and management to produce improved health outcomes. The serious health challenges of access, quality, and cost led to an innovative approach that valued health care effectiveness, cost-efficiency, and quality of care. The drivers of change that influenced population health as we know it today involved many diverse stakeholders, including health policy experts, major nonprofit organizations, national coalitions of health professional organizations, and consumers and patients. Together, they produced national reports, frameworks, and strategies to provide useful models. Given the rise of technology that paralleled the developing population health approach, it is not surprising that much of the major health policy legislation developed between 2000 and 2016 aligned technological advances with improved health care processes. Population health continues to focus on three major health care delivery system changes: expanding the health care delivery options to meet all population needs, transitioning health care from the hospital to the community with an emphasis on health promotion, and providing an innovative volume-to-value payment model that rewards health providers and organizations for improved health outcomes. Today's health sector has combined three approaches—**population**-focused care, **health** for all Americans, and innovative **management** strategies—to form a stable foundation for the next 20 years of health care. **Population health** is the future for today's and tomorrow's health professionals.

Discussion Questions

1. Discuss the population health figure presented in Figure 1.3. Why hadn't the American health system combined these elements before? Why has population health, a new health care delivery approach, become so powerful?
2. Take the time to read Atul Gawandi's article *The Hot Spotters* in the January 24, 2011, issue of the *New Yorker* at https://tinyurl.com/4sakxvtz. The premise of the article ("Can we lower medical costs by giving the neediest patients better care?") aligns exactly with population health's approach of identifying vulnerable populations to improve health outcomes. Today we also hear about "cold spotting." What would this strategy look like, and what would be the purpose? Does it fit within population health?

3. Identify at least three major components of population health that were different and unique from the previous health approaches.
4. Describe why all the following terms are relevant to population health: fee-for-service, medical model, pay-for-performance, accountable care, and value to volume.
5. Over time, the PPACA has provided many innovative ideas and frameworks for improving health outcomes. Discuss the three access and delivery of care innovations that were based in the legislation.
6. Technology served as a solid foundation to support the adoption of population health. Which of these three legislative acts do you think contributed the most to better health delivery processes: HIPPA, HITECH, or MACRA? Please provide one example as part of your rationale.
7. Compare the National Priorities Partnership Model and the Four Pillars of Population Health. How do they differ? What elements do they share?

References

114th Congress. (2016). *H.R. 34: 21st Century Cures Act*. https://www.congress.gov/bill/114th-congress/house-bill/34

Adobe Communications Team. (2019, March 18). *What is control management? Why is it essential?* Workfront Blog. https://www.workfront.com/blog/what-control-management-and-why-it-essential

Ahmad, F., & Anderson, R. (2021). The leading causes of death in the U.S. for 2020. *Journal of the American Medical Association, 325*(18), 1829–1830. https://jamanetwork.com/journals/jama/fullarticle/2778234

American College of Cardiology. (2015, April 28). *Medicare Access and CHIP Reauthorization Act of 2015 (MACRA): What you need to know*. https://www.acc.org/latest-in-cardiology/articles/2015/04/28/15/59/medicare-access-and-chip-reauthorization-act-of-2015-what-you-need-to-know#:~:text=On%20April%2016%2C%202015%2C%20President,quality%20reporting%20programs%20into%20one

American Hospital Association. (n.d.). *What is population health management?* https://www.aha.org/center/population-health-management

Bakshi, S. (2021). The essential role of population health during and beyond COVID-19. *American Journal of Managed Care, 27*(3), 123–128. https://doi.org/10.37765/ajmc.2021.88511

Bialek, R., Moran, J., Amos, K., & Lamers, L. (2020). *Cross-sector collaboration: Making partnerships work for your community public health foundation* (p.36). Public Health Foundation. https://www.phf.org/events/Pages/Cross_Sector_Collaboration_Making_Partnerships_Work_for_Your_Community.aspx

Bleser, W., McStay, F., & Muhlestein, D. (2023). Accountable care in 2023: Evolving terminology, current state, and priorities. *Health Affairs*, February 24, 2023. https://www.healthaffairs.org/content/forefront/accountable-care-2023-evolving-terminology-current-state-and-priorities?utm_medium=email&utm_source=hat&utm_campaign=forefront&utm_content=hat+2+24+2023&utm_term=aco+series&vgo_ee=7zjVhjEBDJ9hKDOcqHBj%2F7TV8qsFUfI%2F1ISxnX2Ui4c%3D

Brenner, J. (2015, February 3). *Healthcare hot spotting—Dr. Jeffrey Brenner.* YouTube, TEDx Free Library of Philadelphia. https://www.youtube.com/watch?v=AGJ7g9ilIvU

Brennan, J., Chan, T., Killeen, J. & Castillo, E. (2015). Inpatient readmissions and emergency department visits within 30 days of a hospital admission. *Western Journal of Emergency Medicine*, 16(7), 1025–1029. https://www.ncbi.nlm.nih.gov/pmc/articles/PMC4703150/

Buehler, J., Snyder, R., Freeman, S., Carson, S. & Ortega, A. (2018). It's not just insurance: The Affordable Care Act and population health. *Public Health Reports*, 133(1), 34–38. https://www.ncbi.nlm.nih.gov/pmc/articles/PMC5805102/

Business Standard. (n.d.). *What is gross national product (GDP)?* https://www.business-standard.com/about/what-is-gross-domestic-product-gdp

Caron, R. (2017). Principles of population health management. In R. Caron, *Population health: Principles and applications for management* (pp. 287–300). HAP/AUPHA.

Carlson, L.M. (2020). Health is where we live, work and play –And in our Zip codes: Tackling social determinants of health. *The Nation's Health*, 50(1), 3. http://www.thenationshealth.org/content/50/1/3.1

Centers for Disease Control and Prevention. (2018, September 14). *Health Insurance Portability and Accountability Act of 1996*. https://www.cdc.gov/phlp/publications/topic/hipaa.html

Centers for Medicare & Medicaid Services. (2017, June 23). *About the CMS Innovation Center*. https://innovation.cms.gov/About/index.html

Chandra, A., Acosta, J., Carman, K. G., Dubowitz, T., Leviton, L., Martin, L. T., Miller, C., Nelson, C., Orleans, T., Tait, M., Trujillo, M., Towe, V., Yeung, D., & Plough, A. L. (2017). Building a national culture of health: Background, action framework, measures, and next steps. *RAND Health Quarterly*, 6(2), 3. https://www.ncbi.nlm.nih.gov/pmc/articles/PMC5568157/

Coburn, D., Denny, K., Mykhalovskiy, E., McDonough, P., Robertson, A., & Love, R. (2003). Population health in Canada: a brief critique. *American journal of public health*, 93(3), 392–396. https://doi.org/10.2105/ajph.93.3.392

Cohen, S. B. (2009, February). *The concentration of health care expenditures and related expenses for costly medical conditions, 2009*. Agency for Healthcare Research and Quality. https://meps.ahrq.gov/data_files/publications/st359/stat359.pdf

Cordani, D. (2020). *Healthcare is on an unsustainable trajectory*. Modern Healthcare, February 29, 2020. https://www.modernhealthcare.com

Elflein, J. (2022). *Major causes of death in the U.S.: 1900 and 2020*. Statista, January 21, 2022. https://www.statista.com/statistics/235703/major-causes-of-death-in-the-us/#:~:text=In%201900%2C%20pneumonia%20and%20influenza,202%20deaths%20per%20100%2C000%20population

Finegold, K., Conmy, A., Chu, R., Bosworth, A., & Sommer, B. (2021). *Issue brief: Trends in uninsured U.S. population 2010–2020*. ASPE/Office of Health Policy, February 11, 2021. https://aspe.hhs.gov/sites/default/files/private/pdf/265041/trends-in-the-us-uninsured.pdf

Gawandi, A. (2011). The hot spotters. *New Yorker, 86*(45), 40–51.

HealthCare.gov. (2010). *Patient Protection and Affordable Care Act*. https://www.healthcare.gov/glossary/patient-protection-and-affordable-care-act/

Healthinsurance.org. (n.d.). *Fee for service. What is fee-for-service?* Healthinsurance.org. https://www.healthinsurance.org/glossary/fee-for-service/

Hewitt, A. (2021). Population health management: A framework for the health sector. In A. Hewitt, J. Mascari, & S. Wagner (Eds.), *Population health management: Strategies, tools, applications, and outcomes* (pp. 3–20). Springer Publishing Company.

HIPAA Journal. (2018). *What is the HITECH Act?* https://www.hipaajournal.com/what-is-the-hitech-act/

Hostetter, M., & Klein, S. (2018). *In focus: Identifying and addressing health disparities among Hispanics*. The Commonwealth Fund, December 27, 2018. https://www.commonwealthfund.org/publications/2018/dec/focus-identifying-and-addressing-health-disparities-among-hispanics#:~:text=Hispanics%20make%20up%20the%20largest,than%20non%2DHispanic%20white%20residents

Institute for Health Improvement. (2022). *The IHI Triple Aim*. http://www.ihi.org/Engage/Initiatives/TripleAim/Pages/default.aspx

Jha, A. (2019, August 6). Population health management: Saving lives and saving money? *Journal of the American Medical Association, 322*(5), 390–391. https://jamanetwork.com/journals/jama/fullarticle/2740704

Kindig, D. (2015). What are we talking about when we talk about population health? *Health Affairs*, April 6, 2015. https://www.healthaffairs.org/do/10.1377/forefront.20150406.046151

Kurani, N., Ortaliza, J., Wager, E., Lucas, F., & Amin, K. (2022). *How has U.S. spending on healthcare changed over time?* Health System Tracker. Peterson-Kaiser Family Foundation, February 25, 2022. https://www.healthsystemtracker.org/chart-collection/u-s-spending-healthcare-changed-time/#:~:text=Health%20spending%20growth%20has%20outpaced%20growth%20of%20the%20U.S.%20economy&text=In%201970%2C%206.9%25%20of%20the,to%2017.7%25%20of%20the%20GDP

Livni, E. (2016). *Regulation nation: What industries are most carefully overseen?* FIND-LAW, February 8, 2016. https://www.findlaw.com/legalblogs/small-business/regulation-nation-what-industries-are-most-carefully-overseen/

Medical Model. (2012). *Farlex partner medical dictionary*. https://medical-dictionary.thefreedictionary.com/medical+model

Mineo, L. (2020). *The lesson is never to be forgotten.* Harvard Gazette, May 19, 2020. https://news.harvard.edu/gazette/story/2020/05/harvard-expert-compares-1918-flu-covid-19/

Nash, D. B. (2012). *The population health mandate: A broader approach to care delivery.* The Four Pillars of Health in a Boardroom Press Special Edition. http://populationhealthcolloquium.com/readings/Pop_Health_Mandate_NASH_2012.pdf

National Academy of Medicine. (2000). *To err is human: Building a safer health system.* National Academies Press.

National Academy of Medicine. (2001). *Crossing the quality chasm: A new health system for the 21st century.* National Academies Press.

National Priorities Partnership. (2008). *National priorities and goals: Aligning our efforts to transform America's healthcare.* National Quality Forum. http://www.qualityforum.org/Setting_Priorities/National_Priorities_Partnership_-_Call_for_Organizational_Nominations.aspx

Numerof, R. (2020). 5 population health statistics bound to change because of COVID-19. *Forbes,* August 19, 2020. https://www.forbes.com/sites/ritanumerof/2020/08/19/5-population-health-statistics-bound-to-change-because-of-covid-19/#5cff63115cf9

Ortaliza, J., McGough, M., Wager, E., Claxton, G., & Amin, K. (2021). *Health spending: How do health expenditures vary across the population?* Kaiser Family Foundation, November 12, 2021. https://www.healthsystemtracker.org/chart-collection/health-expenditures-vary-across-population/#:~:text=Just%201%20percent%20of%20the,for%20health%20services%20in%202019

Pizzi, R. (2015). *Defining population health.* Healthcare IT News, May 23, 2015. https://www.healthcareitnews.com/blog/defining-population-health#:~:text=The%20concept%20of%20population%20health,the%20measurement%20of%20health%20outcomes

Public and Population Health Branch/Strategic Policy Directorate. (July 2001). *The Population Health Template: Key Elements and Actions that Define a Population Health Approach.* Health Canada. https://www.phac-aspc.gc.ca/ph-sp/pdf/discussion-eng.pdf

Riley, R. (2010). *Health starts where we learn.* Robert Wood Johnson Foundation, October 19, 2010. https://www.rwjf.org/en/library/research/2010/10/health-starts-where-we-learn.html

Scommegna, P. (2021). *High premature birth rates among U.S. black women may reflect the stress of racism and health and economic factors.* Population Reference Bureau, January 21, 2021. https://www.prb.org/resources/high-premature-birth-rates-among-u-s-black-women-may-reflect-the-stress-of-racism-and-health-and-economic-factors/

Statista. (n.d.). *Healthcare and military expenditure as a percentage of GDP in select countries worldwide in 2020.* https://www.statista.com/statistics/1175077/healthcare-military-percent-gdp-select-countries-worldwide/

Stiefel, M., & Nolan, K. (2012). *A guide to measuring the Triple Aim: Population health, experience of care, and per capita cost.* Institute for Healthcare Improvement Innovation Series white paper. http://www.ihi.org/resources/Pages/IHIWhitePapers/AGuidetoMeasuringTripleAim.aspx

Tolbert, J., Orgera, K., & Dammico, A. (2020). *Key facts about the uninsured population.* Kaiser Family Foundation, November 6, 2020. https://www.kff.org/uninsured/issue-brief/key-facts-about-the-uninsured-population/

Trading Economics. (2023). *United States—Public spending on education, total (% of GDP).* https://tradingeconomics.com/united-states/public-spending-on-education-total-percent-of-gdp-wb-data.html

Wagner, S. (2018). *Fundamentals of Medical Practice Management.* HAP/AUPHA. (p.256).

World Health Organization (WHO). (1946). *Constitution of the World Health Organization.* https: www.who.int/about/who-we-are/constitution

Credits

Fig. 1.1: Generated with FreeWordCloudGenerator.com.
Fig. 1.2a: Copyright © 2016 Depositphotos/Rawpixel.
Fig. 1.2b: Copyright © 2021 Pexels/SHVETS production.
Fig. 1.2c: Copyright © 2016 Depositphotos/Ondrooo.
Fig. 1.2d: Copyright © 2018 Depositphotos/monkeybusiness.
Fig. 1.2e: Copyright © 2017 Depositphotos/didesign.
Fig. 1.7a: Copyright © 2019 Depositphotos/zzzdim.
Fig. 1.7b: Copyright © 2020 Depositphotos/LanaStock.
Fig. 1.9: Source: Adapted from https://www.statista.com/statistics/1175077/healthcare-military-percent-gdp-select-countries-worldwide/; https://tradingeconomics.com/united-states/public-spending-on-education-total-percent-of-gdp-wb-data.html.
Fig. 1.13a: Source: https://commons.wikimedia.org/wiki/File:1918_flu_in_Oakland.jpg.
Fig. 1.13b: Copyright © 2017 Depositphotos/sudok1.

CHAPTER TWO

Focus on Populations

Community, Public, and Global Health Approaches

Chapter Description

The second chapter introduces three unique perspectives that differ but often complement: population health strategies. Beginning with an introduction to the social-economic model, which serves as a conceptual foundation, each of these three health perspectives is examined for purpose, functions, and unique contributions for improving health care for the American population. The chapter explains (1) the community health approach and the importance of local healthscapes; (2) public health's emphasis on safety net, assessment, and assurance priorities; and (3) global health's impact and increased significance for all populations. Understanding these three unique approaches enables population health managers to reduce duplication in health services and target current gaps in care.

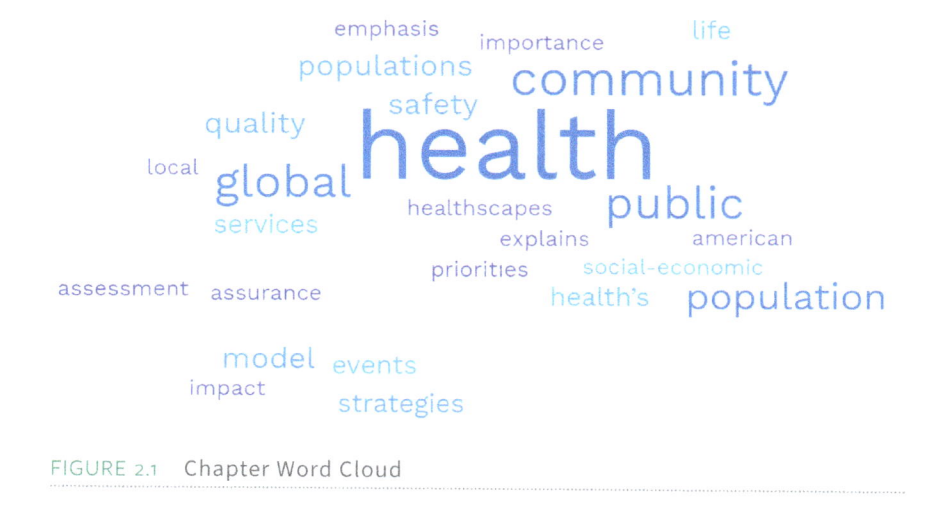

FIGURE 2.1 Chapter Word Cloud

Chapter Objectives

After completing this chapter, students will be able to:

1. Describe the social ecological model as a framework for health
2. Compare and contrast community, public, global, and population health approaches
3. List factors that can influence a community's health
4. Explain public health's role as a safety net provider
5. Summarize the primary functions of global health organizations

Key Words

Community health

Community health worker

Global health

Healthscape

Public health

Quality of life

Socio-ecological model

Workplace health

Community, Public, and Global Health Approaches

What is a **healthscape**? Is it similar to a landscape? The answer is both yes and no. A healthscape is not only the situation where you are, but also the related trends in health care that accompany a particular setting (WordBueno, n.d.). More than just physical location, a healthscape includes the entire health care environment where you live. One of the defining hallmarks of population health is the focus on populations living within these healthscapes. Only population health organizations have the option to strategically select their priority populations, unlike the other major health approaches. **Community**, **public**, and **global health** all have predetermined populations of interest. This chapter describes characteristics of these three health perspectives, highlights the strengths of each, and provides contemporary examples of their successes.

Population health managers use a social-ecological framework to understand and explain the various healthscapes of community, public, and global health populations. A **socio-ecological model** depicts the potential scope of factors that influence health and well-being at each population level (see Figure 2.3).

Each level of the model progresses from a smaller to a larger group as size is a major factor, and health and wellness activities are often designed based on population size. For example, the U.S. Department of Agriculture's (USDA) My Plate campaign was designed for all Americans (USDA, n.d.). The USDA

Chapter Two Focus on Populations | 25

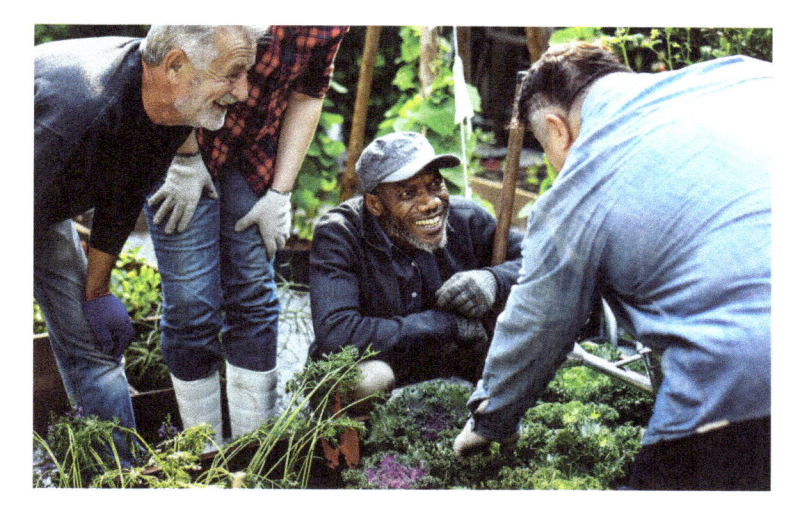

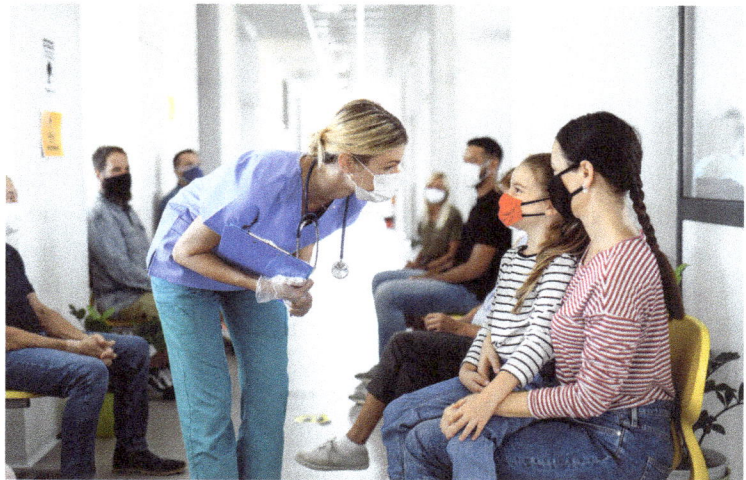

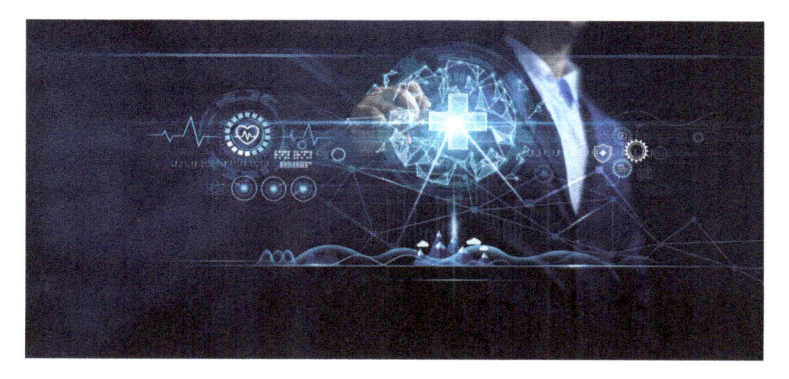

FIGURE 2.2 Community, Public, and Global Health Perspectives: Community Health Gardens, Public Health Vaccines, and Global Health's Impact

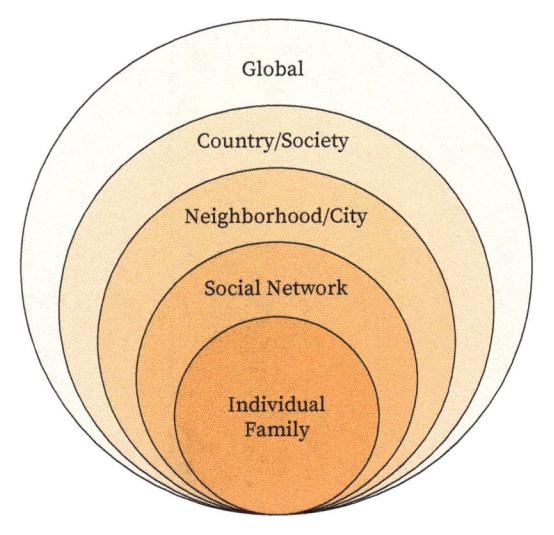

FIGURE 2.3 A Socio-Ecological Framework Model for Priority Populations

developed an easy-to-understand visual aid that appealed to all age groups regardless of their dietary or cultural preferences. Ecological models exist within social contexts and can help identify potential relationships between individuals. Notice that the second level in the model uses the term social network instead of group. A social network represents a special relationship between two or more people while a group is simply two or more individuals. An excellent example of a health approach that targets a subpopulation (e.g., smokers) is the smoking-cessation initiative Tips From Former Smokers (Centers for Disease Control and Prevention [CDC], n.d.). This is a health campaign using a group-level strategy by focusing on smokers and their social networks to serve as a support system for changing behavior. The South End Healthy Boston Coalition is a health intervention example at the city level. This neighborhood health organization includes diverse residents, local leaders, social service providers, and community agencies, which are all aligned to improve not only the health status, but also the safety and quality of life in the South End community (South End Healthy Boston Coalition, n.d.).

Practical Skill: Student Activity

Social networks influence all persons, regardless of age, location, or health status. What is your social network? How many groups do *you* belong to? Remember that groups can be both formal and informal.

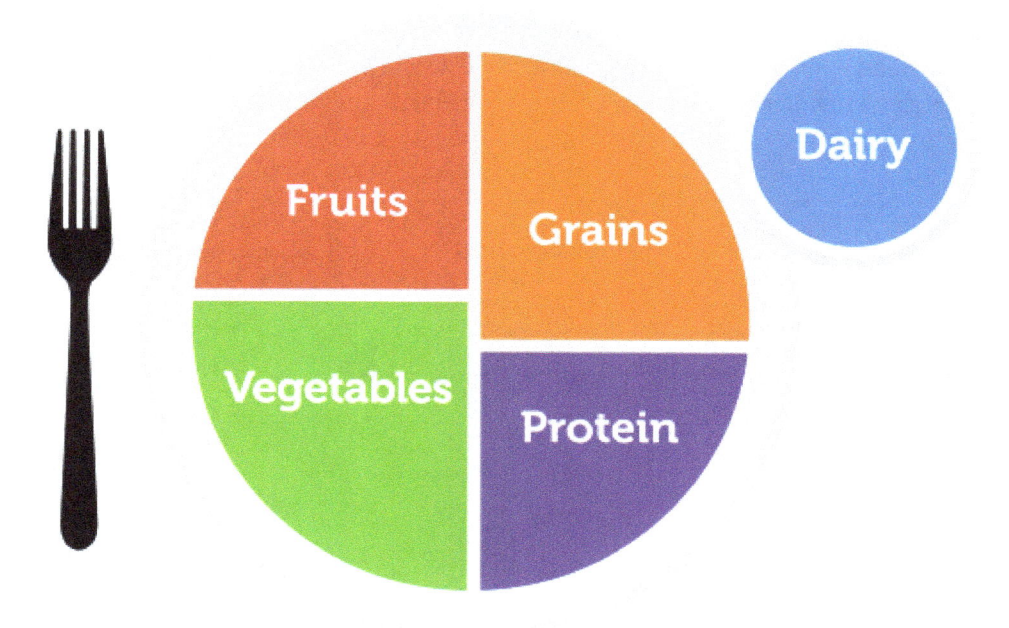

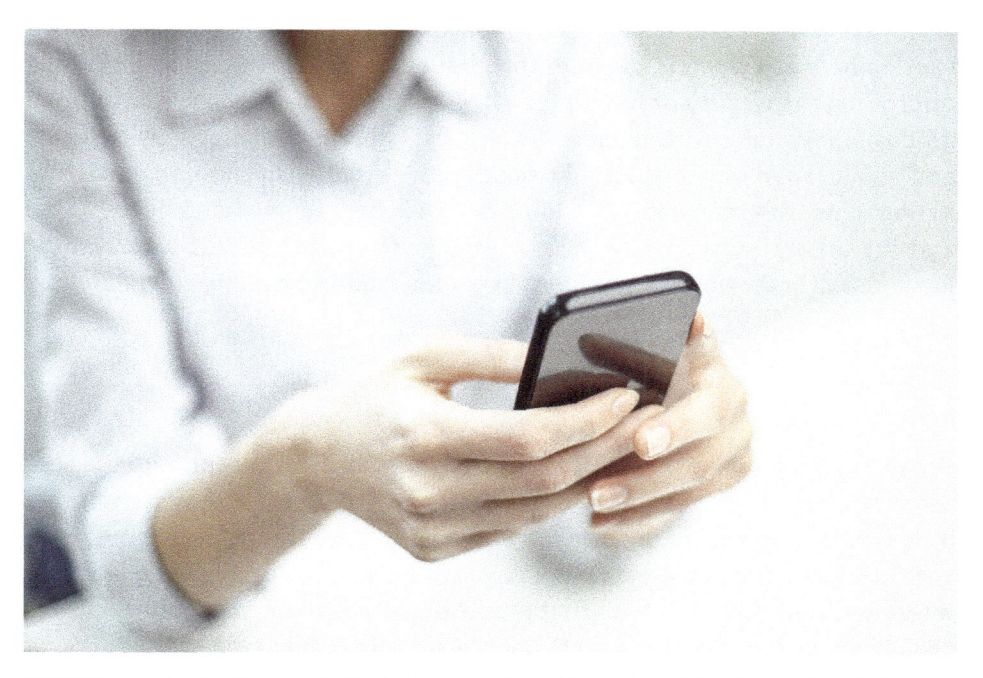

FIGURE 2.4 Socio-Economic Model Intervention Examples: What Is My Plate? Tips From Former Smokers

Community, public, and global health strategies focus on efforts that impact a specified population within a geographic location. Let's also review definitions of each health perspective and then compare with our framework model (see Figure 2.5).

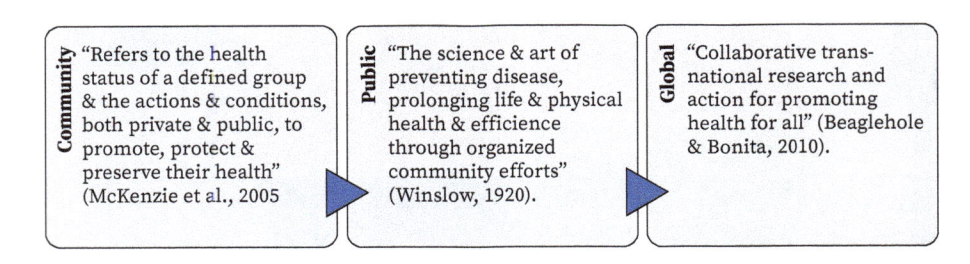

Community	Public	Global
"Refers to the health status of a defined group & the actions & conditions, both private & public, to promote, protect & preserve their health" (McKenzie et al., 2005	"The science & art of preventing disease, prolonging life & physical health & efficiency through organized community efforts" (Winslow, 1920).	"Collaborative transnational research and action for promoting health for all" (Beaglehole & Bonita, 2010).

FIGURE 2.5   Community, Public, and Global Health Definitions

Could you make the connection between the social-ecological model and the three health approach definitions? Together, they should help you visualize the role of each type of population approach.

Not all benefits and advantages of these approaches are obvious, and the overlap between them is considerable, but each of them serves a purpose in improving the quality of health for all. Community health serves a defined group of individuals within a specific locality. Public health moves up the scale and includes not only local public health offices, but also state, regional and national health organizations. Global health is best represented by the WHO and the suborganizations engaged in improving health for all of humanity. Review each of the three descriptions below for a more complete understanding.

Community Health's Population Perspective

Community health is not as well-known as public health, but communities are where we live, work, and play—in other words, they are home. A community is defined as "a group of people who have common characteristics" and those characteristics can include location, race, ethnicity, age, occupation, education, interests, and other diverse attributes (Chegg, n.d.). Often, a community is referenced by its geographic area, but size can also determine a population of interest as in the case of a city or a suburb. Public health populations of interests are defined by each state, and global health has no physical boundary, so they differ from community health.

Since communities vary in size and location, health experts often view community health with a social perspective that helps us better understand the populations by using terms such as specific interests, relationships, concerns, and values (Joint Committee on Health Education and Promotion Terminology, 2012). One common model identifies six socio-ecological characteristics (Seabert et al., 2022). Figure 2.6 shows common socio-ecological attributes, including mutual influence, shared needs, commitment, shared emotional connection, membership, common symbol systems, and shared value of norms.

For example, a community might be a group of residents or a neighborhood who are interrelated in their work, life, and play and share a concern because of common values for the health and welfare of each other. Perhaps they are concerned about the safety of their children walking to school or a lack of playgrounds or greenspaces. They feel one of their neighborhoods has become a haven for drug dealers or that their community is becoming overbuilt with too many homes for the transportation infrastructure. The defining key characteristic can be complex, but the shared linkage is strong enough to form them into an active group seeking well-being for all.

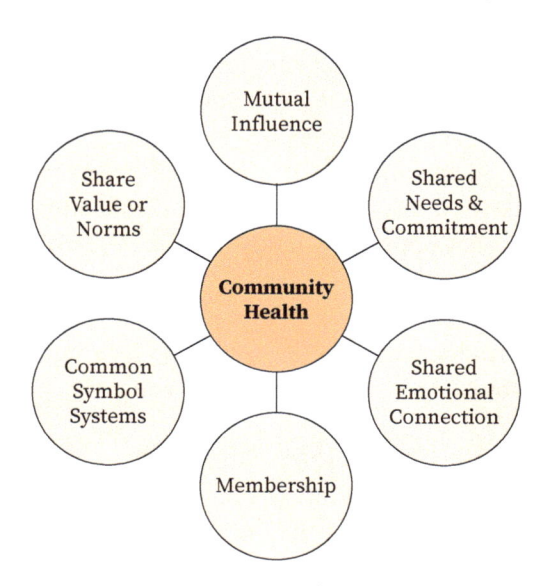

FIGURE 2.6 Community Characteristics From a Socio-Ecological Perspective

Characterizing the Community to Understand the Population

The Lexington Minuteman is a life-sized bronze figure of a colonial farmer with musket, and it stands at the southeast corner of the Lexington Battle Green, facing the route of the British advance. The man atop the fieldstone base was supposed to depict Captain John Parker, leader of the Lexington militia in 1775. The actual Minutemen were an elite subset of this group, young, fit, and able to respond quickly (Lexington Visitors Center, n.d.).

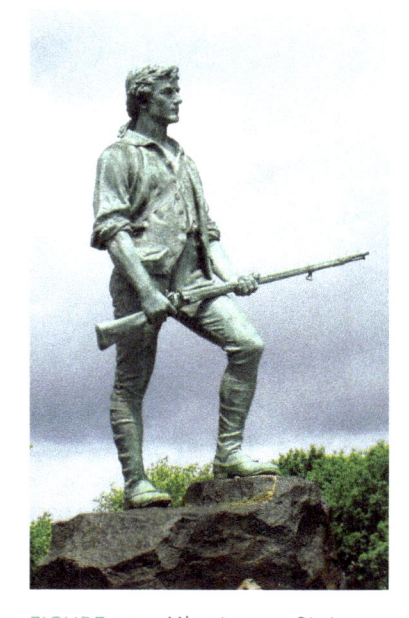

FIGURE 2.7 Minuteman Statue

Complete a quick review of the Lexington, Massachusetts, community (Town of Lexington, n.d.). Can you find one example for each of the six characteristics outlined in Figure 2.6?

Community health, like population health, always seeks to meet the specific needs of the priority population, and often relies on individuals who reside in the area. **Community health workers** (CHWs) are trained individuals (laypersons) who live in the same community and serve as connectors to link group members with available health providers and services (Pérez & Martinez, 2008). CHWs provide outreach to vulnerable community members who may not trust other sources for their health care concerns.

Community Health Workers

CHWs are valuable to the organization of any health system as they can bring understanding and familiarity with the culture and context of the community (Harvey & Fernandez, 2012). Because they are trusted front-line workers, they often advocate and provide outreach to connect at-risk groups with local health promotion programs (American Public Health Association, n.d.). Underserved community members trust CHWs to help advocate for care if they lack certain capabilities as they know CHWs live in their neighborhoods (Eliana, 2022). CHWs may also be known as *Promotores de salud,* or *promotoras,* which is the Spanish term for *community health workers.* The Hispanic community recognizes *promotores de salud* as lay health workers who work in Spanish-speaking communities (CDC, 2019).

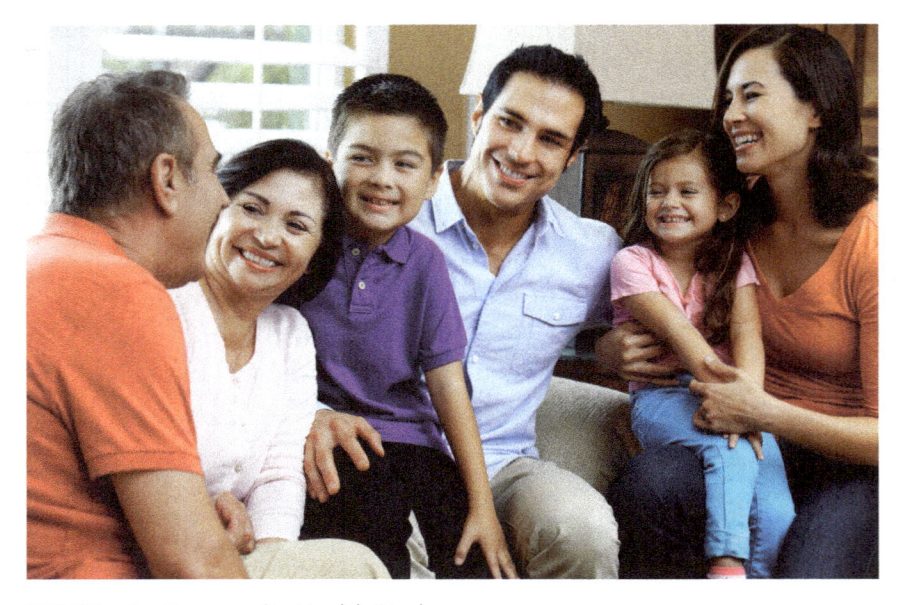

FIGURE 2.8   Community Health Worker

Next, review this short video and learn from CHWs how they define their role.

Source: UAMS Health. (2022, August 12). What is a community health worker? YouTube. https://tinyurl.com/5fbv3uzt

During the COVID-19 pandemic, CHWs provided such important health outreach services that the Health Resources and Services Administration (HRSA) recently announced plans to award 75 grants of up to $3 million each to train 13,000 new and current CHWs and other health support workers to respond to public health needs and emergencies in underserved communities through a network of partnerships (American Health Association [AHA], 2022).

Community Health Priorities

Community health also prioritizes **quality-of-life** issues that are especially important to their resident population. The WHO defines *quality of life* (QOL) as "an individual's perception of their position in life in the context of the culture and value systems in which they live and in relation to their goals, expectations, standards and concerns" (WHO, n.d.). QOL extends beyond just physical health and includes a diverse range of impact factors from economic standing to social belonging. Figure 2.9 presents common QOL indicators. Which of these would you rank as the top priority for your community? Could you rank them in order of importance? Do you think the priorities would change based on the context of the community?

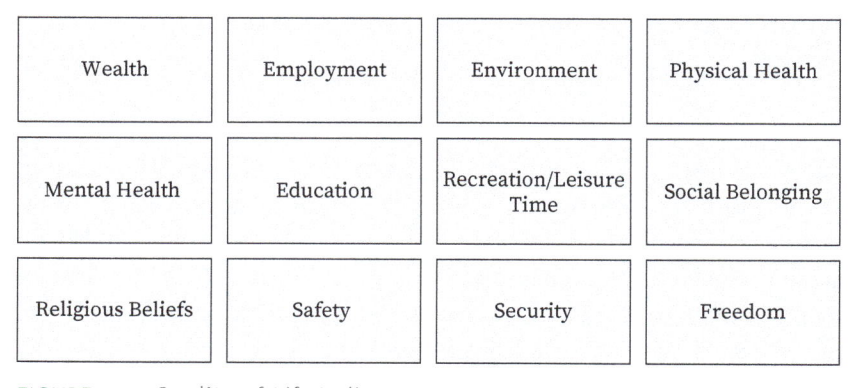

Wealth	Employment	Environment	Physical Health
Mental Health	Education	Recreation/Leisure Time	Social Belonging
Religious Beliefs	Safety	Security	Freedom

FIGURE 2.9   Quality-of-Life Indicators

Quality of Life and Happiness

Were you surprised that one of the indicators included recreation and leisure time? You should also know that QOL measures include results from the World Happiness Report (2022). This QOL metric uses a survey based on the Gallup World Poll to assess which country has the highest levels of GDP, life expectancy, generosity, social support, freedom, and corruption. Notice that these six indicators are like those measures used for the QOL analysis. This data collection protocol for the QOL also includes the analysis of Twitter data. Search for the report and find out the 2021 happiness ranking for the United States. The impact of a community healthscape influences all the World Happiness Report indicators.

Community Health Organizations

Community health is more complex than just a broad focus on the QOL, as it includes local community organizations, health coalitions, and workplace health initiatives. Local community health organizations, which are always nonprofit in nature, can be diverse, such as community grassroots efforts to combat neighborhood drug use to local offices of voluntary health agencies, including national advocacy organizations, such as the American Cancer Society, AHA, and American Lung Association.

Within communities, small local groups form an alliance or coalition to address larger and more complex health problems. One example is the Alliance for Community Health Integration (ACHI), which is in Boston, and a coalition of public health, consumer advocacy, social service, and community organizations working together and addressing health issues such as the impact social determinants of health and health equity (Massachusetts Public Health Association, 2020). Among its diverse members are the Greater Boston Interfaith Organization, Massachusetts Sheltering and Housing Alliance, Greater Boston Foodbank, and Western Massachusetts Health Equity Network. These types of coalitions form when residents realize that small organizations lack the resources to tackle of the most important community health needs.

Workplace Health

Workplace health can be considered a subset of community health and is often associated with employee wellness programs, workplace environmental concerns with safety and unhealthy exposures, and worksite health-related problems that lead to permanent injury or chronic pain. Healthy worksites are much more than just being injury-free, and workplace health also seeks to align meaningful work within life's balance by ensuring employees are healthy and actively engaged in wellness activities.

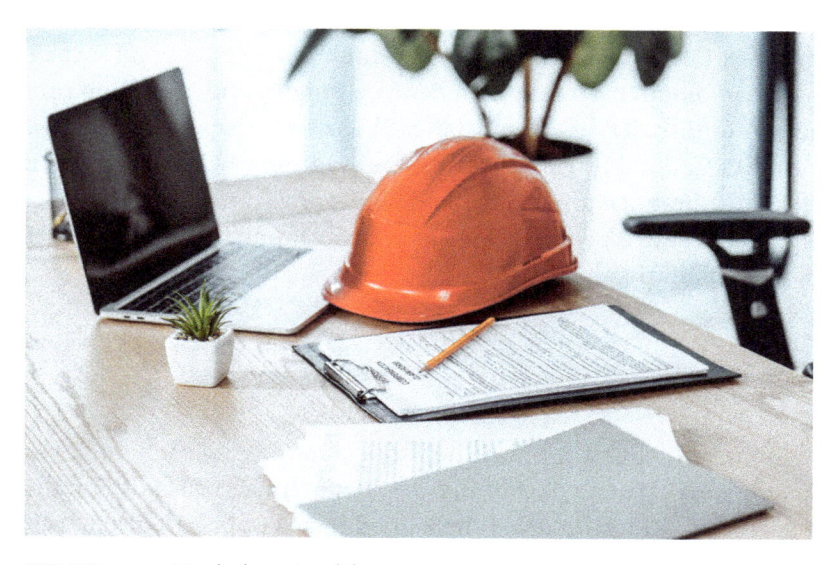

FIGURE 2.10   Workplace Health

Practical Skill: Community and Workplace Health

The Occupational Safety and Health Administration, a part of federal legislation enacted in 1970, ensures safe and healthful working conditions for employees by setting and enforcing standards and providing training, outreach, education, and assistance (U.S. Department of Labor, n.d.). Why is this important? Each day in the United States, at least 12 workers on average die from an injury sustained at work (Seabert et al., 2022). Many more are injured or exposed to lethal work environments.

Which occupations do you think represent dangerous work conditions? Often, we name jobs such as construction, logging, aircraft pilots, and engineers (Industrial Safety and Hygiene News, 2020). However, we forget that other less recognized workplaces are also hazardous, such as nail salons, where employees are exposed to harmful chemicals, and workers employed in the cleaning and hygiene service industry. Did you know that the top three jobs in health care at risk for infections are dentists, critical nurses, and general practitioners (Blain, 2020)?

County and city officials also support community health initiatives by encouraging healthy worksites for employees to attract new companies and positions to their city and suburban areas. Healthy employees support active communities, and investors seek communities with strong infrastructures and growth potential. Employees spend a substantial number of hours at work, and wellness programs can support policies and changes that encourage healthy lifestyles and a balance between work and leisure. Health policies now include smoke-free worksites, the availability of on-site exercise rooms, rest and quiet areas, and cafeterias that serve healthy food choices (Fabius &

Clarke, 2021). Employers who self-insure their workers may offer incentives for ceasing smoking, maintaining a healthy weight, and attending programs designed to combat all types of substance abuse and misuse (Pronk et al., 2010). The Wellness Council of America (n.d.) is a nationally known organization that offers best-practice programs, guidelines, and frameworks to ensure that today's employees are healthy. The shared community goal remains to keep the priority population healthy!

Public Health's Population Perspective

Unlike community health, public health is a nationally mandated sector of American health care. As part of the U.S. Department of Health and Human Services (DHHS), which includes the United States Public Health Service and the Centers for Disease Control and Prevention (CDC, 2018). Public health, as a government entity, has responsibility for the health of all Americans and is legally accountable for the three **core functions** (CDC, 2014):

- **Assessment:** The public health system must continuously and systematically assess the health of the populations to determine the baseline of morbidity (illness) and mortality (death) for communities. This assessment core function helps us to establish what is a "normal" health status for a population.
- **Policy development:** The public health system must work with the community to identify, educate, and solve health problems via a policy approach based in science.
- **Assurance:** The public health system must evaluate the effectiveness of its interventions and ensure a competent workforce to carry out the public health mission.

Public health goals follow a protocol of assessing health status, identifying health problems, developing solutions and appropriate policies, and carrying out its mission effectively. All goals require strategies, and the 10 public health system strategies aligned with the core functions (Public Health National Center for Innovations, 2020). Figure 2.11 presents the relationship between the core function and the 10 public health services.

To comprehend the complexity of public health, consider the CDC's role during the recent pandemic (CDC, 2021), and the impact of protecting a population as large as the approximately 330 million Americans (U.S. Census Bureau, n.d.). This public health organization chart (Figure 2.12) outlines the enormity of the nation's health organizations and its relationships within the health sector.

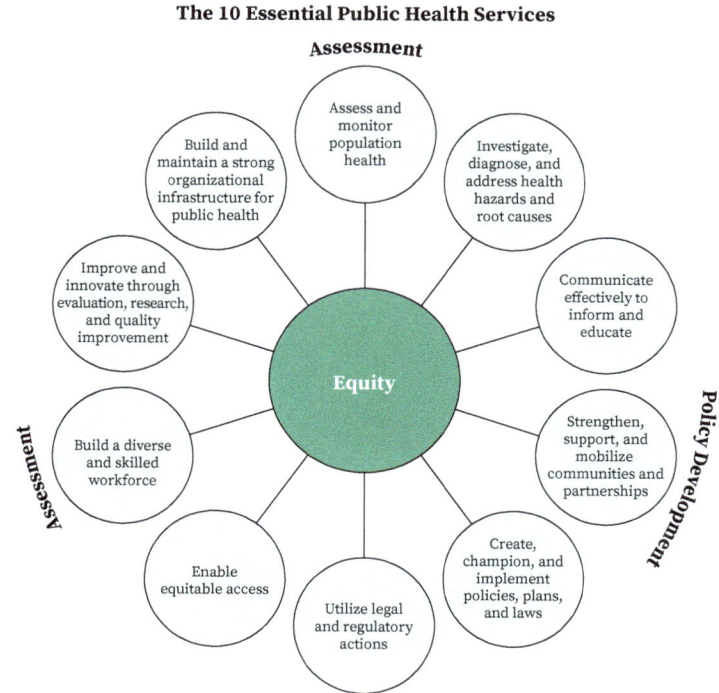

The 10 Essential Public Health Services

Assessment

- Assess and monitor population health
- Investigate, diagnose, and address health hazards and root causes
- Communicate effectively to inform and educate
- Strengthen, support, and mobilize communities and partnerships
- Create, champion, and implement policies, plans, and laws
- Utilize legal and regulatory actions
- Enable equitable access
- Build a diverse and skilled workforce
- Improve and innovate through evaluation, research, and quality improvement
- Build and maintain a strong organizational infrastructure for public health

Center: **Equity**

Axes: Assessment / Policy Development / Assessment

To protect and promote the health of all people in all communities

The 10 Essential Public Health Services provide a framework for public health to protect and promote the health of all people in all communities. To achieve optimal health for all, the Essential Public Health Services actively promote policies, systems, and services that enable good health and seek to remove obstacles and systemic and structural barriers, such as poverty, racism, gender discrimination, and other forms of oppression, that have resulted in health inequities. Everyone should have a fair and just opportunity to achieve good health and well-being.

FIGURE 2.11 The 10 Essential Public Health Services

Federal Agencies			
Government Agencies (Non-public health)	State, Tribal, Local, and Territorial Health Departments	Clinical Care Delivery Systems	International Health Agencies
Media	Community Based Organizations	Private, Nonprofit Associations Philanthropic Organizations	Educational Institutions	Private Industry (Non-sector)

FIGURE 2.12 Public Health Relationships With Community and Other Organizations

Public Health Achievements

Public health will always provide safety net services, but many major public health successes are often overlooked, even though their achievements helped form a foundation for population health. Figure 2.13 presents the top 10 public health's major achievements for the 20th century, and Figure 2.14 highlights the top 10 achievements for the first decade of the 21st century.

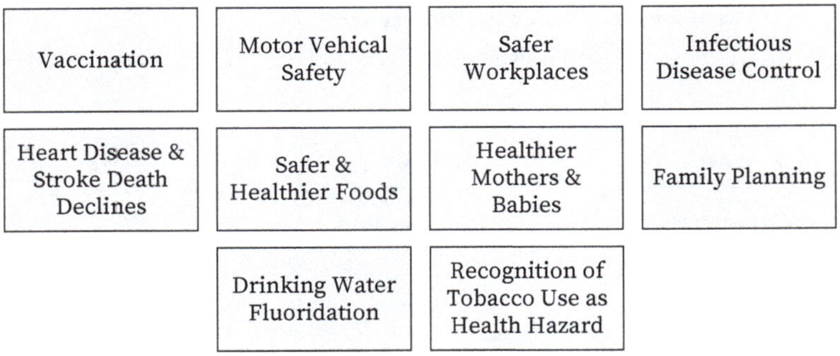

Top 10 Public Health Achievements for the 20th Century

- Vaccination
- Motor Vehical Safety
- Safer Workplaces
- Infectious Disease Control
- Heart Disease & Stroke Death Declines
- Safer & Healthier Foods
- Healthier Mothers & Babies
- Family Planning
- Drinking Water Fluoridation
- Recognition of Tobacco Use as Health Hazard

FIGURE 2.13 Top 10 Public Health Achievements for the 20th Century

Top 10 Public Health Achievements for the First Decade of the 21st Century

- Reductions in Child Mortality
- Vaccine Preventable Diseases
- Access to Safe Water & Sanitation
- Malaria Prevention & Control
- Prevention & Control of HIV/AIDS
- Tuberculosis Control
- Control of Tropical Diseases
- Tobacco Control
- Increased Awareness & Response for Improving Global Road Safety
- Improved Prepardness & Response to Global Health Threats

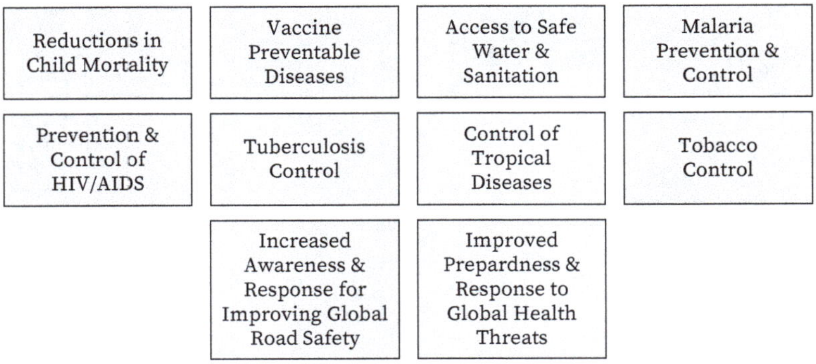

FIGURE 2.14 Top 10 Public Health Achievements for the First Decade of the 21st Century

Practical Skill Student Activity: Public Health Achievements

Which achievement would you consider to be the most valuable in the original list? Which produced the greatest benefit for all Americans? Which achievement would you consider to be the most impactful in the most recent list? How would you describe the differences between the two? What do you predict the public health achievements will be for 2012–2020?

What laws were essential to public health's success? Could you list any? What about seatbelt laws or laws prohibiting smoking in schools and hospitals? For additional information, review the following article titled "Law and Public Health at CDC."

Source: Goodman, R., Moulton, A., Matthews, G., Shaw, F., Kocher, J., Mensah, G., Zaza, S., & Besser, R. (2006). Law and public health at CDC. Morbidity and Mortality Weekly Report, December 22, 2006. https://tinyurl.com/37np9cxs

Healthy People 2030

Public health strategies lacked national impact for all Americans until 1979, when a landmark document, *Healthy People: The Surgeon General's Report on Health Promotion and Disease Prevention*, recommended for the first time a coordinated, health care national strategy (Office of Disease Prevention and Health Promotion [ODPHP], 2021). This report provided baseline evidence for setting health goals and objectives for all populations. Subsequent reports transitioned over the years and now actively address the enormous discrepancy in the distribution and determinants of disease for various at-risk populations. Healthy People 2030 is the latest iteration of our national strategic guidelines for health in the United States.

Healthy People 2030: Building a Healthier Future for All

How comprehensive is Healthy People 2030 (CDC, 2020)? Healthy People 2030 provides 10-year, measurable public health objectives and tools to help track progress toward achieving them and is the fifth edition of America's health agenda. Based on the successes of the previous document, Healthy People 2030, the latest agenda includes vision and mission statements, foundational

1. Attain healthy thriving lives and well-being free of preventable disease, disability, injury, and premature death.

2. Eliminate health disparities, achieve health equity, and attain health literacy to improve the health and well-being of all.

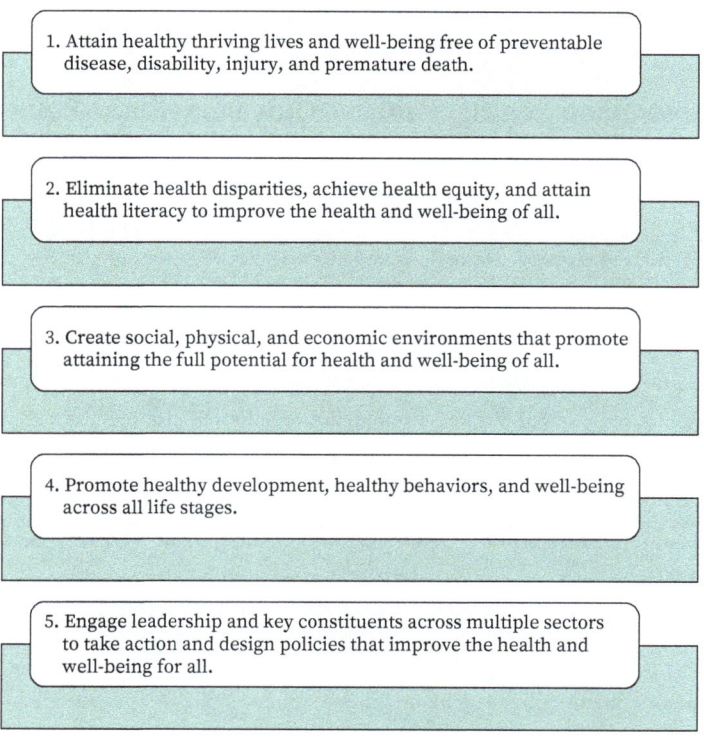

3. Create social, physical, and economic environments that promote attaining the full potential for health and well-being of all.

4. Promote healthy development, healthy behaviors, and well-being across all life stages.

5. Engage leadership and key constituents across multiple sectors to take action and design policies that improve the health and well-being for all.

FIGURE 2.15 Healthy People 2030 Goals

principles, and five major goals. This version of our national public health strategy lists 355 core objectives ranging from reduction of chronic diseases to mitigation of contagious diseases such as COVID-19. Healthy People 2030 provides evidence-supported objectives as well as benchmarks that are valuable metrics for monitoring and state comparisons. The Healthy People 2030 goals serve as guidelines for all collaborative health efforts with all health sectors.

As you would expect, to meet the needs of all populations, the health plan is divided into five topic areas—health conditions, health behaviors, populations, settings, and systems and social determinants of health—and includes more than 350 objectives. Each objective is measurable, and formal reviews (assessments) are conducted at five and 10 years (ODPHP, 2021).

One of the Healthy People 2030 goals that aligns strategically with population health is the national commitment to "eliminate health disparities, achieve health equity, and attain health literacy to improve the health and well-being of all." Population health seeks specifically to provide health promotion and disease prevention efforts to those groups who encounter health disparities. Healthy People 2030 provides objectives, data, resources, frameworks, and definitions to guide health systems efforts toward eliminating health inequities.

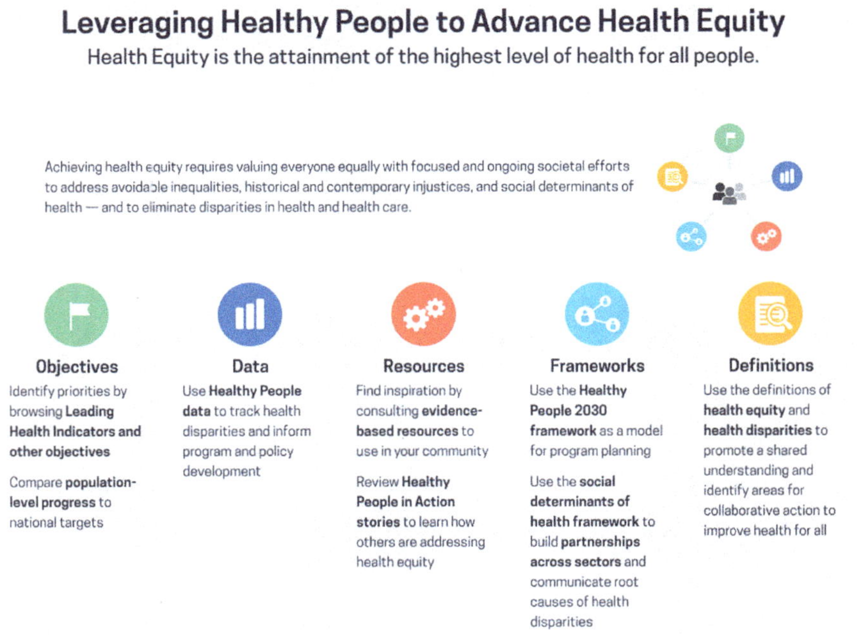

Leveraging Healthy People to Advance Health Equity

Health Equity is the attainment of the highest level of health for all people.

Achieving health equity requires valuing everyone equally with focused and ongoing societal efforts to address avoidable inequalities, historical and contemporary injustices, and social determinants of health — and to eliminate disparities in health and health care.

Objectives
Identify priorities by browsing **Leading Health Indicators** and other objectives

Compare **population-level progress** to national targets

Data
Use **Healthy People** data to track health disparities and inform program and policy development

Resources
Find inspiration by consulting **evidence-based resources** to use in your community

Review **Healthy People in Action** stories to learn how others are addressing health equity

Frameworks
Use the **Healthy People 2030 framework** as a model for program planning

Use the **social determinants of health framework** to build **partnerships across sectors** and communicate root causes of health disparities

Definitions
Use the definitions of **health equity** and **health disparities** to promote a shared understanding and identify areas for collaborative action to improve health for all

FIGURE 2.16 Leveraging Healthy People to Advance Health Equity

Much of today's health sector aligns either directly or indirectly with the public health system. Public health relies on the Healthy People 2030 standards to develop national and local policies and to tailor programs to meet the needs of all Americans. Healthy People 2030 is the blueprint for national health activities during the next 10 years (DHHS, n.d.). State governments decide appropriate public health strategies for their subpopulations, and local public health departments and agencies interact with their geographically assigned and smaller populations to carry out these initiatives.

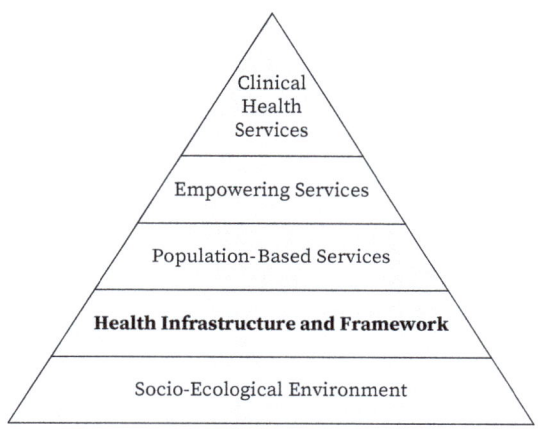

FIGURE 2.17 Sample Public Health Pyramid

Public Health as a Safety Net

What do we mean when we describe public health as a "safety net" health organization? Figure 2.17 presents a simplified version of a public health pyramid, which shows components of a sample health system. Public health, as a safety net organization, functions as the most basic health infrastructure in the country's health system and affects more individuals than other levels of health services in the pyramid. Only socio-ecological environmental factors—which include the social determinants of health—affect more Americans. The pyramid's middle level, identified as population health services, includes activities that are delivered to an entire population, such as water fluoridation and programs such as Special Supplemental Nutrition Program for Women, Infants, and Children (WIC). WIC serves low-income pregnant, postpartum, and breastfeeding women, infants, and children up to age 5 who are at nutritional risk (USDA, 2021).

Note that this is a public health and not a population health pyramid, and the concept of selecting only a priority population based on factors other than geographic location is not an option. The empowering level includes social services that enable and ensure that support systems (e.g., transportation, housing, food security for seniors) are available for certain individuals in need. Public health is less involved at the pyramid's top level as these direct health services are provided by medical and health care providers and a smaller number of the total population will need clinical care.

The Institute of Medicine, now known as the National Academy of Medicine, describes a safety net as comprising those who organize and deliver a significant level of health care and other needed services to uninsured, Medicaid, and other vulnerable patients (Agency for Healthcare Research and Quality, n.d.). Local public health departments provide free vaccinations and other basic services to these at-risk populations but do not provide diagnosis and treatment, which is a key distinction of their health role. Public health also provides many everyday services to all Americans.

The National Association of County and City Health Officials (NACCHO) represents more than 3,000 local health departments across the country (NACCHO, 2022). Members of NACCHO seek to support and advocate for public health agencies by highlighting their essential role in daily life. Review Figure 2.18 as a reminder of the broad and essential responsibilities of a typical local health department.

Local Health Departments Impact Our Lives Every Day

- Chronic Disease
- Infectious Disease
- Food Safety
- Immunization
- Maternal and Child Health
- Emergency Preparedness
- Tobacco Control
- Environmental Health
- Injury and Violence Prevention

Local health departments promote and protect the health of people and the communities where they live and work

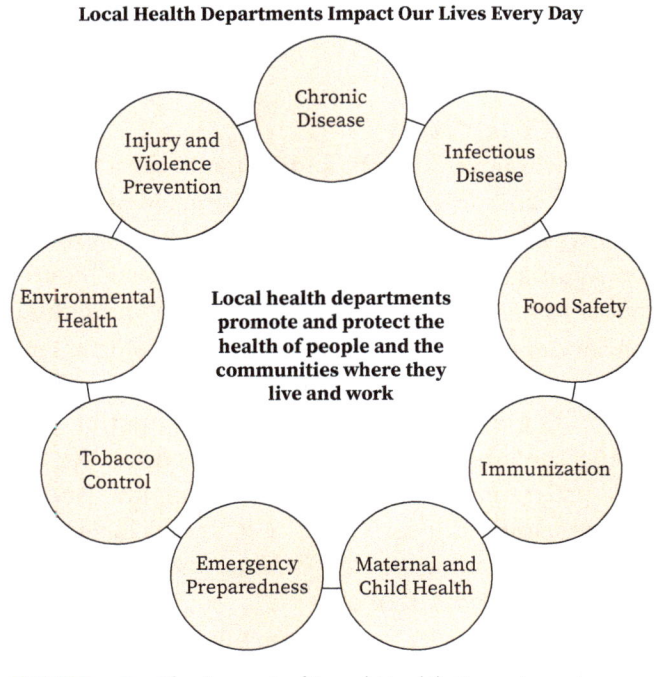

FIGURE 2.18 The Impact of Local Health Departments

Global Health Population Perspective

The World Health Organization

The most well-known global health organization is the WHO, a unit of the United Nations, which coordinates global health and safety by aligning nations, partners, and communities to promote health across all countries. (WHO, 2022a). As you can imagine, only a large multinational health institution would develop a global health initiative with the world's current population tallied at more than 7.9 billion people. Due to the enormous complexity of worldwide health, a successful global effort requires both promoting interdisciplinary collaboration and aligning population-based prevention with individual-level clinic care (Koplan et al., 2009).

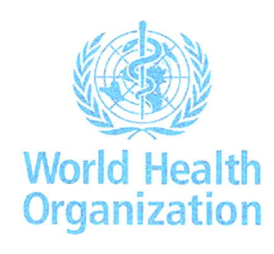

FIGURE 2.19 World Health Organization

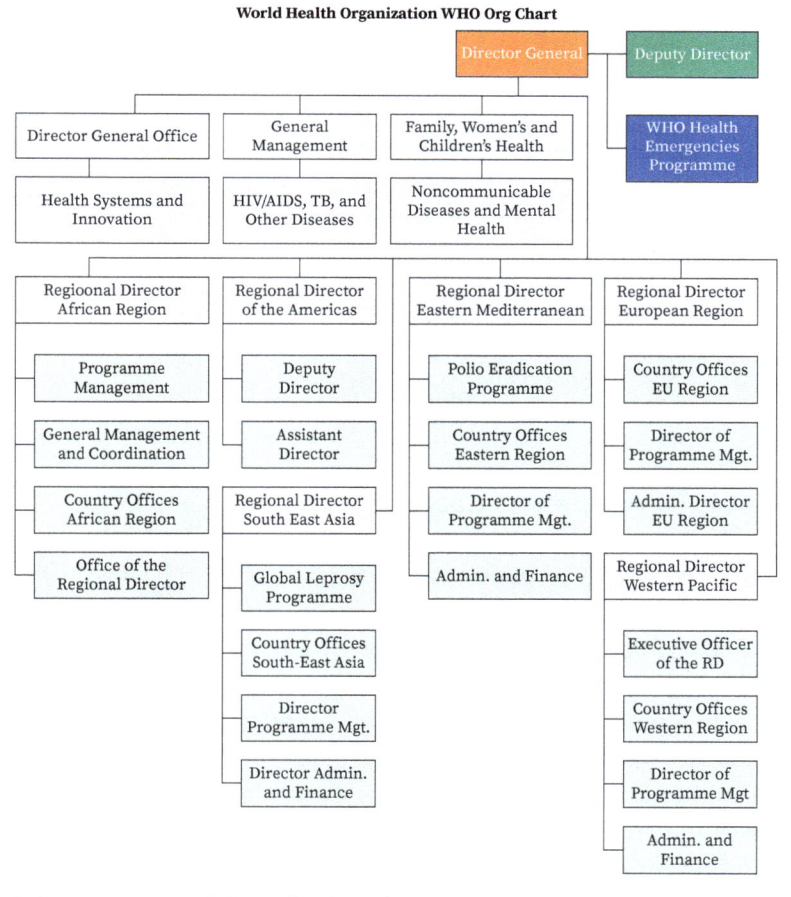

FIGURE 2.20 WHO Organization Chart

An example of the WHO's role as guardian of the world's health status was the official declaration that the novel COVID-19 virus had reached the pandemic stage (Cucinotta & Vanelli, 2020). The organization then launched and coordinated a global synchronized plan to provide vaccines for those countries in need and most vulnerable. The coordination of disease prevention and health promotion requires aligning health organizational cross-sectors by countries, health status and needs, geographic concerns, and national political stability. Refugee and migrant health, increasingly a concern in the 21st century, burdens world health systems and contributes to rising risk for common unhealthy living conditions, which often are major factors for communicable disease transmission (WHO, 2022e).

Six types of major intervention strategies help the WHO prioritize activities and ensure global health (see Figure 2.21).

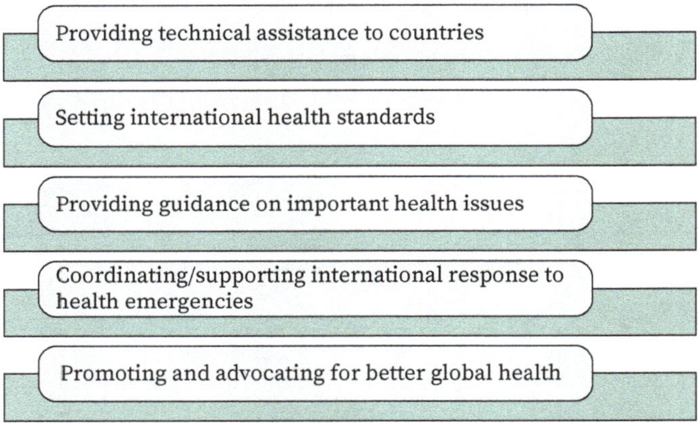

- Providing technical assistance to countries
- Setting international health standards
- Providing guidance on important health issues
- Coordinating/supporting international response to health emergencies
- Promoting and advocating for better global health

FIGURE 2.21   WHO Intervention Strategies for Global Health

Sustainable Development Goals

The WHO has more than 150 member nations and is led by an appointed director-general whose responsibility is to implement the latest set of initiatives and activities outlined in the WHO's sustainable development goals (SDGs). These 17 goals will help ensure the best QOL for the world's population. Today, the WHO continues to improve the world's health by supporting the United Nations' 2030 Agenda for Sustainable Development, adopted in 2015 (WHO, 2022b). This universal plan for world peace, prosperity, and health includes 17 SDGs (United Nations, n.d.). Health has a primary place, as Goal 3 is to "[E]nsure healthy lives and promote well-being for all at all ages." The WHO assumes Goal 3 accountability for meeting 13 health-specific targets as part of this global effort (WHO, 2022b).

Chapter Two Focus on Populations | 43

Practical Skill: Population Health Activity

Review the history of the SDGs and then watch the informative video. Do you know all 17 SDGs?

Source: United Nations. (n.d.). The 17 goals. https://tinyurl.com/553mwprv

Would you rank them in the same order?

Global health must address common health threats that include communicable disease outbreaks (e.g., measles, Ebola, SARS, COVID-19), bioterrorism built on the deliberate release of agents (e.g., virus, bacteria) to cause death in people, animals, or plants, rising violence and crimes in health care settings, and human trafficking (Szydlowski et al., 2022).

Climate Change

The single largest health threat facing humanity is climate change as experts have predicted that approximately 250,000 additional deaths per year will occur between 2030 and 2050 due to malnutrition, malaria, diarrhea, and heat stress related to climate change (WHO, 2021).

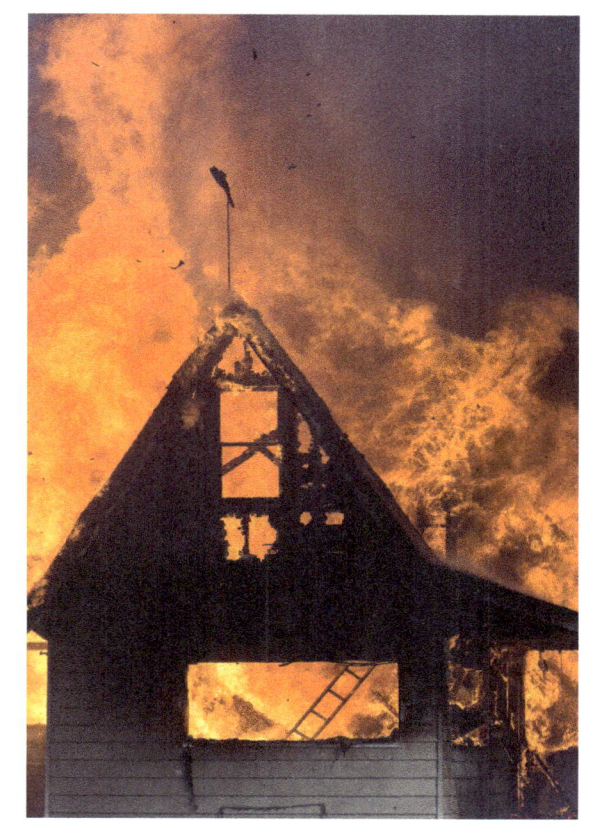

FIGURE 2.22 Climate Change Crisis in the United States

> **Practical Skill: Assessing the Impact of Climate Change for Community, Public, and Global Health Actions**
>
> One of the most dramatic impacts of climate change in the United States has been the increased incidence of wildfire, primarily in California. View the video. Have wildfire disasters continued to increase in the past few years? Is this a global, public, or community health issue?
>
> *Source: PBS. (2020, September 7).* California wildfires illustrate the consequences of climate change. *https://tinyurl.com/bddtntbn*
>
> Now, you can comprehend the tremendous burden of the WHO as it copes with environmental disasters that decrease life expectancy across the world.

These complex activities require an enormous workforce of more than 8,000 employees representing a variety of positions, including public health experts, scientists, doctors, epidemiologists, and, of course, managers who are deployed across the globe and trained to monitor daily health status and provide large-scale and rapid emergency crisis responses (WHO, 2022c). The global health approach truly encompasses the mission of improving QOL for all.

Summary

Ensuring quality of life for all Americans requires diverse approaches and sustained collaborations. Community, public, and global health offer valuable strengths and strategies to positively affect populations across the country. Unlike in population health, these approaches serve geographically defined populations, and each differs in mission, strategies, and scope. Community health events may be tailored to unique QOL issues compared to public health's focus on safety net services and prevention of disease. Global health's impact continues to increase as the recent pandemic and climate change events trigger growing concerns and crises that directly affect the United States. Together, these entities offer a coordinated effort to improve health, especially for those who are most vulnerable and in need of support.

Discussion Questions

1. Why does the socio-ecological environmental model best illustrate potential relationships available for population health?
2. Provide at least three specific benefits of using a community health worker as part of a local community hospital or organization.
3. Describe the benefits for employers to participate in workplace health initiatives.
4. Which public health safety net activity do you feel to be the most important? Why?
5. Healthy People 2030 serves as the nation's blueprint for health. List each of the five major goals and identify how it relates to population health.
6. The WHO sponsors the SDGs. Which of these goals has the potential to affect the United States most significantly? Share your top three goals.
7. Americans are concerned about climate control. Which climate change example would you use to illustrate our current climate crisis?

References

Agency for Healthcare Research and Quality. (n.d.). *Topic: Safety net*. https://www.ahrq.gov/topics/safety-net.html

American Hospital Association. (2022, April 15). *Organizations can apply for ARPA grants to train community health workers*. https://www.aha.org/news/headline/2022-04-15-organizations-can-apply-arpa-grants-train-community-health-workers

American Public Health Association. (n.d.). *Community health workers*. https://www.apha.org/apha-communities/member-sections/community-health-workers

Aronica, K., Crawford, E., Licherdell, E., & Noah, J. (n.d.). *Core principles of the ecological model—Individual, interpersonal, organizational, community, and public policy*. Lumen Learning. https://courses.lumenlearning.com/suny-buffalo-environmentalhealth/. https://courses.lumenlearning.com/suny-buffalo-environmentalhealth/chapter/core-principles-of-the-ecological-model/

Beaglehole, R., & Bonita, R. (2010). What is global health? *Global Health Action*, *3*, doi: 10.3402/gha.v3i0.5142

Blain, R. (2020, October 23). *Top 10 most dangerous jobs at risk for infection*. https://www.humanresourcesonline.net/top-10-most-dangerous-jobs-for-infection-risk-2

Centers for Disease Control and Prevention. (2014). *The public health system and the 10 essential public health services—PowerPoint*. https://www.cdc.gov/publichealthgateway/publichealthservices/essentialhealthservices.html

Centers for Disease Control and Prevention. (2015). *Components of the public health system description.* https://www.cdc.gov/publichealthgateway/funding/rfaot13/pyramid_description.html

Centers for Disease Control and Prevention. (2018). *About CDC: Our history—Our story.* https://www.cdc.gov/about/history/index.html

Centers for Disease Control and Prevention. (2019). *Promotores de salud/Community health workers.* https://www.cdc.gov/minorityhealth/promotores/index.html

Centers for Disease Control and Prevention. (2021, February 4). *CDC in action: Working 24/7 to stop the threat of COVID-19.* https://www.cdc.gov/budget/documents/covid-19/CDC-247-Response-to-COVID-19-fact-sheet.pdf

Centers for Disease Control and Prevention. (n.d.). *Tips from former smokers.* https://www.cdc.gov/tobacco/campaign/tips/quit-smoking/index.html

Centers for Disease Control and Prevention. (2022) *Violence prevention: The social-ecological model: A framework for prevention.* https://www.cdc.gov/violenceprevention/about/social-ecologicalmodel.html

Chegg. (n.d.). *Quiz 1 intro to health.* https://www.chegg.com/flashcards/quiz-1-intro-to-health-edc0730e-6fcd-4be3-8fb1-107c13ae57c4/deck

Cucinotta, D., & Vanelli, M. (2020, March 19). WHO declares COVID-19 a pandemic. *Acta Biomedica, 91*(1), 157–160. doi: 10.23750/abm.v91i1.9397

Dahlberg, L., & Krug, E. (2002). Violence: a global public health problem. In E. Krug, L. Dahlberg, J. Mercy, A. Zwi, & R. Lozano (Eds.), *World report on violence and health* (pp. 1–21). World Health Organization.

Eliana. (2022). *Community health worker training.* Talence. https://chwtraining.org/everything-you-need-to-know-about-chw-roles/#:~:text=Peer%20educator%2C%20peer%20support%20worker,patient%20navigator%2C%20family%20support%20worker

Fabius, R., & Clarke, J. (2021). Building cultures of health and wellness within organizations. In D. Nash, A. Skoufalos, R. Fabius, & W. Oglesby (Eds.), *Population health: Creating a culture of wellness.* Jones and Bartlett Learning.

Harvey, S. R., & Fernandez, M. E. (2012). Identifying the core elements of effective community health worker programs: A research agenda. *American Journal of Public Health, 102*(9), 1633–1637. https://doi.org/10.2105/AJPH.2012.300649

Industrial Safety and Hygiene News. (2020). *Top 25 most dangerous jobs in the United States.* https://www.ishn.com/articles/112748-top-25-most-dangerous-jobs-in-the-united-states

Invictus. (2022, February 7). *Top 10 most dangerous jobs according to OSHA.* https://www.invictuslawpc.com/most-dangerous-jobs-osha/

Joint Committee on Health Education and Promotion Terminology. (2012). Report of the 2011 Joint Committee on Health Education and Promotion Terminology. *American Journal of Health Education, 43*(2), 1–19.

Koplan, J., Bond, T., Merson, M., Reddy, K., Rodriguez, M., Sewankambo, N. & Wasserheit, J. (2009). Towards a common definition of global health. *Lancet, 373*(9679), P1993–P1995. https://www.thelancet.com/journals/lancet/article/PIIS0140-6736(09)60332-9/fulltext

Lexington Visitors Center. (n.d.). *Minuteman statue*. https://www.tourlexington.us/attractions/pages/minuteman-statue

Massachusetts Public Health Association. (2020). *The Alliance for Community Health Integration (ACHI)*. https://mapublichealth.org/achi/

McKenzie, J., Pinger, R., & Kotecki, J. (2005). *An introduction to community health*. Jones and Bartlett Publishers.

National Association of County and City Health Officials. (2017). *Local health departments impact our lives every day*. https://www.naccho.org/uploads/downloadable-resources/transition-appendix-A-Infographic.pdf

National Association of County and City Health Officials. (2022). *About NACCHO: What makes NACCHO the organization it is today*. https://www.naccho.org/about

Office of Disease Prevention and Health Promotion. (2021). *Healthy People 2030: Building a healthier future for all*. U.S. Department of Health and Human Services. https://health.gov/healthypeople

Pérez, L., & Martinez, J. (2008). Community health workers: Social justice and policy advocates for community health and well-being. *American Journal of Public Health, 98*(1), 11–14.

Pronk, N., Lowry, M., Kottke, T., Austin, E., Gallagher, J., & Katz, A. (2010). Association between optimal lifestyle adherence and short-term incidence of chronic conditions among employees. *Population Health Management, 13*(6), 289–295.

Public Broadcasting System. (2020, November 10). *ZIP codes can predict your health*. https://www.pbs.org/video/nov-10-2020-zip-codes-predict-your-health-5cvrlq/

Public Health National Center for Innovations. (2020). *10 essential public health services*. https://phnci.org/uploads/resource-files/EPHS-English.pdf

Seabert, D., McKenzie, J. & Pinger, R. (2022). *McKenzie's an introduction to community & public health* (10th ed.). Jones & Bartlett Learning.

South End Healthy Boston Coalition. (n.d.). *About us*. http://sehbc.blogspot.com/p/about-us.html

Szydlowski, S., Babela, R., Poku, B., Anderson, T., Krcmery, V., Fried, B. Akinci, F., Gifford, B., Ullmann, S., Bhadelia, A., & Knaul, F. (2022). Future trends in global health. In M. Counte, B. Ramirez, D. West, & W. Aaronson (Eds.), *The global healthcare manager: Competencies, concepts, and skills* (pp. 452–455).

Town of Lexington. (n.d.). *Lexington history resources*. https://www.lexingtonma.gov/854/Lexington-History-Resources

United Nations. (n.d.). *The seventeen goals*. https://sdgs.un.org/goals

U.S. Census Bureau. (n.d.). *U.S. and world population clock*. https://www.census.gov/popclock/

U.S. Department of Agriculture. (2021, July 27). *About WIC: The special supplemental nutrition program for women, infants, and children.* https://www.fns.usda.gov/wic/about-wic

U.S. Department of Agriculture. (n.d.). *What is My Plate?* https://www.myplate.gov/eat-healthy/what-is-myplate

U.S. Department of Labor. (n.d). *About OSHA.* https://www.osha.gov/aboutosha

Wellness Council of America. (n.d.). *WELCOA: Wellness Council of America.* https://www.welcoa.org/

Winslow, E. (1920). The untilled fields of public health. *Science, 51*(1306), 23–33.

WordBueno. (n.d.). *Healthscape.* https://wordbueno.com/word/healthscape

World Happiness Report. (2022). *World happiness report 2023.* https://worldhappiness.report/

World Health Organization. (2022a). *Frequently asked questions.* https://www.who.int/about/frequently-asked-questions

World Health Organization. (2022b). *Sustainable development goals.* https://www.who.int/health-topics/sustainable-development-goals#tab=tab_1

World Health Organization. (2022c). *Who we are.* https://www.who.int/about/who-we are#:~:text=Our%20team%20of%208000%2B%20professionals,%2C%20epidemiologists%2C%20scientists%20and%20managers

World Health Organization. (2022d). *WHO brochure: Working for better health.* https://www.who.int/about/what-we-do/who-brochure

World Health Organization. (2022e). *Refugees and migrants.* https://www.thelancet.com/journals/lancet/article/PIIS0140-6736(09)60332-9/fulltext

World Health Organization. (2023.). *Climate Change.* https://www.who.int/health-topics/climate-change#tab=tab_1

World Health Organization. (n.d.) *WHOQOL: Measuring quality of life.* https://www.who.int/toolkits/whoqol

Credits

Fig. 2.1: Generated with FreeWordCloudGenerator.com.
Fig. 2.2a: Copyright © 2017 Depositphotos/Rawpixel.
Fig. 2.2b: Copyright © 2020 Depositphotos/halfpoint.
Fig. 2.2c: Copyright © 2022 Depositphotos/ipopba.
Fig. 2.3a: Source: Adapted from A) https://www.cdc.gov/violenceprevention/about/social-ecologicalmodel.html; https://www.scielo.br/j/csc/a/3hrn64cpBqBFb9mNfP-4KGXr/?lang=en; B) Etienne G. Krug, et al. "World Report on Violence and Health," https://apps.who.int/iris/bitstream/handle/10665/42495/9241545615_eng.pdf. Copyright © 2002 World Health Organization.
Fig. 2.4a: Source: https://www.myplate.gov/eat-healthy/what-is-myplate.
Fig. 2.4b: Copyright © 2015 Depositphotos/Syda_Productions.

Fig. 2.7: Copyright © by Henry Hudson Kitson (CC BY-SA 3.0) at https://commons.wikimedia.org/wiki/File:Minute_Man_Statue_Lexington_Massachusetts_cropped.jpg.

Fig. 2.8: Copyright © 2013 Depositphotos/monkeybusiness.

Fig. 2.10: Copyright © 2019 Depositphotos/IgorVetushko.

Fig. 2.11: Adapted from "The 10 Essential Public Health Services," https://phnci.org/uploads/resource-files/EPHS-English.pdf. Copyright © 2020 by The Public Health National Center for Innovations.

Fig. 2.12: Adapted from Denise Seabert, James F. McKenzie, and Robert R. Pinger, "Organizations That Help Shape Community and Public Health," McKenzie's *An Introduction to Community & Public Health*. Copyright © 2021 by Jones and Bartlett Learning.

Fig. 2.13: Source: MMWR Weekly, vol. 48, vol. 12.

Fig. 2.14: Source: https://www.cdc.gov/media/releases/2011/p0623_publichealth.html.

Fig. 2.15: Source: https://health.gov/healthypeople/about/healthy-people-2030-framework.

Fig. 2.16: Source: https://health.gov/sites/default/files/2022-04/HP2030_Advance-Health-Equity-Graphic.jpg.

Fig. 2.17: Adapted from A) T. Frieden, "A Framework for Public Health Action: The Health Impact Pyramid" *American Journal of Public Health*, vol. 100, no. 4. Copyright © 2010 American Public Health Association; B) L. Michele Issel, Rebecca Wells, and Mollie Williams, "Context of Health Program Development and Evaluation in *Health Program Planning and Evaluation*," Health Program Planning and Evaluation, pp. 21–22. Copyright © 2022 Jones Bartlett Learning.

Fig. 2.18: Source: Adapted from https://www.naccho.org/uploads/downloadable-resources/transition-appendix-A-Infographic.pdf.

Fig. 2.19: Copyright © by World Health Organization (WHO).

Fig. 2.20: Source: http://www.orgcharting.com/world-health-organization/.

Fig. 2.21: Denise Seabert, James F. McKenzie, and Robert R. Pinger, McKenzie's *An Introduction to Community & Public Health*, p. 34. Copyright © 2021 by Jones and Bartlett Learning.

Fig. 2.22: Copyright © 2015 Depositphotos/jamiehooper.

CHAPTER THREE

Public Health Skills for Population Health

Chapter Description

This chapter describes essential public health tools and skills used for coordinating population health care. Three types of epidemiological analyses—descriptive, analytical, and managerial—provide vital data to assess a population's health status. Common health indicators also include measures for the frequency of diseases (cases, prevalence, and incidence) and specific rates for assessing exposures and outcomes such as morbidity and mortality rates. Population health relies on standardized rates to identify at-risk populations and learn which health programs need to be developed and offered to prevent further disease. *Managerial epidemiology* refers to the application of epidemiological findings to refine population health decision-making when organizing care and health promotion activities for specific populations.

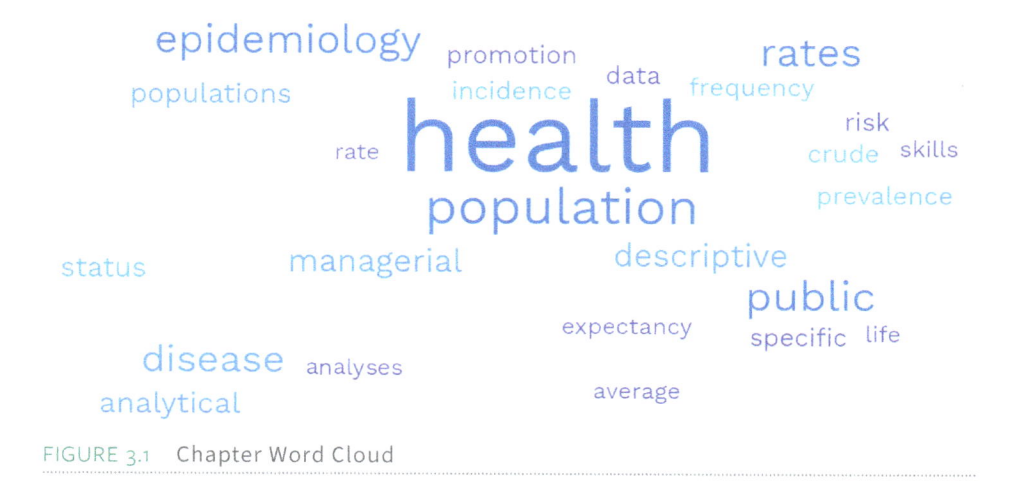

FIGURE 3.1 Chapter Word Cloud

Chapter Objectives

After completing this chapter, students will be able to:

1. Discuss public health strategies applicable to population health
2. Describe the importance of average life expectancy as a population outcome
3. Explain the importance of the public health triangle
4. Identify public health measurements (indicators) and their relevance for identifying at-risk populations
5. Demonstrate basic rate calculations and show application to population health
6. Define and explain descriptive, analytic, and managerial epidemiology

Key Words

Attack rate

Average life expectancy

Case

Centers for Disease Control and Prevention (CDC)

Chronic disease

Communicable disease

Community health needs assessment

Crude rates

Endemic, epidemic, and pandemic

Epidemiology: Descriptive, analytical, and managerial

Incidence and prevalence

Indicator

Rate

Specific rates

World Health Organization (WHO)

Public Health Strategies for Population Health

The history of American public health begins with the early years of our nation and has been shaped by the necessity to prevent and control disease in the entire population (Institute of Medicine, 1988). It is difficult to imagine our country without sanitation facilities, clean water, or safe food, but these challenges existed for many years. Over the years, public health responded to the public's most immediate health needs to ensure Americans have a long-life expectancy and high quality of life. See each of the public health roles presented in Figure 3.2.

If you review these six phases carefully, you will notice a definite shift from protecting Americans from communicable diseases to promoting healthy lifestyles that prevent chronic diseases. Public health and population health are aligning with the common goal of improving the quality of life for all.

Over the years, public health's contribution to improving health care for Americans has resulted in remarkable successes. A benchmark that measures

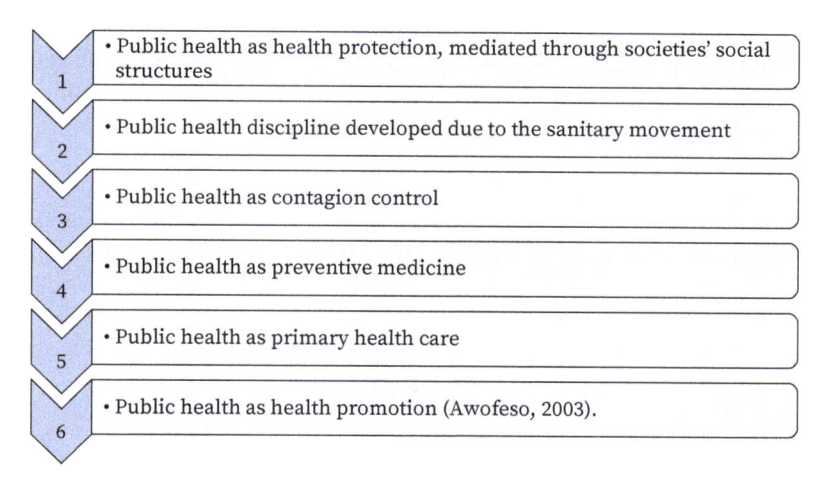

Chapter Three Public Health Skills for Population Health | 53

1. Public health as health protection, mediated through societies' social structures
2. Public health discipline developed due to the sanitary movement
3. Public health as contagion control
4. Public health as preventive medicine
5. Public health as primary health care
6. Public health as health promotion (Awofeso, 2003).

FIGURE 3.2 Six Transitional Phases of Public Health

public health's successful outcomes for the American population is the **average life expectancy** indicator. The average life expectancy, which is the average remaining years an individual of a particular age can be expected to live, increased for Americans by more than 25 years in the past 100 years (Schanzenbach et al., 2016). In 1900, the average American was not expected to live until age 50, and now a baby born in 2021 is expected to live until age 76.6 (McPhillips, 2022).

Public Health Tools for Population Health

Exploring Epidemiology

Understanding previous public health achievements and the outcomes metric, average life expectancy, helps frame the necessity for obtaining up-to-date and reliable data for every population. However, health is a dynamic state, and identifying sub-populations most at risk

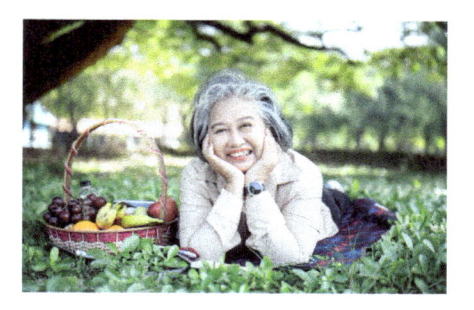

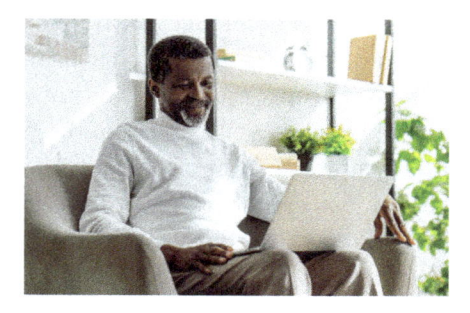

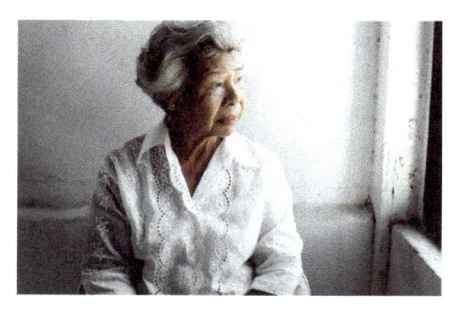

FIGURE 3.3 Seniors Today

requires additional computational skills. Public health national assessments contribute significant data to help inform population health decision-making. An essential population health tool is **epidemiology**.

Let's begin by reading this short newspaper quote:

> *"The Wall Street Journal* reports that 25 million children under age 5, compared to 300 million adult Americans, have access to at least one COVID-19 vaccine."
>
> Source: Wainer, D. (2022, June 7). *Pfizer and Moderna won't get a shot in the arm from toddlers.* Wall Street Journal, B12.

What did you learn from this information? You should be able to identify the number (i.e., count) of American children compared to adults who may or may not have received the vaccine. We do not know where these children are located, which vaccine was available to them, or whether their parents intended for them to receive the vaccine. Before health professionals attempt to identify a population's vulnerabilities, a review of descriptive and analytical data can provide evidence of potential risk factors and overall health status. Both population health and public health rely on the science of epidemiology (Caron, 2017a).

Epidemiology is the study of the distribution and determinants of health-related states or events in specified populations and the application of this study to the control of health problems (Turnock, 2021). Population health professionals know that using only counts, percentages, or frequencies alone often does not offer enough information to provide a solid foundation for a health promotion plan that will be effective. For example, suppose that 25% of the population report flu-like symptoms. That information does not tell us the age, gender, place, time frame, or flu severity of the population at risk. To answer these questions, we need to understand the Public Health Triangle and apply the tools of descriptive epidemiology.

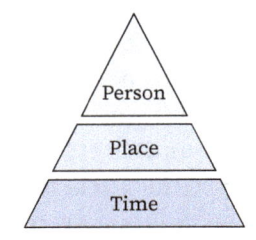

FIGURE 3.4 The Public Health Triangle: Person, Place, and Time

When reporting any population data, it is important to identify the person (population), place (location), and time (time frame). For example, 25 cases of flu were reported among residents older than age 65 living in a local Boston nursing home last week. Population health professionals use this type of data to monitor specific populations.

Descriptive Epidemiology

Descriptive epidemiology can identify patterns among cases and in populations by time, place, and person (CDC, n.d.). There are multiple ways an epidemiologist can explain these patterns, frequency (distribution) and the potential causes, risk factors, exposures, or contributing agents (determinants) of the disease. For example, diseases are often first described as either **communicable**—meaning infectious or potentially even contagious, or lifestyle—which refers to **chronic** conditions such as heart disease, type 2 diabetes mellitus, or other conditions that have been associated with negative health behaviors such as excessive smoking, alcohol consumption, or sedentary lifestyles (United Nations Chronicle, n.d.). Of course, we know that genetic predispositions can also cause these diseases as well. But these designations do not tell us the number of individuals within our population with the disease or condition. Descriptive studies seek to answer the questions about who, when, where, and how many.

Let's review other basics of epidemiology—the count, frequency, and percentage.

- Count—Use of numerical numbers
- Frequency—A total of the count
- Percentage (%)—The amount in each hundred (100)

Frequency of disease within a population can be expressed using three common terms: ***epidemic***, ***endemic***, and ***pandemic***. As local health continues to rapidly be affected by global impacts, the frequency of disease remains especially relevant (see Table 3.1 below).

TABLE 3.1   Terms for Frequency of Disease in Populations

Epidemiological Term	Definition
Epidemic	An unexpectedly large number of cases of an illness, a specific health-related behavior, or another event in a particular population
Endemic	A disease that occurs at an expected level in a population or at a certain location
Pandemic	An outbreak of disease over a wide, geographical area such as a continent or multiple continents

Source: Seabert, D., McKenzie, J., & Pinger, R. (2022). McKenzie's an introduction to community and public health (10th ed.). Jones and Bartlett Learning.

Calculating Disease Rates in Populations

Public health provides us with important and valuable tools for measuring health status and a common first choice is to determine a rate of disease or illness. A simple ***case*** refers to an individual who is diagnosed with a disease or a condition. Each person is a case. But a ***rate*** is the number of events or cases that occur in a given population in a given period of time. Rates are invaluable for population health, and the two most common crude rates are mortality rates (number of deaths) and morbidity rates (number of people who are sick). **Crude rates** are simply those that refer to the entire population. We can examine the occurrence of diseases within a population using two standard rates: **prevalence** and **incidence**. See Table 3.2 for their definitions expressed as equations.

TABLE 3.2   Prevalence and Incidence Rate Equations

Name of Rate	Definition of Rate (Equation)
Prevalence	Number of individuals with health-related events or cases of a disease/Total population at the same period
Incidence	Number of new health-related events or cases of a disease/Population at risk during the same period

Source: Seabert, C., McKenzie, J., & Pinger, R. (2022). McKenzie's an introduction to community and public health (10th ed). Jones and Bartlett Learning.

Practical Skill: Crude Rates

In fictitious X county, the population is comprised of 50,000. A total of 200 individuals have tested positive for ABC in the week of October 10–17, 2xxx. Calculate the prevalence rate for X county.

$$\frac{200 \text{ (Number of cases)}}{50{,}000 \text{ (total population)}} = .004 \times 1{,}000 = 4$$

Answer: The prevalence rate is four cases of ABC per 1,000 in X county for October 10–17, 2xxx.

Notice that both rates rely on similar equations with the number of cases in the numerator and the total population in the same period. Can you spot the difference between these two important rates? A prevalence rate is much easier to calculate as the denominator is simply the total population at the same time period. But an incidence rate requires the epidemiologist to know "the population at risk" for the denominator and not just the total population. This means that the population at risk has been exposed to a certain risk factor.

Measuring Health Status

When an unknown disease emerges, public health officials often calculate an **attack rate**, which is a special incidence rate, for that population and a single disease outbreak (Friis, 2018). It is one of the few rates expressed as a percentage,

Chapter Three Public Health Skills for Population Health | 57

which is unique compared to an incidence or prevalence rate. The equation for an attack rate is provided below.

Case example: On a flight from Australia to the United States, 38 individuals reported severe symptoms of food poisoning, with diarrhea and nausea being most common. Once the plane landed, public health officials interviewed all subjects and found the following outcomes: 130 of the 275 passengers and five of the flight crew (n = 10) reported severe symptoms. Calculate the attack rate for this unknown cause of illness.

TABLE 3.3 Attack Rate Equation

Name of Rate	Definition of Rate (Equation)
Attack rate	$\dfrac{\text{Number of people ill}}{\text{Number of people ill plus well}} \times 100$ in a specific period

Was your answer 37%? If not, recheck your calculations and the equation.

Crude and Specific Rates to Characterize Priority Populations

Calculating standard rates provides valuable evidence on the frequency of disease. Population health programs begin by assessing crude rates such as mortality (death) and morbidity (sickness) and then move to calculate specific rates that further define the characteristics of a priority population or even a subpopulation. Table 3.4 presents two examples of crude rates that are applicable for population health. *Crude* (raw) rates refer to those in which the denominator is the total population.

TABLE 3.4 Examples of Common Rates

Crude Rates	Definition (Equation)
Mortality rate	$\dfrac{\text{Number of deaths within a given period}}{\text{Population size}} \times 100{,}000$
Birth rate	$\dfrac{\text{Number of live births within a given period}}{\text{Population size}} \times 100{,}000$

Source: Caron, R. (2017b). Public health foundations for population health managers. In A. Hewitt, J. Mascari, & S. Wagner (Eds.), Population health management: Strategies, tools, applications, and outcomes *(pp. 30–31). HAP/AUPHA.*

If your priority population represents a specific age group, for example seniors, then a crude rate does not provide specific enough data. **Specific rates** are frequently calculated for age, gender, and specific cause of death

(Friis & Sellers, 2013). One of the most important specific rates, the single cause of death, is the infant mortality rate (shown in Table 3.3), which requires knowing the exact number of deaths for children younger than age 1 year. This rate is often used to compare health status among countries to assess the quality of life. Review Table 3.5 for specific rate equations.

TABLE 3.5   Examples of Specific Rate Equations

Specific Rate Example	Definition (Equation)
Age	Age-specific death rate = $\dfrac{\text{Number of deaths among residents Ages 35–50 in an area in a year}}{\text{Total population ages 35–50 in a given population in the same year}} \times 100{,}000$
Gender	Female death rate = $\dfrac{\text{Number of female deaths}}{\text{Number of persons in a population at a given period}} \times 100{,}000$
Single illness or cause of death: Infant mortality rate	Infant mortality rate = $\dfrac{\text{Number of deaths in a year of children Younger than age 1 year}}{\text{Number of live births in the same year}} \times 1{,}000$

Source: Caron, R. (2017b). Public health foundations for population health managers. In A. Hewitt, J. Mascari, & S. Wagner (Eds.), Population health management: Strategies, tools, applications, and outcomes (pp. 30–31). HAP/AUPHA.

Crude rates do not consider the age range for an entire population. The infant mortality rate shown in Table 3.5 requires knowing the exact number of deaths for children younger than age 1 year. A crude rate is not specific enough to tell us the birth rate for women ages 18 to 33. Rates used to make comparisons across groups and over time when groups differ in age structure are referred to as ***adjusted rates*** (Friis & Sellers, 2013). The rates are statistically adjusted by age and size of cohort.

Practical Skill: Practice Activity

A student is researching state cancer deaths for females ages 20 to 35 diagnosed with breast cancer. List *all* the potential types of rates the student would need to calculate to provide a descriptive epidemiological overview.

Analytical Epidemiology

Frequency and rates of disease provide initial data on the status of a population, but they do not identify risk factors or causation of disease or injury.

Chapter Three Public Health Skills for Population Health | 59

Analytical epidemiology uses calculations and analyses to develop hypotheses concerning relationships between risk factors and disease. The most well-known example of an analytical analysis was the study designed to establish cigarette smoking (a risk factor) as being associated (showed a relationship) with lung cancer (Seabert et al., 2022). Analytical epidemiology often requires the use of observational or experimental study designs (see Figure 3.5).

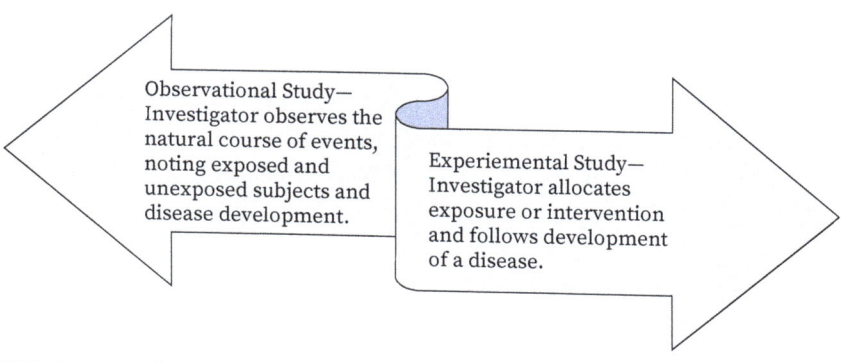

Observational Study—Investigator observes the natural course of events, noting exposed and unexposed subjects and disease development.

Experiemental Study—Investigator allocates exposure or intervention and follows development of a disease.

FIGURE 3.5   Observational and Experimental Study Options

Population health planners use this type of information to identify the importance of certain risk factors. For example, one type of observational study is known as a *cohort study*, when researchers track a cohort (specific population) over time and make comparisons based on a health condition or disease. This type of cohort study is often referred to as a *population-based cohort study*. Another type of cohort study occurs when researchers compare cohorts with and without different exposures (Friis, 2018). For example, an exposure-based study could be used to compare a group exposed to secondhand smoke and a second group not exposed to secondhand smoke in their workplaces. Analytical epidemiology requires a comparison group before a rate can be calculated. What is the

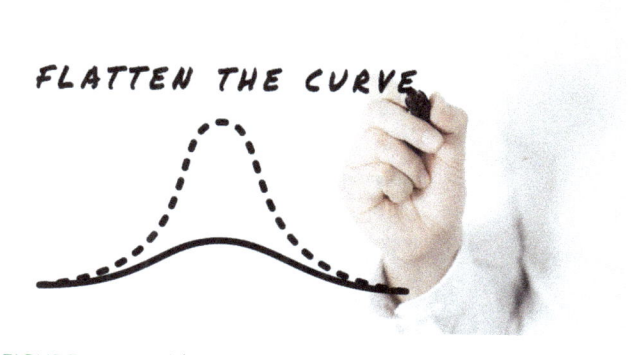

FIGURE 3.6   Epidemiology: Flatten the Curve Chart

value of analytic studies for population health? These studies clearly identify the at-risk sub-population from within the larger population. With this information, health planners can align health promotion and disease prevention efforts before disease occurs in these specific groups.

Managerial Epidemiology

Population health leverages epidemiological information in several ways from identifying at-risk groups to designing health promotion programs to prevent negative health behaviors. Managerial epidemiology refers to the application of epidemiology to both health care decision-making (Fleming, 2013) and

Practical Skill: Managerial Epidemiology Application

How would we use this population health skill? Let's assume you are a population health manager responsible for 10,000 individuals in an at risk-population. A recent analysis indicated 200 of 10,000 in the population contracted COVID-19 in the past year. Although all 200 individuals had been notified and offered opportunities to receive the vaccine for free, only 100 participated. Your epidemiological analysis data aligned with clinical data indicates that the 100 who did not receive the vaccine have multiple comorbidities, and the social determinants of health data also indicates these individuals live alone. Combining the epidemiological analyses, electronic health record, and social determinants of health risk score indicates the need for a stronger vaccine intervention with this population. This example of managerial epidemiology shows the ultimate value is the ability to improve health outcomes and quality of life.

Population health managers may rely on epidemiologists to provide essential calculations and indicators of health status. Their role, as decision-makers, is to understand and interpret descriptive, analytical, and managerial epidemiological findings to inform decisions that will affect multiple and diverse populations.

One last point to remember when reviewing epidemiological data and examining interpretations of the information, is the significant difference between the CDC and the World Health Organization (WHO). Each organization follows a specific mission, either national or worldwide, and its own definitions and data collection and analysis processes. Take the time to review the video below.

Source: The Infographics Show (2020). WHO vs. CDC—What do they actually do? YouTube. https://tinyurl.com/z6dv9xdw

management problems (Rohrer, 2013). Population health uses managerial epidemiological skills to answer the following types of questions:

- Who is the population, and what is their health status?
- Which population health needs should be addressed in this care setting?
- What types of health care services and which location should be selected to address this population's health needs (Oleski, 2001)?

Managerial epidemiology applies results from analytical and clinical measures and interprets findings to inform decision-making when identifying populations at risk and to select the appropriate health promotion activities and efforts for health promotion and population well-being.

Summary

Public health has drastically improved the health of Americans in the past 100 years with numerous achievements to prolong life expectancy. The field has evolved over six distinct stages to reach the current era of health promotion, which aligns with population health goals. Epidemiology is a valuable public health tool that enables skilled population health professionals to assess the health status of their priority populations and to plan health promotion initiatives to prevent further disease. Three branches of epidemiology useful to population health are descriptive, analytical, and managerial. Descriptive analyses focus on the determinants and distribution of disease by assessing overall exposure to risk factors and frequency of cases in large populations. Descriptive data includes cases, frequency of disease metrics, prevalence, and incidence data, and many of the standard crude rates that focus on mortality and morbidity. Analytical epidemiology requires a comparison group whether using case-control or cohort studies. Analytical analyses discover relationships between risk factors, exposures and disease or health status. Managerial epidemiology benefits population health decision-making by providing population health status and outcomes data that can be applied to population risk segmentation and tailored health promotion efforts.

Discussion Questions

1. Provide an example of an endemic, an epidemic, and a pandemic disease.
2. What is the difference between a crude and disease-specific (cancer) rate?
3. Why are prevalence rates more useful than incidence rates for measuring chronic diseases?

4. Explain the three diverse types of epidemiology: descriptive, analytical, and managerial. Be sure to include an example.
5. Discuss why the infant mortality rate is the universal rate used for comparing a country's health status.

References

Awofeso, N. (2003, May). What's new about the "new public Health"? *American Journal of Public Health*, 93(5), 705–709. doi:10.2105/ajph.93.5.705

Caron, R. (2017a). Epidemiology: The basic science of public health. In R. Caron (Ed.), *Population health: Principles and applications for management* (pp. 28–56). HAP/AUPHA.

Caron, R. (2017.). Public health foundations for population health managers. In A. Hewitt, J. Mascari, & S. Wagner (Eds.), *Population health management: Strategies, tools, applications, and outcomes* (pp. 30–31). HAP/AUPHA.

Centers for Disease Control and Prevention. (n.d.). Chapter 1: Introduction to analytical epidemiology. In *Public health practice: An introduction to epidemiology and biostatistics* (3rd ed.). https://www.cdc.gov/csels/dsepd/ss1978/lesson1/section7.html

Centers for Disease Control and Prevention. (1999, April 2). 10 great public health achievements—United States 1900–1999. *MMWR Weekly*, 48(12), 241–243. https://www.cdc.gov/mmwr/preview/mmwrhtml/00056796.htm

Centers for Disease Control and Prevention. (2020). *Healthy People 2030*. National Center for Health Statistics. https://www.cdc.gov/nchs/healthy_people/hp2030/hp2030.htm

Centers for Disease Control and Prevention Online Newsroom. (2011, June 23). *CDC identifies top global public health achievements in first decade of 21st century*. https://www.cdc.gov/media/releases/2011/p0623_publichealth.html

Fleming, S. T. (2013). Managerial epidemiology: It's about time! *Journal of Primary Care & Community Health*, 3(2), 138–139. doi: 10.1177/2150131912375132

Friis, R. (2018). *Epidemiology 101* (2nd ed.). Jones and Bartlett Learning.

Friis, R. H., & Sellers, T. A. (2013). *Epidemiology for public health practice* (5th ed.). Jones & Bartlett Learning.

Goodman, R., Moulton, A., Matthews, G., Shaw, F., Kocher, J., Mensah, G., Zaza, S., & Besser, R. (2006, December 22). Law and public health at CDC. *Morbidity and Mortality Weekly Report*, Centers for Disease Control and Prevention. https://www.cdc.gov/mmwr/preview/mmwrhtml/su5502a11.htm

Institute of Medicine (US) Committee for the Study of the Future of Public Health. (1988). 3, A history of the public health system. In *The future of public health*. National Academies Press. https://www.ncbi.nlm.nih.gov/books/NBK218223/

McPhillips, D. (2022, April 8). *U.S. life expectancy continues historical decline with another drop in 2021 study finds*. CNN Health. https://www.cnn.com/2022/04/07/health/us-life-expectancy-drops-again-2021/index.html#:~:text=CNN%20Store-,US%20 life%20expectancy%20continues%20historic%20decline,drop%20in%202021%2C%20study%20finds&text=Life%20expectancy%20in%20the%20US,to%2076.6%20years%20in%202021

Office of Health Promotion and Disease Prevention. (2021, August 23). *History of Healthy People*. U.S. Department of Health and Human Services. https://health.gov/our-work/national-health-initiatives/healthy-people/about-healthy-people/history-healthy-people

Oleski, D.M. (Ed.) (2001). *Epidemiology and the delivery of health care services* (2nd ed.), Kluwer Academic/Plenum Publishers.

Rohrer, J. (2013). Managerial epidemiology. *Journal of Primary Care & Community Health, 3*(2), 82. doi: 10.1177/2150131913375551

Schanzenbach, D. W., Nunn, R., & Bauer, L. (2016, June). *The changing landscape of American life expectancy*. The Hamilton Project. https://www.hamiltonproject.org/assets/files/changing_landscape_american_life_expectancy.pdf

Seabert, D., McKenzie, J., & Pinger, R. (2022). *McKenzie's an introduction to community and public health* (10th ed.). Jones and Bartlett Learning.

Statista. (2022). *Life expectancy (from birth) in the United States, from 1860 to 2020*. https://www.statista.com/statistics/1030079/life-expectancy-united-states-all-time/

Turnock, B. (2021). *Epidemiology and disease control in essentials of public health* (2nd ed.). Jones and Bartlett Learning.

United Nations Chronicle. (n.d.). *Lifestyle diseases: An economic burden on the health services*. https://www.un.org/en/chronicle/article/lifestyle-diseases-economic-burden-health-services#:~:text=Lifestyle%20diseases%20share%20risk%20factors,metabolic%20syndrome%2C%20chronic%20obstructive%20pulmonary

Wainer, D. (2022, June 7). Pfizer and Moderna won't get a shot in the arm from toddlers. *Wall Street Journal*, B12.

Credits

Fig. 3.1: Generated with FreeWordCloudGenerator.com.
Fig. 3.3a: Copyright © 2022 Depositphotos/Anatta_Tan.
Fig. 3.3b: Copyright © 2019 Depositphotos/AndrewLozovyi.
Fig. 3.3c: Copyright © 2017 Depositphotos/Rawpixel.
Fig. 3.6: Copyright © 2020 Depositphotos/kLuka.

CHAPTER FOUR

Population Health Frameworks

Chapter Description

This chapter describes the most important models and guidelines used when organizing health care for populations. While previous chapters discussed the role and need for population health, Chapter 4 introduces the "how" to improve health outcomes. Population health frameworks represent perspectives from industry, government, philanthropic foundations, and public and community health. The original Triple Aim®, sponsored by the Institutes of Health, has served as guidance for many other models, including the industry example, the Population Health Alliance Framework. The Culture of Health model features a quality-of-life vision and details the collective actions needed by community organizations. Two public and community frameworks, the Collective Impact

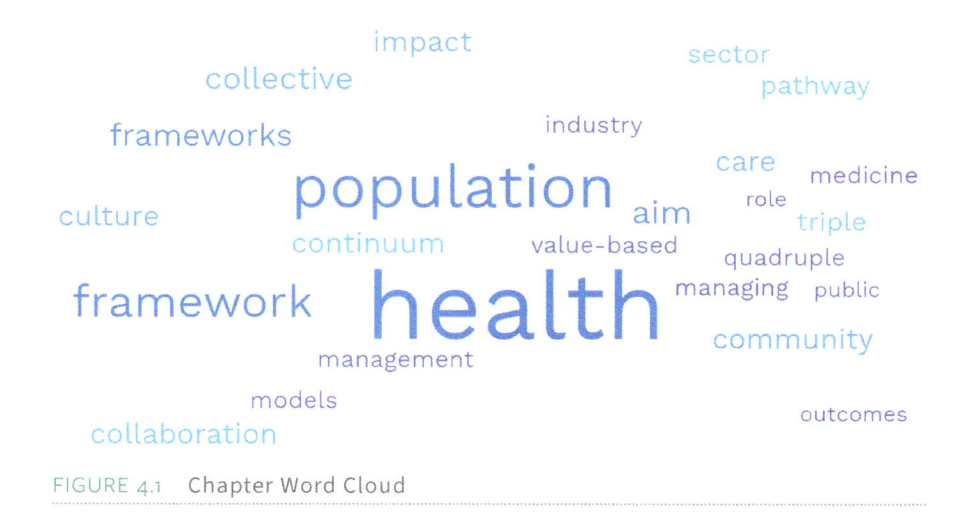

FIGURE 4.1 Chapter Word Cloud

Framework, and the Continuum of Collaboration, highlight the development of strong intersectoral relationships, which are also seen in the American Hospital Association's (AHA) Pathway to Population Health. Each framework has been widely adopted by the national health sector.

Chapter Objectives

After completing this chapter, students will be able to:

1. Identify the components of the Triple Aim and the Quadruple Aim
2. Discuss the Culture of Health vision and explain the four Action Areas
3. Describe the Pathway to Population Health's four portfolios
4. Explain the Population Health Alliance's (PHA) Population Health Management Framework process flow
5. Provide a rationale for why value-based care and precision medicine were added to the PHA's framework
6. Provide examples of each relationship level on the Continuum of Collaboration
7. Identify the six initiative criteria outlined in the Collective Impact Framework

Key Words

Triple Aim	Continuum of Collaboration	Pathways to Population Health
Quadruple Aim	Culture of Health	Precision medicine
Collective Impact Framework	PHA Population Health Management Framework	Value-based care

Managing the Health of Populations

As presented in Chapter 2, community, public, and global health approaches share both commonalities and differences with population health. The major distinction will always be population health's emphasis on managing the health of populations for quality of outcomes and cost. The term managing implies a way of planning, conducting, directing, and controlling business (Koontz & O'Donnell, 1968). The operational frameworks presented in this chapter provide outlines for applying core activities and implementing strategies that directly affect care delivery. These guidelines differ from previously mentioned frameworks such as the National Priorities Partnership (NPP, 2008), and the four pillars of health (Nash, 2012) that only described the various components of a population health management system. This chapter introduces the how-to for operationally focused health population models.

Key Frameworks for Managing Populations: The Two Visions

The Triple Aim Vision

When it was introduced in 2008, the original Triple Aim offered a much-needed solution for the conundrum of unmet health needs and rising expenses by focusing simultaneously on three key aims of health care delivery: access, quality, and cost (Berwick et al., 2008). Although the framework of aligning the three key elements almost seems simplistic today, it was an incredibly innovative idea to integrate all three health care operations together. Now, we recognize that this framework effectively linked payors, providers, and patients together and formed the foundation of population health management (see Figure 4.2).

The Institute for Health Improvement (IHI) built on these original health goals by further transforming the model into active strategies that would play a crucial role in improving health care outcomes. The three strategies were designed to ensure (a) the creation of the right foundation for population management, (b) that services were managed at a scale for the populations, and (c) that a learning system would be established to drive and sustain the work overtime (Whittington et al., 2015). Figure 4.3 depicts a schematic of the IHI's iron triangle.

The **Triple Aim**, one of the most important population health models, clarified that all three factors be pursued at the same time,

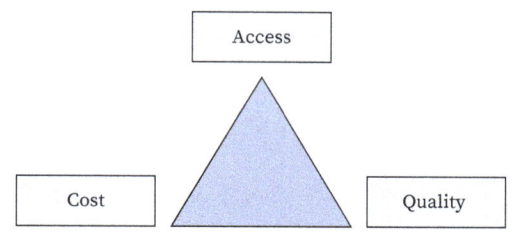

FIGURE 4.2   The Original Triple Aim

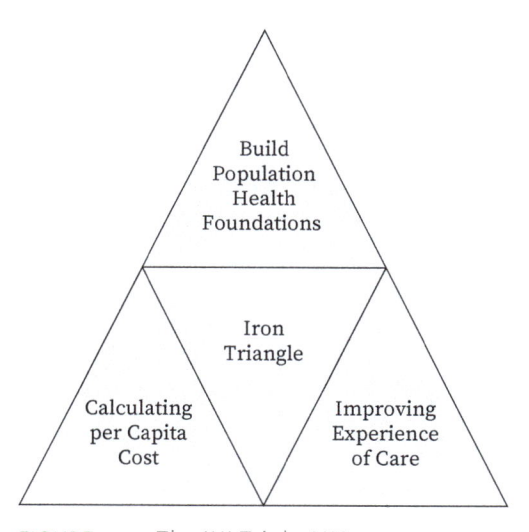

FIGURE 4.3   The IHI Triple AIM

which necessitated a new health care delivery approach—not one based on the medical model of one person at a time with fee-for-service payment. Each of the three strategies that form this "iron triangle" altered how health care delivery is provided to populations, including the development of a new type of health organization: the accountable care organization (ACO). The ACO serves as the initial operational model that required the use of alternative payment systems and introduced the value-over-volume requirements. Chapter 11 provides a full explanation of the ACO model, and Chapter 10 describes in detail the various alternative payment systems that permit a value-over-volume approach.

Over the years, the Triple Aim has been revised to reflect broader goals of enhancing patient experience, improving population health, and reducing costs.

Practical Skill: The Burnout Phenomenon in the Health Care Workforce

As students consider entering the health care work arena, it is worth noting the truly negative impact of "burnout" on all health care personnel, including physicians, nurses, and even hospital CEOs. First, review the article describing the phenomenon of health care burnout and then the second article, which presents an overview of the cost to the health system. What are your suggestions? What needs to be done that will allow the goals of Triple Aim to be reached? Can you provide three strategies or find a solution?

Source: Reith, T. P. (2018). Burnout in United States healthcare professionals: A narrative review. Cureus, 10*(12), e4681. https://tinyurl.com/tvrtr824*

Source: Lagasse, J. (2022, November 28). Cost of burnout-related physician turnover totals $5 billion annually. Healthcare Finance. *https://tinyurl.com/hskemtf6*

Health professionals have suggested that a fourth goal be added to address the workforce experience (Bodenheimer & Sinsky, 2014). Given today's demanding work environment, the rate of health practitioner burnout and loss of morale have significantly increased, and the joy of work has decreased (Feely, 2017). An emphasis on the well-being of health providers would help retain valuable personnel and reduce the multiple staff shortages facing the health sector today (Glickman, 2022).

Other health researchers suggest that the quadruple aim would benefit from an emphasis on productivity to further align the four goals of population health (Arnetz et al., 2020). In this case, the idea of ***productivity*** refers to the individual outcomes required to create results, which places additional pressure on the workforce. If the health organization chooses to adopt an efficiency focus, this step would allow for positive results because when changes occur, the process improves and therefore increases overall workplace **efficiency**. These types of changes reflect a stronger population health management function at work.

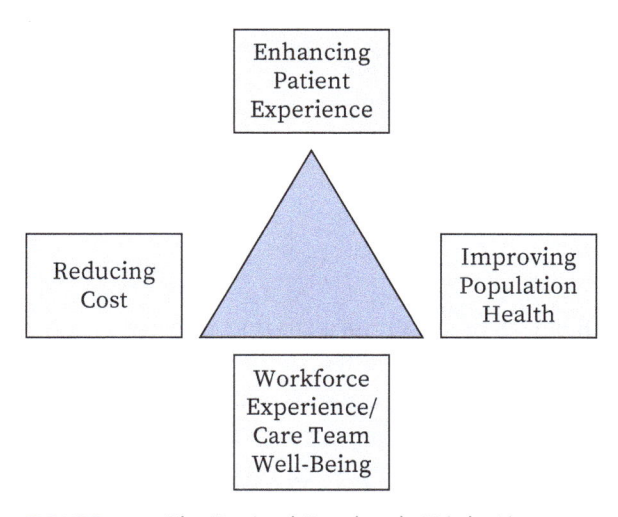

FIGURE 4.4   The Revised Quadruple Triple Aim

Today, the modified Triple Aim and **Quadruple Aim** model, which was developed as part of the Institutes of Health's focus on quality, continues to form the core goals and serve as a vision for population health.

The Cultural of Health Framework: A Population Health Vision for Communities

Sponsored by a national nonprofit health organization, the Culture of Health Action Framework identified a vision of population health for the community and became so widely known that it helped elevate the concept of health for all to be a valued national priority. This detailed model expanded on strategies and activities from community, public, and global health approaches to form a strong action framework and pathway (Chandra, 2017). The **Culture of Health** model was the first to emphasize that health is influenced by where we live, learn, work, and play (see Figure 4.4).

Action Area 1
Making Health a Shared Value

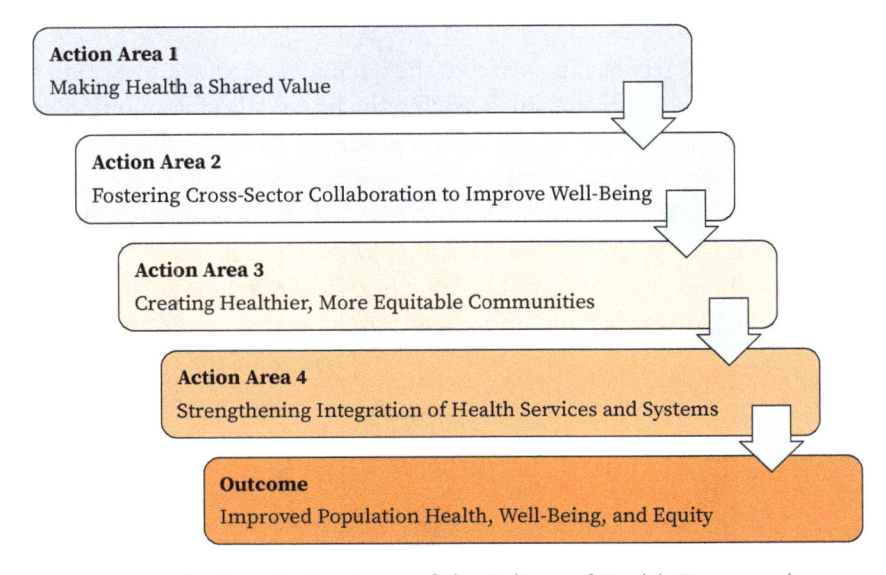

Action Area 2
Fostering Cross-Sector Collaboration to Improve Well-Being

Action Area 3
Creating Healthier, More Equitable Communities

Action Area 4
Strengthening Integration of Health Services and Systems

Outcome
Improved Population Health, Well-Being, and Equity

FIGURE 4.5   The Four Action Areas of the Culture of Health Framework

This national model includes action steps that appeal to all types of community organizations and industry sectors. The Culture of Health framework describes a process for developing community solutions, beginning with developing the all-important first step of reaching consensus on the value of health for all. Steps 2 and 4 describe strategies for recruiting program partners and ensuring that any future initiatives address health equity. For health sector partners, Step 4 is a call to action for strengthening the health system to meet contemporary needs. The framework also includes a fifth step that outlines the processes for improvement and assessment to ensure sustainability of any program.

Collaboration Frameworks for Managing Population Health

The Continuum of Collaboration

Public and community models and guidelines designed to build and improve community health relationships offer benefits for implementing population health. One example, the **Continuum of Collaboration** is a framework that emphasizes four relationship levels: networking, coordinating, cooperating, and collaborating (Himmelman, 2002; Association of State Public Health Nutritionists, 2017).

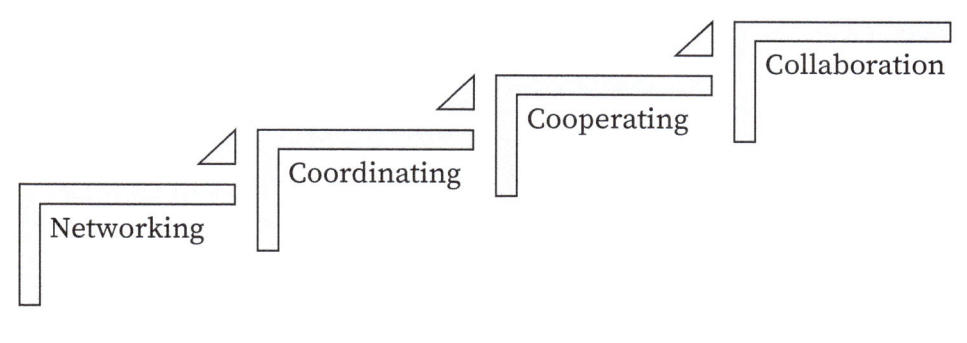

FIGURE 4.6   The Continuum of Collaboration

As you review the model, note that each additional step requires a stronger commitment between the partnering agencies. Not all community initiatives require true collaboration, and cooperating activities would be sufficient. During the COVID-19 pandemic, local hospitals, public health agencies, and other community organizations partnered to find necessary resources such as personal protective equipment (PPE), deliver food boxes, and find housing for patients when hospitals became overwhelmed (Bathija, 2021). This partnership is an example of the collaborative relationship level because all these organizations were needed to find the essential resources and complete the supply chain.

The Collective Impact Framework

A similar relationship approach, the **Collective Impact Framework**, suggests that combining influence factors from multiple levels and change agents from within levels will produce a greater social product than any single entity could manage alone (Kania & Kramer, 2011). *Collective impact* can be defined as "a network of community members, organizations, and institutions who advance equity by learning together, aligning, and integrating their actions to achieve population and systems level change" (Collective Impact Forum, n.d.). Both public and community organizations would be part of producing quality health care if involved in a collective impact project. Each collective impact project must include these five conditions in the initiative (see Figure 4.7).

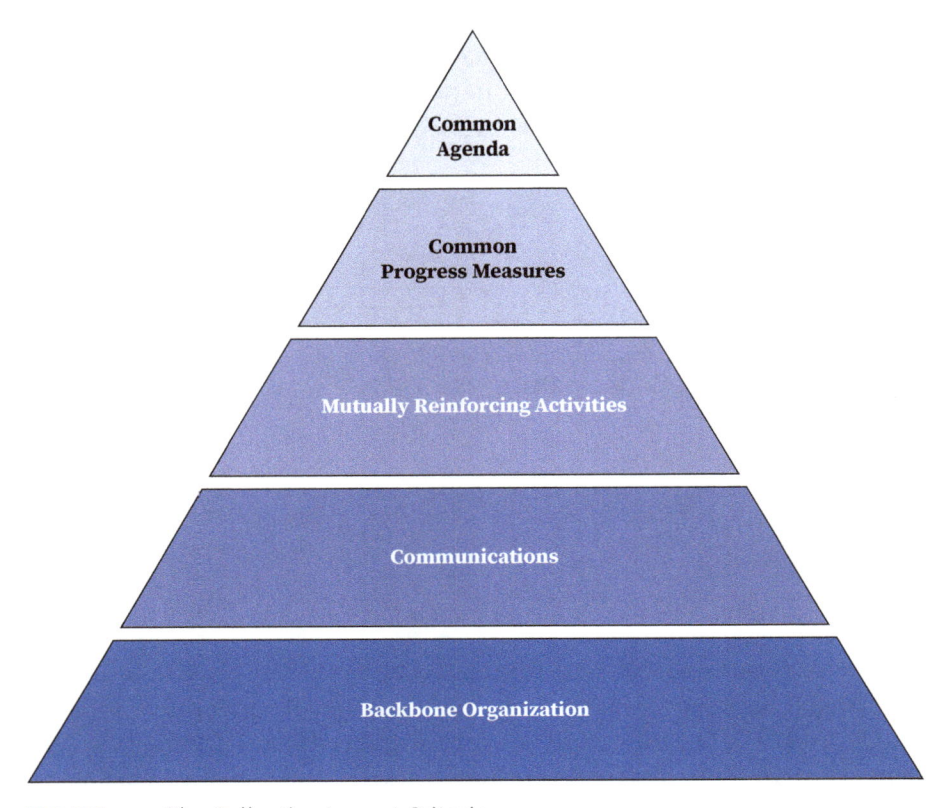

```
                    Common
                    Agenda

              Common
              Progress Measures

          Mutually Reinforcing Activities

              Communications

            Backbone Organization
```

FIGURE 4.7   The Collective Impact Criteria

Practical Skill: Collective Impact

Try assessing your understanding of the Collective Impact Framework by reviewing the Wilmington Collective Community Impact Study (Karpyn et al., 2018).

Instructions:

1. Access the following URL: https://tinyurl.com/5n6mdykx

2. Review the article and identify each of the five conditions necessary for collective impact.
3. Was the Wilmington Collective Impact Intervention successful?

Implementing Multisectoral Population Health Initiatives

Pathways to Population Health Framework

The Triple Aim identified population health goals, and additional frameworks have strongly emphasized requiring collaboration between all health sector stakeholders, especially health payors, providers, and patients (consumers). To ensure hospitals and health systems followed a successful transition to the population health model, the AHA, in partnership with other major health organizations, developed a strategic guidance framework document titled *The Pathways to Population Health: An Invitation to Healthcare Change Agents* (Saha et al., 2017). The document first outlined the foundational concepts of the pathway. Figure 4.8 presents **Pathways to Population Health** foundation statements.

1	2	3	4	5	6
Health and well-being develop over a lifetime.	Social determinants drive health and well-being outcomes throughout the life course.	Place is a determinant of health, well-being, and equity.	The health system needs to address the key demographic shifts of our time.	The health system can embrace innovative financial models and deploy existing assets for greater value.	Health creation requires partnership because health care only holds a part of the puzzle.

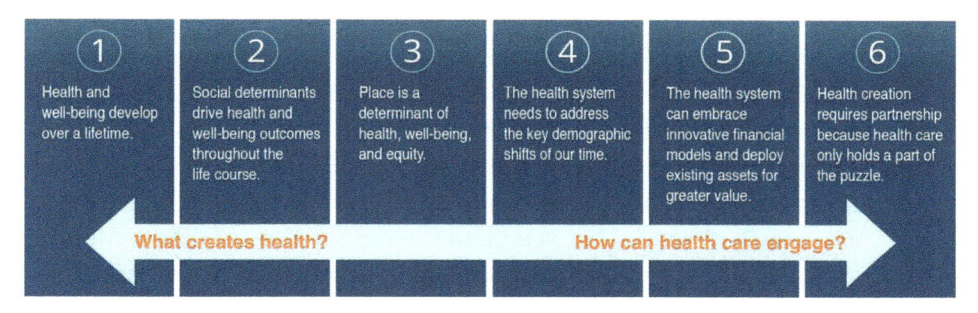

← What creates health?   How can health care engage? →

FIGURE 4.8 Six Foundational Concepts of Pathways to Population Health

The first three steps focus on the meaning of health, potential risk factors, and the importance of place or home as a contributor to overall health status. The remaining steps are specific strategic activities for the health system to (4) address the key demographic shifts of our time, (5) embrace financial models and deploy existing assets for greater value, and (6) create partnerships with other entities because health only holds part of the puzzle. These last major activity steps clearly align with Triple Aim's focus on serving populations at risk, managing costs, and creating a positive health outcome for all. Do you see any similarities to the Culture of Health model?

The Pathway to Population Health strategy organized the areas of work into two categories and then further separated them into four portfolios of activities for ease of hospital and health system adoption (see Figure 4.9).

The first portfolio category, identified as Population Management, highlights the health sector's responsibility of providing and managing the physical, mental, social, and/or spiritual health and well-being for all populations.

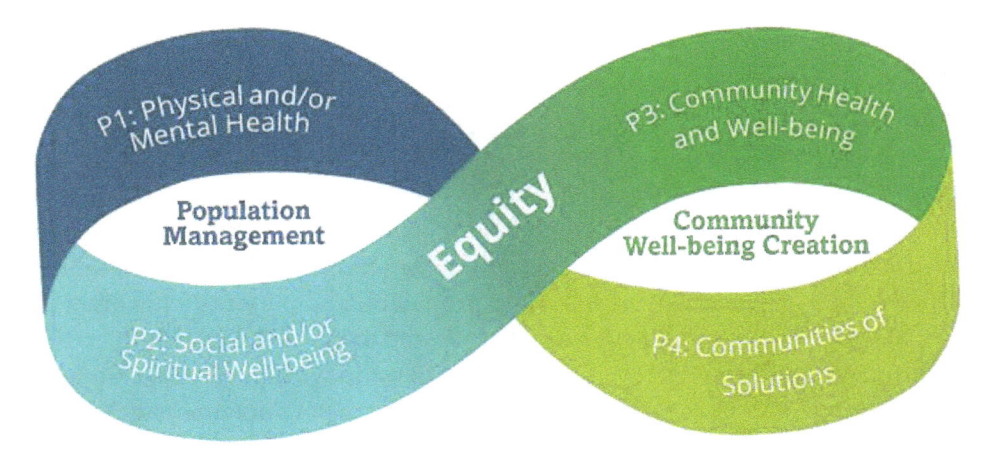

FIGURE 4.9 The Portfolios of Population Health Framework

Portfolios 1 and 2 encompass the actual delivery of health care with an equal focus on social and spiritual well-being. Portfolios 3 and 4, which include community of health and well-being and the communities of solutions, underscore the strategic importance of the health sector's alignment with community and other industry sector partners. The innovative strategy of communities of solutions is the long-term focus to build a successful health system for all and a recognition that population health will continue to evolve and change over time. Continuously threaded between and around these portfolios is the concept of equity. Health care equity demands that population health prioritizes strategies that remove complex and deeply embedded root causes of health inequities and disparities such as poverty, discrimination, lack of good jobs, equal education opportunities, and safe and secure homes and environments. Was equity a concept in the Culture of Health model?

Individual hospitals and/or health systems and communities can select among the four portfolios' strategies and activities to target specific populations at risk and/or risk factors to improve overall health. See Table 4.1.

Portfolios 1 and 2 provide examples based on both clinical (diabetes outcomes) and preventive (screenings and peer supports) tasks needed for quality health and well-being. In Portfolio 3, an example highlights a multisectoral partnership program that developed solutions for food insecurity in at-risk neighborhoods. Portfolio 4 expands on the multisectoral partnership concept on a larger scale by highlighting a collaborative initiative example where stakeholders chose to prioritize minority-owned local businesses as purchase partners.

Population Health Alliance Framework

Other industry organizations also recognized the need for developing the step-by-step processes of population health management. The PHA, the

Chapter Four Population Health Frameworks | 75

TABLE 4.1   Portfolios of Population Health Strategies

	Portfolio 1: Physical and/or Mental Health	Portfolio 2: Social and/or Spiritual Well-Being	Portfolio 3: Community Health and Well-Being	Portfolio 4: Communities of Solutions
Type of population	Defined	Defined	Place-based and defined	Place-based and defined
Focus of work	Proactively address mental and/or physical health for the population for which your organization is responsible (e.g., patients, employees)	Proactively address social and spiritual drivers for the population for which your organization is responsible (e.g., patients, employees)	Improvement of health, well-being, and equity focused on specific topics across a place-based or defined population	Whole community transformation with a focus on long-term structural changes needed for a thriving, equitable community
Example activities	Manage diabetes outcomes for a primary care panel, integrate mental health into primary care	Screen for and address social determinants of health in partnership with community social-service agencies; establish peer-to-peer support	Engage in a multisectoral partnership to address food insecurity in key neighborhoods	Engage in a multisectoral partnership to create long-term structure, policy, and systems changes (e.g., preferred purchasing from minority-owned local businesses)

Source: Saha, S., Loehrer, S., Cleary-Fisherman, M., Johnson, K., Chenard, R., Gunderson, G., Goldberg. R., Little, J., Resnick, J., Cutts, T., & Barnett, K. (2017). Pathways to population health: An invitation to health care change agents. *Institute for Healthcare Improvement. http://www.ihi.org/Topics/Population-Health/Documents/PathwaystoPopulationHealth_Framework.pdf.*

health industry's multistakeholder professional and trade association, provides frameworks and guidance to member organizations that are involved with implementing population health concepts (PHA, n.d.a). These industry members include major stakeholders such as national health plans, health systems, employer solutions, academia, biopharma, and health-related technology companies.

The PHA defines a *population health management* program as one that addresses health needs at all points along the continuum of health and well-being through participation of, engagement with and targeted interventions for the population." (PHA, n.d.b). Based on this definition, it is not a surprise that the "person" is at center of this framework. The **PHA Population Health Management Framework** (PHA-PHMF) is a process that places the person at the center of population health and shows the various management activities in a sequential order. Because this framework focuses on management, it also includes two major PHM strategies: value-based care and precision medicine (PHA, n.d.b).

The PHA-PHMF aligns with all the population health processes and provides the following benefits:

- First, it addresses all the important stakeholders, including payors, providers, and patients, who are placed at the center of the model.
- Second, it offers a process for meeting the health needs of a priority population at all stages along the entire continuum of health and wellness.
- Third, it allows for context by referencing the community as a major stakeholder and the importance of culture and environment.
- Fourth, it recently added two influential factors to affect population health in the future: value-based care and precision medicine.

The model begins with three action strategies that are applicable to any priority population: (a) identification and monitoring of the population's health status, (b) conducting a health assessment (either a public health or a hospital's community health assessment), and (c) completing a risk stratification, which is a systematic process for identifying and predicting a patient's risk levels. (Risk segmentation and stratification will be covered in detail in Chapter 9.)

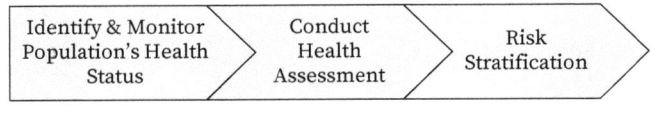

FIGURE 4.10 Initial Population Health Management Framework Action Steps

As presented next in the framework, the care continuum includes multiple categories of care: health promotion and wellness, health risk assessment, care coordination and advocacy, and disease/case management. These population health levels of care inform us what type of tailored intervention is needed as well as which community resources should be involved in the care process and ensure that cultural and environmental considerations are an integrated priority. The final framework section identifies the assessment measures and monitors cost-efficiency as well as health outcomes (e.g., psychosocial, behavioral change, clinical), which measure productivity, satisfaction, and quality of life.

The PHA-PHMF simplifies population health administrative and operational processes into four action steps, as seen in Table 4.2.

The two-way flow of information shows an interactive relationship between all components of the framework, which is necessary to ensure a multisectoral initiative is coordinated and can integrate all aspects of population health. All the action steps, activities, and strategies are aligned to ensure the population health care delivery process produces successful health outcomes.

Chapter Four Population Health Frameworks | 77

TABLE 4.2   Simplified PHA-PHMF Workflow

Strategy	Operational Action Steps
Assessment *Knowing your population*	• Population monitoring • Population identification • Health assessments
Stratification *Discovering vulnerabilities and strengths*	• Risk stratification—Low, moderate, high • Health/promotion wellness option • High-risk management strategies • Care coordination/advocacy planning • Disease/case management treatment and follow-up
Person-centered interventions *Tailoring to you*	• Community resources • Cultural and environmental impacts • Organizational capabilities
Impact evaluation *Assessing for population health improvement*	• Positive clinical outcomes and health status • Financial outcomes linked to health value • Psychosocial outcomes (cultural/environmental progress) • Behavior change—Person-centered development • Efficiency and effectiveness, satisfaction, and quality of life

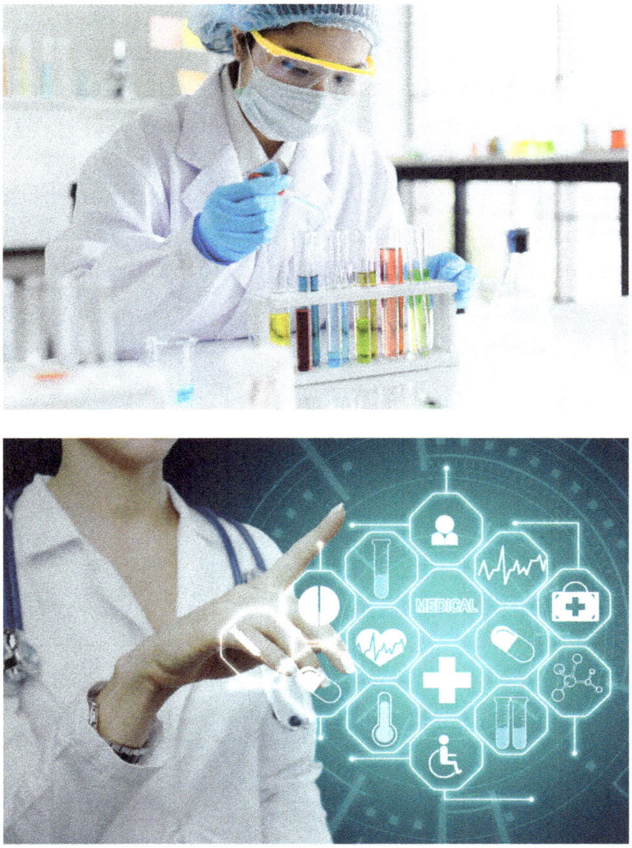

FIGURE 4.11   Precision Medicine and Value-Based Care

Precision Medicine as Key to Value-Based Care

Also included in the PHA-PHMF are two important impact factors: value-based care and precision medicine. **Value-based care** refers to the shift to population-focused care with positive health outcomes per unit of cost as a value (Porter, 2010). (Note that Chapter 1 introduced the volume-to-value discussion, and Chapter 10 covers value-based care in depth.) As the health industry evolves away from the medical model and fee for service for each health encounter, value-based care will ensure that both the patient and the provider are rewarded for quality-of-care outcomes. This overarching feature of value-based care is why it has a prominent place in the PHA-PHMF.

The AHA (2021) describes **precision medicine** as a tailoring of medical treatment to the individual characteristics of each patient. Precision medicine, which is sometimes referred to as *personalized medicine*, focuses on integrating data from an individual's genetics, environment, and lifestyle to customize and personalize treatments (AHA, 2021). One example can be seen in the development of personalized drugs appropriate for each person (Olden & Erwin, 2023). However, if precision medicine focuses on the individual, how will this concept ever work with population health, which focuses on large groups?

A COVID-19 example illustrates how these two influential factors can combine to improve health care dramatically while also being cost-effective (see Figure 4.12). COVID-19 affected minority populations disproportionately compared to the rest of the American population. The benefit of precision medicine is that it produces an improved disease-specific, treatment pathway, such as COVID-19, by combining personalized pharmacologic options and other new biological therapies. In other words, it can transform how health care providers

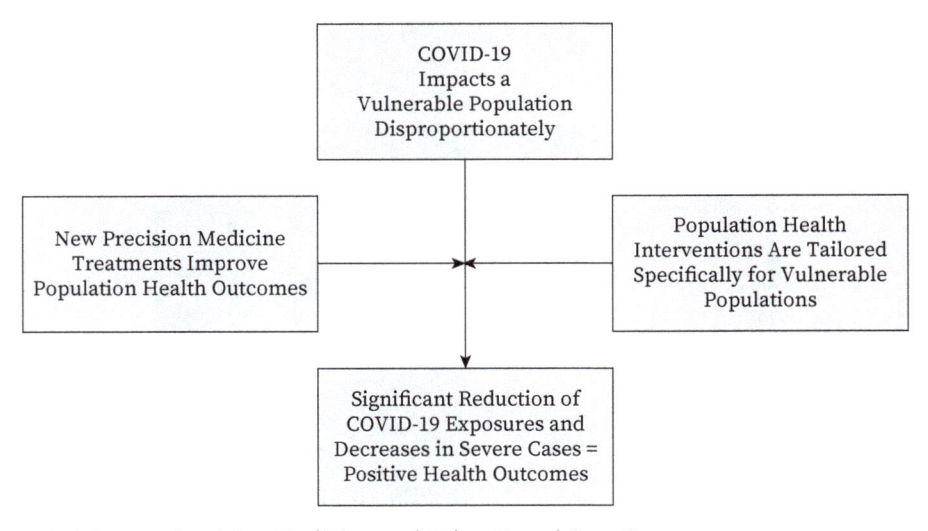

FIGURE 4.12 Precision Medicine and Value-Based Care Synergy

treat a disease. Population health determines the risk factors for priority populations and tailors' intervention programs that also focus on social determinants of health, including culture issues and inclusion factors. COVID-19 health outcomes improved significantly due to the cooperation of these two strategies (Hoppszallern, 2021). Precision medicine not only led to better care and personalized pharmacologic options (AHA, 2021) but saved lives as well.

Neither of these two contemporary approaches would have been as successful alone as they are combined. Imagine what this means for you. In the future, your care may be based not only on recommendations for your age, gender, or disease diagnosis but also your unique genetic vulnerabilities and strengths and the right value-based care plan. Precision medicine and value-based care are complementary concepts and valuable additions to population health.

Summary

Population health's primary goal will always be the improvement of health for all Americans. In recent years, major frameworks and models have emerged to provide specific objectives and strategies to attain that goal. The Iron Triangle not only identified but specified that access, cost, and quality had to occur within all processes to ensure health sector success. The Culture of Health model infused the value of health concept into every community, and the Continuum of Collaboration and the Collective Impact framework demonstrated viable and successful community relationship options useful for impacting today's health care. The AHA's Pathway to Population Health highlighted the role of multisectoral relationships and underscored the necessity for health systems and individual hospitals to align with other local stakeholders to ensure sustainable health outcomes. The PHA-PHMF supplied an up-to-date industry template that identified a complete process for managing population health and its integration with all health sector organizations. Future population health professionals will follow these frameworks as they engage with their priority populations.

Discussion Questions

1. The routinely referenced framework for population health management is the Triple Aim—now known as the Quadruple Aim—with multiple articles published on its impact. However, its goals are not as well known, but they still serve as a valid and solid foundation today. List the three goals and give an example of a population health process, product, or activity that represents the fulfillment of that goal.

2. Just as the Triple/Quadruple Aim served as the foundation for population health strategies for health sector organizations, the Culture of Health provided the essential framework for communities and the nation to embrace an innovative approach to health care. The Culture of Health outlined four action areas for improvement across the county (see Figure 4.4). Action areas have been translated into specific programs: evidence for action, health data for action, policies for action, and systems for action. Watch the video *Building a Culture of Health: In Our Time* to learn more about each program. Identify the purpose of each of the four programs.

    Source: Robert Wood Johnson Foundation. (n.d.). Building a culture of health: In our time. *https://tinyurl.com/yewbyt8w*

3. Community and public health organizations routinely pool their resources as a strategy to improve population health. The Continuum of Collaboration (Figure 4.6) shows each stage of the various relationship types. Each stage increases the complexity, intensity, and formality that lead to greater accountability. Review page 8 of *Community Health Partnerships Tools and Information for Development and Support* to learn detailed information about each of the four stages. Describe the relationship for each level of accountability between the partner organizations.

    Source: National Business Coalition on Health and the Community Coalitions Health Institute. (n.d.). Community health partnerships tools and information for development and support. *https://tinyurl.com/2nfzr3c8*

4. While the Continuum of Collaboration easily defines relationships between common community and public health partners, the Collective Impact framework describes the five conditions and criteria essential for ensuring that quality health care is produced. Identify each of the five criteria and their purpose.

5. The AHA and other partners developed a strategic guidance framework document, *The Pathways to Population Health: An Invitation to Healthcare Change Agents*, to ensure the health sector was equally involved in implementing population health strategies. The four program areas for the Pathways to Population Health framework were called *portfolios*. Identify each of the four portfolios and give an example of a program or activity that reflects population health strategies.

Source: Saha, S., Loehrer, S., Cleary-Fisherman, M., Johnson, K., Chenard, R., Gunderson, G., Goldberg. R., Little, J., Resnick, J., Cutts, T., & Barnett, K. (2017). Pathways to population health: An invitation to health care change agents. *Institute for Healthcare Improvement. https://tinyurl.com/4hmcka5u*

References

American Hospital Association. (2021, March 22). *Personalized and population-level interventions key to value-based care*. https://www.aha.org/sponsored-executive-dialogues/2021-04-22-precision-medicine-and-population-health

Arnetz, B.B., Goetz, C.M., Arnetz, J.E. et al. (2020). Enhancing healthcare efficiency to achieve the Quadruple Aim: an exploratory study. *BMC Res Notes* 13, 362 (2020). https://doi.org/10.1186/s13104-020-05199-8

Association of State Public Health Nutritionists. (2017, November 16). *ASPHN collaboration primer*. https://asphn.org/wp-content/uploads/2017/10/collaboration-primer.pdf

Bathija, P. (2021, March 25). *Joining hands for greater impact: How hospitals are partnering to support their communities through COVID-19*. https://www.aha.org/news/blog/2021-04-25-joining-hands-greater-impact-how-hospitals-

Berwick, D., Nolan, T., & Whittington, J. (2008). The Triple Aim: Care, health, and cost. *Health Affairs, 27*(4), 759–769. doi: 10.1477/hlthaff.27.4.759

Bodenheimer, T., & Sinsky, C. (2014). From Triple to Quadruple Aim: Care of the patient requires care of the provider. *Annals of Family Medicine, 12*(6), 574–576. https://doi.org/10.1470/afm.1714

Chandra, A., Acosta, J., Carman, K.G. et al., (2017). Building a national culture of health: Background, action framework, measures, and next steps. *Rand Health Quarterly, 6*(2), 3. https//:www.ncbi.nlm.nih.gov/pmc/articles/PMC5568157

Collective Impact Forum. (n.d.). *What is collective impact?* https://collectiveimpactforum.org/what-is-collective-impact/

Culture of Health (2022). *Culture of health prize—2020–2021* Video. Robert Wood Johnson Foundation. https://www.rwjf.org/en/library/features/culture-of-health-prize.html

Culture of Health Action Framework. (2022). *Taking action*. Robert Wood Johnson Foundation. https://www.rwjf.org/en/cultureofhealth/taking-action.html

Feeley, D. (2017, November 28). *The Triple Aim or the Quadruple Aim? Four points to help set your strategy.* Institute for Health Improvement. http://www.ihi.org/communities/blogs/the-triple-aim-or-the-quadruple-aim-four-points-to-help-set-your-strategy

Glickman, E. (2022, January 10). *Workplace shortages, burnout strain hospital HR staff.* https://rise.articulate.com/share/Xp7j0GajpgMBEUs448kRAYtSzDgwNqZp?utm_source=newsletter&utm_medium=email&utm_content=Link%20to%20Academic%20Integrity%20Module&utm_campaign=provost-weekly#/

Himmelman, A. T. (2002, January). *Collaboration for a change: Definitions, decision-making model, roles, and collaboration process guide.* Himmelman Consulting.

Hoppszallern, S. (2021). *Precision medicine and population health: Personalized and population-level interventions key to value-based care.* American Hospital Association and Illumina. https://www.aha.org/system/files/media/file/2021/04/Illumina_PrecisionMedicine_dialogue_042521.pdf

Institute for Health Improvement. (2022). *The IHI Triple Aim*. http://www.ihi.org/Engage/Initiatives/TripleAim/Pages/default.aspx

Kania, J., & Kramer, M. (2011, Winter). Collective impact. *Stanford Social Innovation Review*. https://ssir.org/articles/entry/collective_impact

Karpyn, A., Wolgast, H., & Tracy, T. (2018, November 8). Realizing collective impact for community health: A Wilmington case study. *Delaware Journal of Public Health, 4*(5), 8–14. https://www.ncbi.nlm.nih.gov/pmc/articles/PMC8452445/

Koontz, H., & O'Donnell, C. (1968). *Principles of management: An analysis of managerial functions.* McGraw Hill Publishing Book Company.

Lagasse, J. (2022, November 28). *Cost of burnout-related physician turnover totals $5 billion annually.* Healthcare Finance. https://www.healthcarefinancenews.com/news/cost-burnout-related-physician-turnover-totals-5-billion-annually

Nash, D. B. (2012). *The population health mandate: A broader approach to care delivery.* The Four Pillars of Health in a Boardroom Press Special Edition. http://populationhealthcolloquium.com/readings/Pop_Health_Mandate_NASH_2012.pdf

National Priorities Partnership. (2008). *National priorities and goals: Aligning our efforts to transform America's healthcare.* National Quality Forum. http://www.qualityforum.org/Setting_Priorities/National_Priorities_Partnership_-_Call_for_Organizational_Nominations.aspx

Olden, P., & Erwin, C. (2023). *Management of healthcare organizations: An introduction* (4th ed.). ACHE Management Series. Health Administration Press.

Porter, M. E. (2010, December). What is the value of health care? *New England Journal of Medicine*, *464*(26), 2277–2281. doi: 10.1056/NEJMp1011024

Population Health Alliance. (n.d.a). *About PHA*. https://populationhealthalliance.org/about/

Population Health Alliance. (n.d.b). *PHA Framework*. https://populationhealthalliance.org/research/understanding-population-health/

Reith, T. P. (2018). Burnout in United States healthcare professionals: A narrative review. *Cureus, 10*(12), e4681. https://doi.org/10.7759/cureus.4681

Saha, S., Loehrer, S., Cleary-Fisherman, M., Johnson, K., Chenard, R., Gunderson, G., Goldberg. R., Little, J., Resnick, J., Cutts, T., & Barnett, K. (2017). *Pathways to population health: An invitation to health care change agents*. Institute for Healthcare Improvement. http://www.ihi.org/Topics/Population-Health/Documents/PathwaystoPopulationHealth_Framework.pdf

Whittington, J. W., Nolan, K., Lewis, N., & Torres, T. (2015). Pursuing Triple Aim: The first 7 years. *Milbank Quarterly*, *94*(2), 264–400. https://doi.org/10.1111/1468-0009.12122 https://www.ncbi.nlm.nih.gov/pmc/articles/PMC4462878/#:~:text=Policy%20Points,In%202008%2C%20researchers%20at%20the%20Institute%20for%20Healthcare%20Improvement%20(IHI,to%20reduce%20the%20per%20capita

Credits

Fig. 4.1: Generated with FreeWordCloudGenerator.com.

Fig. 4.5: Adapted from "The Four Action Areas of the Culture of Health Framework," https://www.rwjf.org/en/insights/blog/2015/11/measuring_what_matte.html. Copyright © 2015 by Robert Wood Johnson Foundation.

Fig. 4.7: Source: Adapted from https://www.cleverfiles.com/howto/collective-impact.html.

Fig. 4.7a: Copyright © 2021 Depositphotos/zizou07.

Fig. 4.8: Copyright © by Saha et al. (CC BY-SA 4.0) at https://www.ihi.org/Topics/Population-Health/Documents/PathwaystoPopulationHealth_Framework.pdf.

Fig. 4.9: Copyright © by Saha et al. (CC BY-SA 4.0) at https://www.ihi.org/Topics/Population-Health/Documents/PathwaystoPopulationHealth_Framework.pdf.

Table 4.1: Copyright © by Somava Saha, et al. (CC BY-SA 4.0) at http://www.ihi.org/Topics/Population-Health/Documents/PathwaystoPopulationHealth_Framework.pdf.

Fig. 4.11a: Copyright © 2020 Depositphotos/Tong_Nawarit.

Fig. 4.11b: Copyright © 2019 Depositphotos/peshkov.

PART II

Health

Part II of this text examines the foundations of health and describes their impact on individual wellness, social determinants of health, and positive lifestyle behaviors needed to ensure health for all populations. Chapter 5 focuses on individual health choices and health risk assessments as well as health promotion and disease prevention activities used to attain wellness and well-being. The Health in All Policies framework highlights community health strategies that can improve all aspects of daily life. Chapter 6 covers the impact of the social determinants of health, which can lead to issues of food insecurity and access to care. The chapter provides a discussion on disparities, health equity, diversity, and inclusion strategies. The Upstream, Midstream, and Downstream framework introduces students to opportunities and situations in which health professionals can eliminate health care bias and improve health equity. Chapter 7 challenges students to examine their own healthy behaviors and everyday health decision-making processes as consumers. The Health Belief Model and Transtheoretical Theory provide step-by-step action strategies that can be adopted to change negative health behaviors. This chapter also shares behavior economic examples that use "nudges" and "influencers" to help patients overcome negative lifestyles and make positive health decisions. Population health relies on behavior change theories, behavior economic strategies, and targeted interventions that reduce the negative impact of social determinants of health to create positive health programming for all.

CHAPTER FIVE

Health Promotion and Wellness for All Populations

Chapter Description

The fifth chapter introduces the essential population health strategies of health promotion, disease prevention, and wellness. Population health emphasizes the five components of individual health along with the goal of attaining high-level wellness for all populations. To ensure that all Americans benefit for this strategy, health care delivery systems need to transition from the traditional primary, acute, and nursing home care of previous generations to the expanded Continuum of Care. This chapter also describes the use of personal health risk assessments as a valuable tool that assesses current wellness status and provides motivation for future healthy lifestyle behavior changes. At a societal level, the Health in All Policies framework provides advocacy guidance for population health interventions that key public and diverse community stakeholders can initiate to improve quality of life.

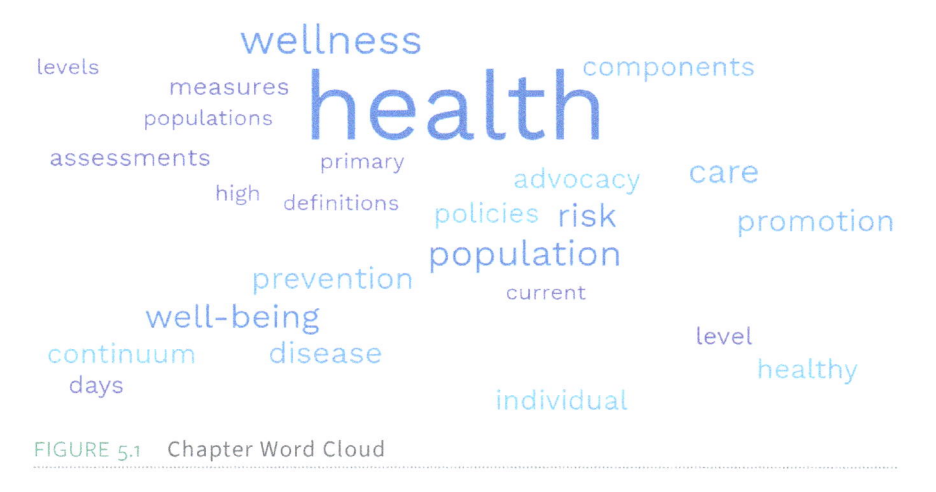

FIGURE 5.1 Chapter Word Cloud

Chapter Objectives

After completing this chapter, students will be able to:

1. Describe the current definitions for health, wellness, and well-being
2. Identify the five components of individual health
3. Complete an individual health risk assessment
4. Discuss and provide an example of the Continuum of Care model
5. Identify the Healthy Days Measures
6. Explain the importance of the Health in All Policies model

Key Words

Advocacy	Health advocacy	Health risk assessment	Levels of prevention (primary, secondary, tertiary)
Components of health	Health in All Policies	Healthy Days Measures	Well-being
Continuum of Care	Health promotion		
Disease prevention	Health promotion programs	High-level wellness	Wellness
Health			

Exploring Health Definitions

There is a familiar folk saying that goes "If you haven't got your health, you haven't got anything" that appeared in the popular comedy *The Princess Bride* more than 35 years ago (*The Princess Bride*, 1987). Health status does define your quality of life. The World Health Organization's (WHO) description of **health**—"a state of complete physical, mental and social well-being and not merely the absence of disease or infirmity" (WHO, 1946)—emerged as the first globally acknowledged health definition. Today, we know that the WHO's definition has been expanded to include both a spiritual and an emotional or behavioral health component. See Figure 5.2 for the current definitions of these five components of individual health.

Two of these definitions can be easily confused: mental health and emotional health. *Mental health*, as defined above, refers to cognitive functions, not to how an individual interacts with others. *Emotional health* most closely represents the concept of behavioral health. A contemporary definition describes *behavioral health* as the "scientific study of the emotions, behaviors and biology relating to a person's mental well-being, their ability to function in everyday life and their concept of self" (Array Behavioral Health, n.d.). You will find this misunderstanding exists in the health sector as the term *behavioral health* is becoming more prominent than *emotional health*.

Chapter Five Health Promotion and Wellness for All Populations | 89

Physical Health	• Ability to perform daily tasks without undue fatigue, refers to the integrity of the individual.
Social Health	• Ability to interact well with people and the environment. Having satisfying interpersonal relationships.
Mental Health	• Ability to learn, one's intellectual capacity.
Emotional Health	• Ability to control emotions so that one feels comfortable expressing them when appropriate and does not express them inappropriately.
Spiritual Health	• Belief in some unifying force. For some, it is nature, for others, it is scientific laws, and for others, it is a godlike force.

FIGURE 5.2 Components of Individual Health

Practical Skill: Checkback Activity

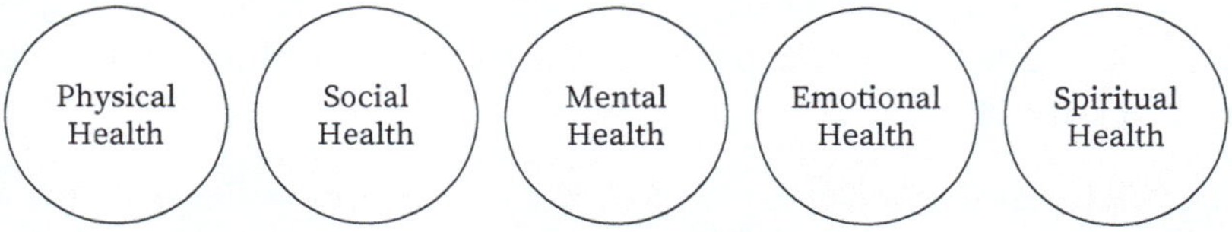

(Physical Health) (Social Health) (Mental Health) (Emotional Health) (Spiritual Health)

FIGURE 5.3 The Five Components of Health

Ask your classmates how they would rate their health status today using these five health components. Use a scale of 1 to 10 with 10 being perfect health. Students might report they have a rating of 7 or 8 and attribute the score to feeling fatigued from studying or experiencing too much stress in their lives. Other students might rate themselves as 9, saying that they have only slight cold symptoms today. Everyone assesses their own health status daily, which supports the concept that health is dynamic—it fluctuates continually.

High-Level Wellness and Well-Being

The concept of health that envisions a balanced state of the five interrelating components is known as **wellness,** and, as you can imagine, it is not easily attained. Canadian health promotion and community health experts years ago developed the "wellness" model that describes a more holistic definition of health (Ottawa Charter, 1986). **High-level wellness** can best be described as the desirable balance and integration among the five **components of health**. Figure 5.4 depicts high-level wellness as a desirable balance and alignment among the five components of health.

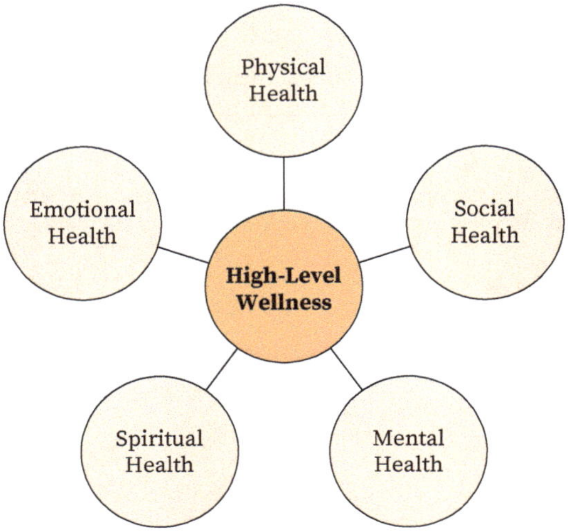

FIGURE 5.4   High-Level Wellness: Total Alignment of Individual Health Components

Review the following two definitions. Which one do you think best represents *your* concept of wellness?

- The Wellness Council of America (WELCOA) defines **wellness** as "the active pursuit to understand and fulfill your individual human needs—which allows you to reach a state where you are flourishing and able to realize your full potential in all aspects of life" (WELCOA, n.d.).
- The concept of **well-being** is described as a personal "state of being comfortable, healthy and happy" (Wellbeing People, 2018).

If you are sensing that *well-being* is broader and more expansive than *wellness*, you would be correct. A recent publication by the Robert Wood Johnson Foundation titled *Well-Being: Expanding the Definition of Progress* provides global examples of well-being developed by practitioners, researchers, and innovators from around the world (Plough, 2020). The authors conclude the key to global wellness is ensuring equity so that everyone has a just opportunity to be as healthy as possible. We all seek to live a long and healthy life with the goal that the length of time a person spends sick or disabled can be reduced and that the maximum lifespan is achieved (Stibich, 2019).

Chapter Five Health Promotion and Wellness for All Populations | 91

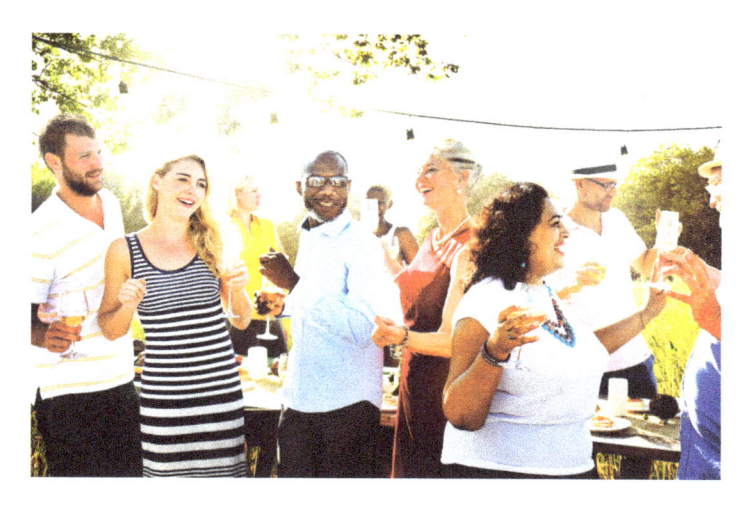

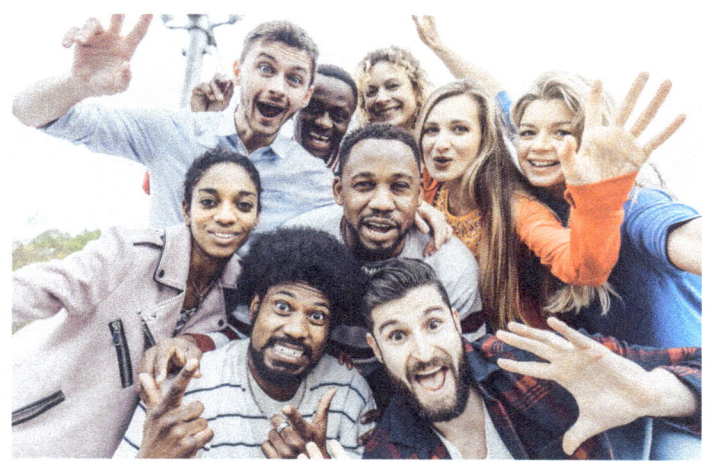

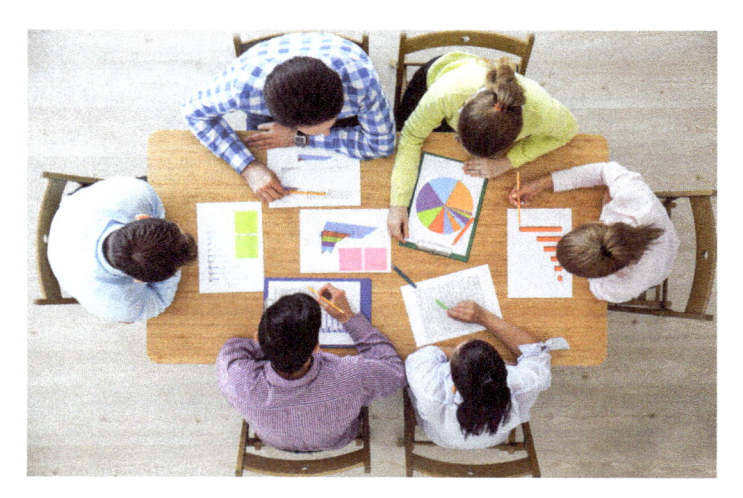

FIGURE 5.5 Diverse Healthy Environments

As depicted in the images above, we all live, work, and play in different circumstances, and these factors can also significantly affect our health status. The determinants of health can include physical, biological, social, cultural, and behavioral factors (Last, 2001). In addition to our individual genetic makeup, populations are diversely affected by external factors such as the social and physical environment, lifestyle behaviors, and medical care outcomes (Hayes & Delk, 2018). These influential factors are referred to as the major contributors of population health outcomes.

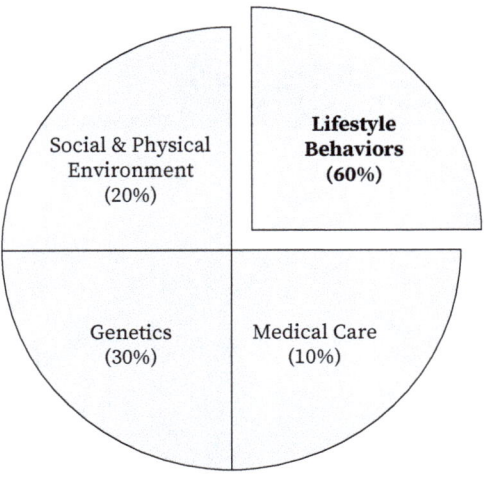

FIGURE 5.6   Major Contributors of Population Health Outcomes

Were you surprised to see that personal genetics contribute only 30% to your health outcomes? Did you expect that medical care contributes only 10% toward your overall health status? Figure 5.6 clearly illustrates that your own lifestyle behaviors are twice as important to your overall health status as compared to your genetic makeup. Socio-economic (SEC) factors, including where you live and your income, are a major component of assessing a population's health risk. To be more inclusive, SEC factors can be replaced by the concept of social determinants of health (SDOH), which are much more than just assessing income and educational levels. SDOH are especially important for managing a population's health and will be discussed in detail in the next chapter.

Health Assessments for Population Health

Healthy Days Measures

Now that we know which factors can influence our health status, how do we assess *health-related* quality of life? One of the first population health assessment tools developed was **Healthy Days Measures**, which are four simple questions that ask each person to rate their perceived state of health (Centers for Disease Control and Prevention [CDC], 2018).

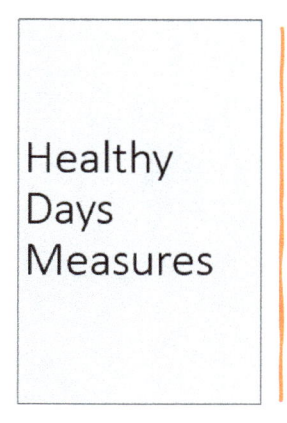

Healthy Days Measures	Would you say that in general your health is excellent, very good, good, fair or poor?
	Now thinking about your physical health, which includes physical illness and injury, how many days during the past 30 days was your physical health not good?
	Now thinking about your mental health, which includes stress, depression, and problems with emotions, how many days during the past 30 days was your mental health not good?
	During the past 30 days, approximately how many days did poor physical or mental health keep you from doing your usual activities, such as selfcare, work, or recreation?

FIGURE 5.7   Healthy Days Measures

Simply calculate your score by subtracting the number of unhealthy days from healthy days. What was your score? This simple questionnaire has been completed by millions of Americans over the years. Because these data can be aggregated for large and small populations and compared over time, population health organizations have found Healthy Days Measures useful for (a) identifying health disparities, (b) tracking population trends, and (c) adopting a measure that is universally compatible with the WHO's definition of health.

Health Risk Assessments

The average American does not think about the five components of individual health, the four major contributors of their health status, or the number of days that are healthy in a month. We know that if the public seeks medical information on a symptom or a disease, they will use an internet search engine to locate the desired information. When searching for basic health information, you might encounter a pop-up quiz asking you to assess your health risk with a few short questions. These pop-ups are marketing tools and used to create interest for purchasing a product (Blunt, 2022). However, when visiting a primary care provider, you will be asked to complete a brief questionnaire, usually digitally, about your health conditions and status that is based on a valid and reliable health assessment tool. Formal questionnaires, such as these, are referred to as individual **health risk assessments** (HRAs). The information within them can provide a snapshot of one's general health status. The data from thousands of individuals can be aggregated to determine various disease risks across a population. HRAs help identify those patients or consumers who would benefit from participation in a specific type of health promotion program (McAlearney, 2003).

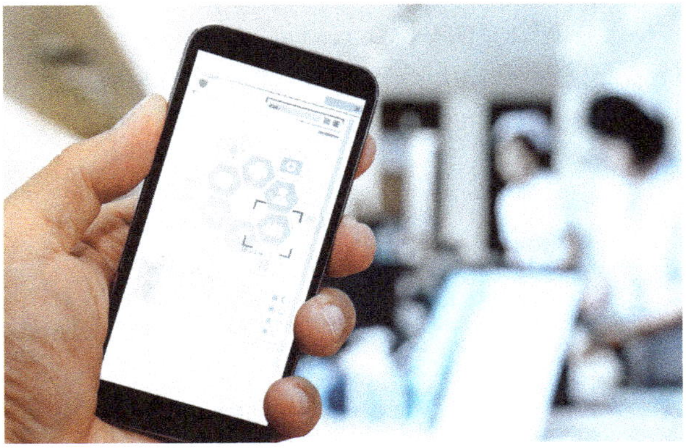

FIGURE 5.8 Health Risk Assessment Mobile Apps

Practical Skill: Checkback Activity

HRAs, which are usually questionnaires/surveys, can be completed in person or digitally and function as screening tools to identify and monitor health status (PDHI, 2022). The CDC has defined the minimum requirements for the Medicare health risk assessment in *A Framework for Patient-Centered Health Risk Assessments* (CDC, 2015). One of the most validated HRAs used as a quality-of-life baseline tool is the 36-Item Short Form Health Survey (RAND, n.d.), which is based on a 1990s medical outcomes research study (McAlearney, 2003). Today, the 12-Item Short Form Survey (SF-12) is used frequently by health providers as a brief health assessment that measures both physical and mental health status.

Access the following link to see the SF-12 questionnaire and review the questions: https://tinyurl.com/28nn6599

Access the following link to complete the online survey and receive a summary document of your health risks (S-12 OrthoToolkit, 2021): https://tinyurl.com/yeymua4v

What did you discover? Were there significant differences between these two risk assessments? Which one provided you with the most useful information?

Population Health Applications of Health Promotion and Disease Prevention

Population health reimagined traditional health care by transitioning from a medical model with a focus on the individual and clinical treatment to an inclusive all-population perspective that integrated **health promotion** and **disease prevention** activities across the **Care Continuum**. With the adoption of HRAs and their essential role at beginning of the health care delivery process, health providers and professionals routinely have opportunities to affect at-risk populations before severe disease emerges.

Compare these definitions of *health promotion* and *disease prevention*. Can you detect both commonalities and differences in the perspectives?

If you decided that health promotion strategies are extremely broad and include outreach activities, you would be correct. **Health promotion programs and activities** are defined as "any type of planned combination of educational, political, environmental, regulatory or organizations mechanisms that support actions and conditions of living conducive to the health of individuals, groups, and communities" (Joint Committee on Health Education and Promotion Terminology, 2012). The goal is to reach as many individuals within a priority population as possible. If you also noticed that the **levels of prevention** follow more of a (a) prevent, (b) diagnosis, and (c) treatment clinical model, then you were also correct. For

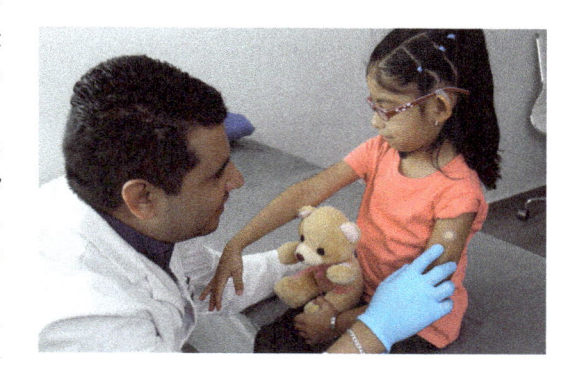

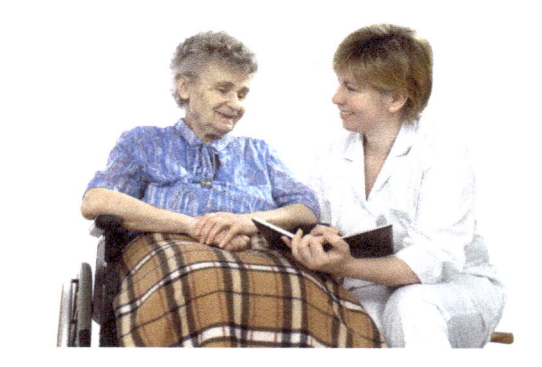

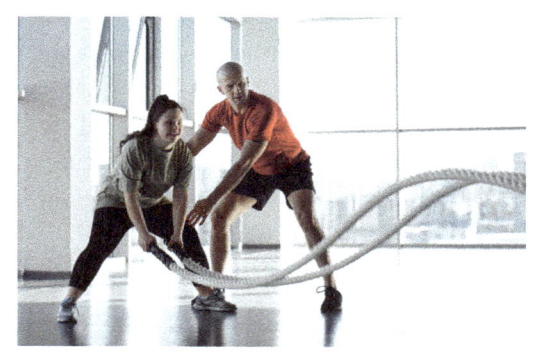

FIGURE 5.9 Health Promotional Events

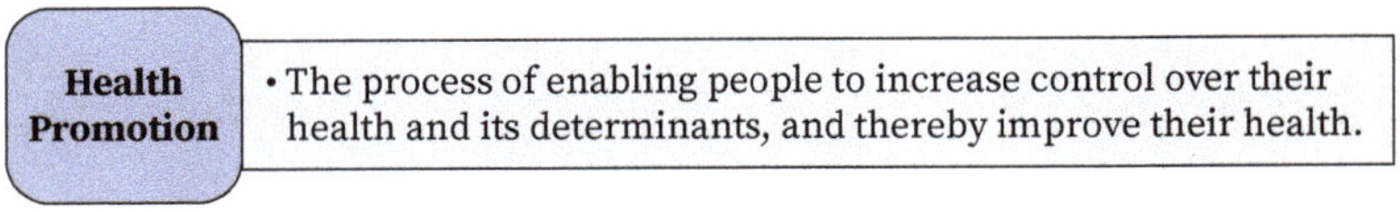

Health Promotion: The process of enabling people to increase control over their health and its determinants, and thereby improve their health.

FIGURE 5.10   Defining Health Promotion

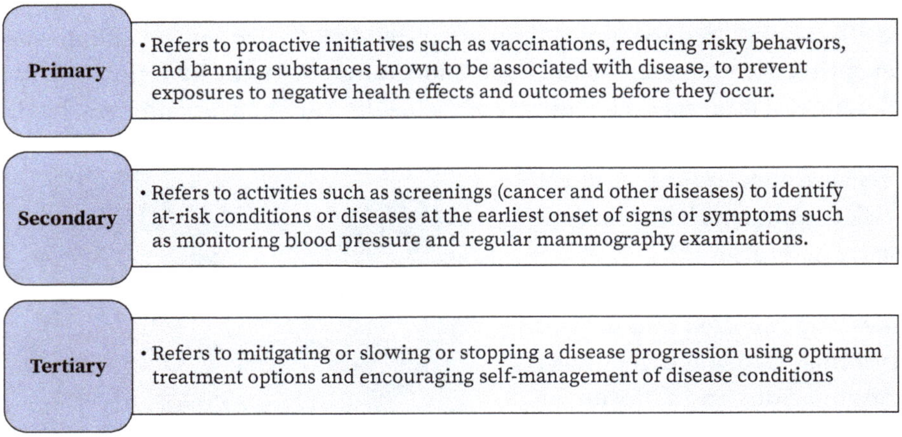

Primary: Refers to proactive initiatives such as vaccinations, reducing risky behaviors, and banning substances known to be associated with disease, to prevent exposures to negative health effects and outcomes before they occur.

Secondary: Refers to activities such as screenings (cancer and other diseases) to identify at-risk conditions or diseases at the earliest onset of signs or symptoms such as monitoring blood pressure and regular mammography examinations.

Tertiary: Refers to mitigating or slowing or stopping a disease progression using optimum treatment options and encouraging self-management of disease conditions

FIGURE 5.11   Defining Levels of Prevention

example, if you wanted to prevent or limit disease outcomes, you would expect to see a process of vaccination, screenings, and follow-up to disease treatment with self-management. Notice that the actual treatment for acute conditions is not part of the three levels of prevention.

Population Health: The Role of Advocacy

Health promotion efforts tailored for at-risk and vulnerable populations often require advocacy efforts (Parvanta et al., 2018). **Advocacy** refers to activities that influence public opinion and attitudes that directly affect people's lives. Organizations and individuals can advocate alone or join groups to support a common health cause. The purpose of **health advocacy** efforts can be to change individual behavior or a population's lifestyles or encourage development of positive health policies. The American Hospital Association (AHA) recently released the organization's 2023 advocacy agenda, which focuses on four primary goals:

- Ensuring access to care and providing financial relief
- Strengthening the health care workforce
- Advancing quality, equity, and transformation
- Enacting regulatory and administrative relief (AHA, 2023)

Population health initiatives would clearly align with advocacy activities to improve access to care and advance quality and equity.

Public health agencies regularly sponsor advocacy efforts that support population health initiatives tailored towards vulnerable populations. As part of public health's three-part mandate, an emphasis is required to focus on improving population health using health promotion and disease prevention communication frameworks. The Office of Disease Prevention developed several initiatives to advocate for COVID-19 testing and vaccination during the pandemic, including the ***WECANDOTHIS*** campaign, which encouraged community residents to join a group to spread resources about the disease and free vaccinations (U.S. Department of Health and Human Services, n.d.; see Figure 5.12).

COVID-19 Community Corps

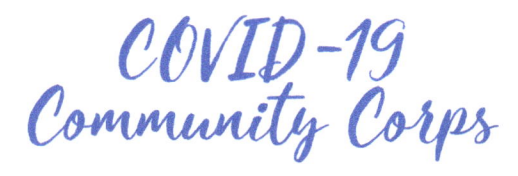

FIGURE 5.12 COVID-19 Community Corps

Other health promotion campaigns succeeded in targeting specific vulnerable populations (National Institutes of Health and Office of Disease Prevention, n.d.; see Figure 5.13).

COLLEGE AIM CollegeAIM
National Institute on Alcohol Abuse and Alcoholism (NIAAA)
https://www.collegedrinkingprevention.gov/collegeaim/

SAFE TO SLEEP Safe to Sleep® Campaign
***Eunice Kennedy Shriver* National Institute of Child Health and Human Development (NICHD)**
https://safetosleep.nichd.nih.gov/

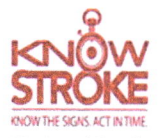

KNOW STROKE KNOW THE SIGNS. ACT IN TIME. Know Stroke
National Institute of Neurological Disorders and Stroke (NINDS)
https://www.stroke.nih.gov/about/

FIGURE 5.13 Public Health Campaigns Examples of Health Promotion and Disease Prevention Initiatives

Each of these advocacy campaigns tailored their messages to specific at-risk populations—including adolescents, parents, and individuals with high blood pressure or heart disease—and serve as examples of health advocacy efforts to improve the health of all Americans.

Expanding the Continuum of Care

To effectively include both health promotion and disease prevention activities, population health professionals recognized that the current continuum of care needed to be expanded. A ***Continuum of Care*** refers to care over time and was commonly thought of in terms of the phases of illness (Health Information Management System Society, 2014; National Cancer Institute, n.d.). The original Continuum of Care primarily included only three basic phases: (a) primary care (primary care provider visit), (b) acute care (hospital/treatment), and (c) nursing home care (follow-up). Today, the Continuum of Care framework is more than primary care and acute care. Population health care services expanded in both directions to encompass preventive care (health advocacy, health promotion, and disease prevention), and post-acute care (rehabilitation, home care, palliative, and hospice) services. As an unintended consequence of the COVID-19 pandemic, we can now also add the concept of virtual care or telehealth to the continuum as this technology emerged as a viable care option during the pandemic (NYU Langone Health/NYU School of Medicine, 2020). Chapter 12 is devoted to an explanation of virtual care.

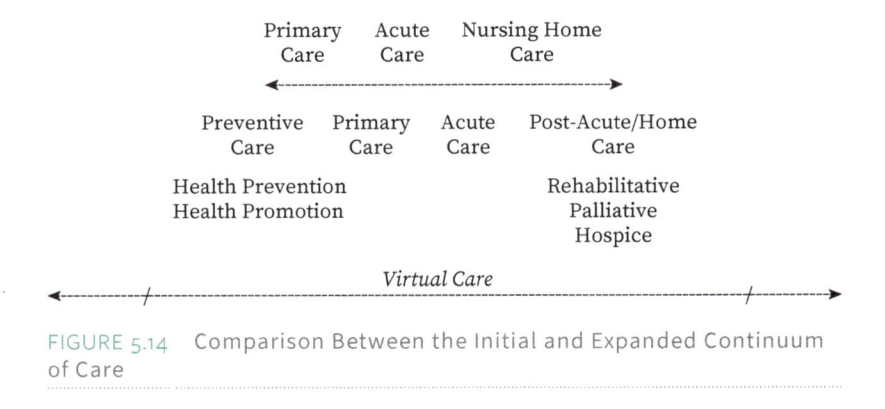

```
              Primary    Acute    Nursing Home
               Care      Care         Care
              <----------------------------------->

           Preventive  Primary   Acute   Post-Acute/Home
              Care      Care     Care         Care

           Health Prevention              Rehabilitative
           Health Promotion                 Palliative
                                             Hospice

                            Virtual Care
           <------+----------------------------------------+------>
```

FIGURE 5.14 Comparison Between the Initial and Expanded Continuum of Care

This expansion increased the type of services available across the continuum to better meet patients,' consumers,' and population's health needs beyond the treatment phase. Now, the entire health sector emphasizes preventive care to proactively delay the development of lifetime chronic diseases.

Health in All Policies

The Culture of Health promoted the best-in-community examples of how to create healthy places to work, live and play, and yet many of the primary causes of health disparities and inequities are beyond the scope of any single organization or even group of health systems to alleviate. Within America today, neighborhoods exist that do not have access to fresh food, who lack safe and secure places to play and shop and face daily pollution in the air they breathe.

Health in All Policies (HIAP) is a collaborative approach to improving population health by incorporating health considerations into decision-making across various sectors and policy issues (Office of the Associate Director for Policy and Strategy, 2016). The HIAP approach adopted by communities and municipalities is a universal strategy to alleviate these types of situations and, even more importantly, ensure harmful impacts do not occur in the future. Health promotion strategies need to address environmental issues and promote policies that protect and ensure that all future community, state, and national policies support health for all.

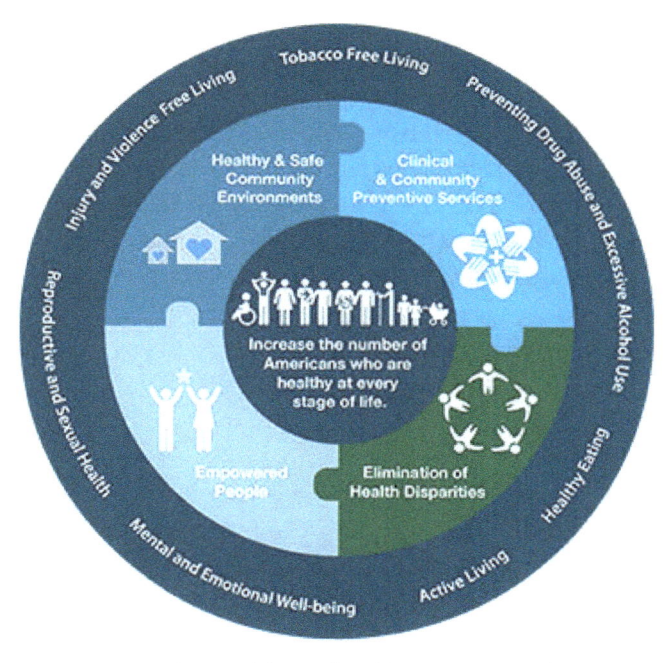

FIGURE 5.15   The Health in All Policies Framework

The four major sections of HIAP approach list distinct types of partnerships: clinical and community preventive services, elimination of health disparities, empowered people, and healthy and safe community environments. Not every industry sector needs to be involved in all these initiatives. The benefit of the HIAP appears in the outer circle with the identification of health policies for change (see Figure 5.16).

Tobacco Control	Preventing Drug & Substance Abuse	Healthy Eating
Active Living	Mental & Emotional Well-Being	Reproductive & Sexual Health
	Injury and Violence Free Living	

FIGURE 5.16   Health in All Policies: Areas for Change

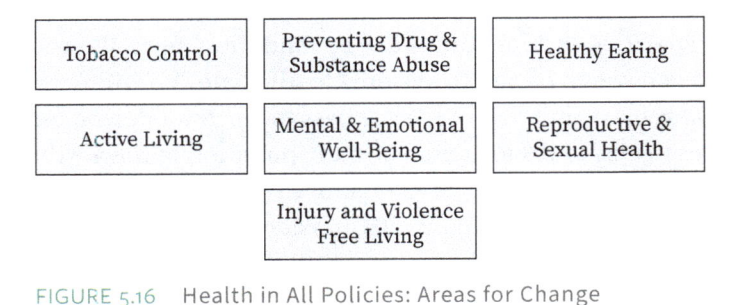

Which of the above options should your neighborhood or college campus prioritize? Which health sector partners would be needed to change policies? Ensuring active living requires safe and secure green spaces for all individuals. What organizations would be involved? Do we need local industries to set aside land for green spaces to accompany any plant or company expansions? Do we need to expand school and public no-smoking zones to become universal drug-free zones?

The CDC sponsors a HIAP website with available resources for all communities and organizations at https://www.cdc.gov/policy/hiap/index.html (CDC, n.d.). The WHO supported this perspective with a clarifying statement in 2013 that emphasized the need for all public policies to adopt an approach that both avoided harmful health impacts and addressed health equity and disparities (Kieny, 2013).

Summary

Everyone wants to be healthy. Applying the concepts of wellness and well-being, along with understanding the four components of individual health, enables population health to improve the quality of life for all populations. Health promotion programs such as healthy eating and tobacco cessation and disease prevention activities of vaccination and screenings form essential foundations for many population health interventions. Today, these concepts are integrated throughout the Continuum of Care to provide populations multiple options and wellness opportunities throughout the lifespan. The HIAP framework provides guidelines to continue shifting from the medical model to a population-based approach. Positive outcomes documented by the Healthy Days Measures and population HRAs encourage health professionals to move beyond hospital-only acute care and actively seek collaborations within the community.

Discussion Questions

1. In Chapter 2, the text discusses relevant issues to community health, but the focus on individual health, wellness, and well-being is just as relevant to population health. Population health must address all five components and not just physical health so that all populations attain high-level wellness. Imagine your population health organization served 100,000 individuals. Which of the five components of health would be the most difficult to support? Provide an example.
2. As described in Figure 5.6, lifestyle behaviors are the largest contributors to health status. One strategy population health uses to increase positive health behaviors is to encourage personal health promotion and disease prevention strategies and activities. People can adopt health promotion activities (the process of enabling people to increase control over their health and its determinants) or help advocate for better health policies. Review the AHA's advocacy agenda's goals. Provide an activity or example that would improve the health of Americans for each goal.
3. Describe the levels of prevention and give an example of how population health encourages disease prevention.
4. To ensure the integration of health promotion and provide patient-centered care throughout the lifespan, population health has focused on expanding the Continuum of Care. How would you describe the changes that have expanded the Continuum, and why do you think they were needed?

References

American Hospital Association. (2023). *AHA advocacy agenda 2023*. https://www.aha.org/advocacy-agenda?utm_source=newsletter&utm_medium=email&utm_campaign=aha-today&mkt_tok=NzEwLVpMTC02NTEAAAGJu8yGHyfUeys7eETHl81OT5tImfsj-eGY8Jhmbv5oHzYuEqTQobA2QE2VFoUM948mp3r5QvTtdINYVGlR2-vE2IFjwVvN-Heyb4LY4hpi_HXa-GrA

Array Behavioral Care. (n.d.). *Defining behavioral health*. https://arraybc.com/defining-behavioral-health

Blunt, W. (2022, June 23). *A step-by-step guide for using quizzes in digital marketing*. Shortstack. https://www.shortstack.com/blog/using-quizzes-in-digital-marketing/

Centers for Disease Control and Prevention. (n.d.). *Health in All Policies*. https://www.cdc.gov/policy/hiap/index.html

Centers for Disease Control and Prevention. (2015). *A framework for patient-centered health risk assessments*. Office of the Associate Director for Policy and Strategy. https://www.cdc.gov/policy/hst/hra/

Centers for Disease Control and Prevention. (2018, October 31). *How does the CDC measure health-related quality of life?* https://www.cdc.gov/hrqol/methods_measures.htm?

Culture of Health. (2022). *Building a culture of health*. Robert Wood Johnson Foundation. https://www.rwjf.org/en/cultureofhealth.html

Fos, P., Fine, F., & Zuniga, M. (2018). Medical management in population health care. In *Managerial epidemiology: For health care organizations* (10th ed). Jossey-Bass.

Hayes, T., & Delk, R. (2018). *Understanding the social determinants of health*. American Action Forum, September 4, 2018. https://www.americanactionforum.org/research/understanding-the-social-determinants-of-health/

Health Information Management System Society. (2014). *Definition: Continuum of Care*. http://s3.amazonaws.com/rdcms-himss/files/production/public/2014-05-14-DefinitionContinuumofCare.pdf

Joint Committee on Health Education and Promotion Terminology. (2012). *Report of the 2011 Joint Committee on Health Education and Promotion Terminology*. American Association of Health Education.

Kieny, M.-P. (2013). *Closing the health equity gap: Policy options and opportunities for action*. https://www.afro.who.int/sites/default/files/2017-06/SDH-closing-health-equity-gap-policy-opportunities-for-action-WHO2013.pdf

Last, J. M. (2001). *Dictionary of epidemiology* (4th ed). Oxford University Press.

McAlearney, A. (2003). *Population health management: Strategies to improve outcomes*. Health Administration Press/Association of University Programs in Health Administration.

National Cancer Institute. (n.d.). *Continuum of Care*. National Cancer Institute Dictionary of Cancer Terms. https://www.cancer.gov/publications/dictionaries/cancer-terms/def/continuum-of-care

National Institutes of Health and Office of Disease Prevention. (n.d.). *Public health campaigns*. https://prevention.nih.gov/research-priorities/dissemination-implementation/nih-public-health-campaigns

NYU Langone Health/NYU School of Medicine. (2020, April 30). Telemedicine transforms response to COVID-19 pandemic in disease epicenter. *ScienceDaily*. www.sciencedaily.com/releases/2020/04/200430150220.htm

Office of the Associate Director for Policy and Strategy. (2016). *Health in All Policies*. https://www.cdc.gov/policy/hiap/index.html

Ottawa Charter. (1986). *Ottawa charter 1986*. World Health Organization. https://www.who.int/publications/i/item/ottawa-charter-for-health-promotion http://www.who.int/healthpromotion/conferences/previous/ottawa/en/

Parvanta, C., Nelson, D., & Harner, R. (2018). *Public health communication: Critical tools and strategies*. Jones and Bartlett Learning.

Chapter Five Health Promotion and Wellness for All Populations | 103

PDHI. (2022, March 2). *Health risk assessment for Medicare annual wellness visit.* https://www.pdhi.com/health-assessment/health-risk-assessment-for-medicare-annual-wellness-visit/

Plough, A. L. (2020). *Well-being: Expanding the definition of progress.* The Robert Wood Johnson Foundation Culture of Health Series. Oxford Press.

The Princess Bride. (1987). *If you haven't got your health, you haven't got anything.* Video. https://www.youtube.com/watch?v=fUKO_Y6RqEk

RAND. (n.d.) *36-item short form survey instrument.* RAND. https://www.rand.org/health-care/surveys_tools/mos/36-item-short-form.html

Stibich, M. (2019, November 25). *Compression of morbidity and reducing suffering.* Verywell Health. https://www.verywellhealth.com/compression-of-morbidity-2223626#:~:text=Reducing%20Age%2DRelated%20Suffering&text=Compression%20of%20morbidity%20is%20a,means%20%22being%20unhealthy%22

U.S. Department of Health and Human Services. (n.d.). *COVID-19 public education campaign: COVID-19 community corps.* https://wecandothis.hhs.gov/resource/older-adults-toolkit

Wellbeing People. (2018, July 20). *What does well-being actually mean?* https://www.wellbeingpeople.com/2018/07/20/what-does-wellbeing-actually-mean/#:~:text=Well-being%20%5B%20noun%20%5D%20%E2%80%93%20the%20state,being%20comfortable%2C%20healthy%20or%20happy

Wellness Council of America. (n.d.). *WELCOA's definition of wellness.* https://www.welcoa.org/resources/definition-of-wellness/#:~:text=Wellness%20is%20the%20active%20pursuit,in%20all%20aspects%20of%20life

World Health Organization. (1946). *Constitution of the World Health Organization.* https://www.who.int/about/who-we-are/constitution

Credits

Fig. 5.1: Generated with FreeWordCloudGenerator.com.
Fig. 5.5a: Copyright © 2015 Depositphotos/Rawpixel.
Fig. 5.5b: Copyright © 2019 Depositphotos/Kzenon.
Fig. 5.5c: Copyright © 2019 Depositphotos/ALotOfPeople.
Fig. 5.8: Copyright © 2017 Depositphotos/everythingposs.
Fig. 5.9a: Copyright © 2023 Depositphotos/arlette_lg.
Fig. 5.9b: Copyright © 2011 Depositphotos/alexraths.
Fig. 5.9c: Copyright © 2020 Pexels/Cliff Booth.
Fig. 5.11: Source: Adapted from A) https://www.emro.who.int/about-who/public-health-functions/health-promotion-disease-prevention.html; B) Peter J. Fos, et al., "Medical Management in Population Health Care," *Managerial Epidemiology: For Health Care Organizations,* pp. 150–151. Copyright © John Wiley & Sons, Inc.
Fig. 5.12: Source: https://wecandothis.hhs.gov/.
Fig. 5.13a: Source: https://www.collegedrinkingprevention.gov/collegeaim/.

Fig. 5.13b: Source: https://safetosleep.nichd.nih.gov/.
Fig. 5.13c: Source: https://www.stroke.nih.gov/about/.
Fig. 5.15: Source: https://www.cdc.gov/policy/hiap/index.html.

CHAPTER SIX

Social Determinants of Health

Impact on Population Health

> ## Chapter Description

Chapter 6 describes two major influences on the health status of all Americans. First, the social determinants of health (SDOH) are known to the U.S. health care system; in fact, their long-standing role, importance, and direct impact on marginalized communities of color remain major challenges. Second, motivated by the drastic health outcomes for vulnerable populations stemming from COVID-19, health systems in collaboration with public health initiatives have targeted health care disparities as a changeable driver of health status. This chapter describes SDOHs, their immense impact on at-risk populations, and subsequent health disparity issues. Population health goals and interventions focus on reducing and eliminating negative social drivers of health factors and

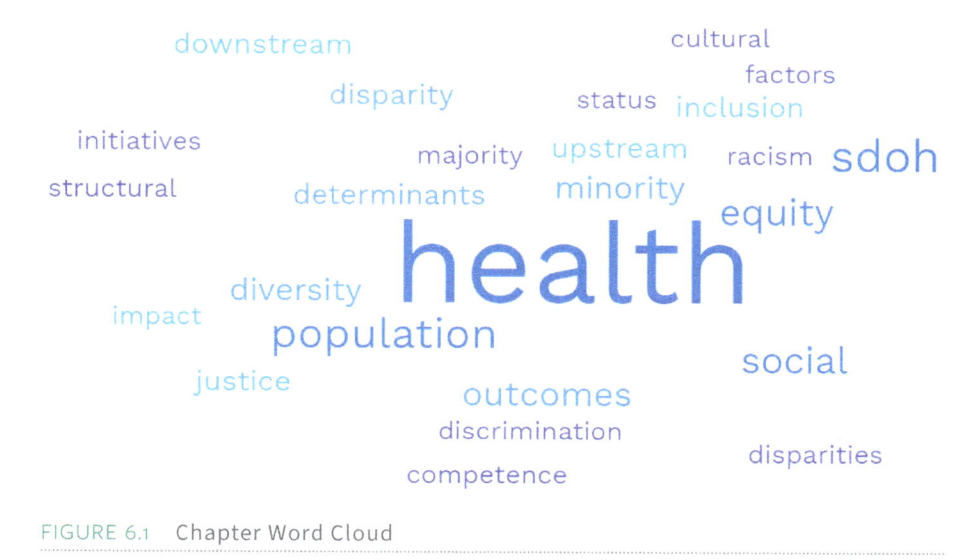

FIGURE 6.1 Chapter Word Cloud

encourage collaborations among other community organizations to address and improve health outcomes. The application of health equity, disparity, and social justice initiatives and efforts to close the health equity gap remains an integral component of population health.

Chapter Objectives

After completing this chapter, students will be able to:

1. Describe the SDOH
2. Identify the diverse impacts of SDOH on quality of life
3. Discuss upstream, midstream, and downstream population health factors and outcomes
4. Define the concepts of diversity, inclusion, and majority and minority health
5. Explain health inequities and their relationship to health disparity
6. Provide examples of both social justice and structural racism
7. Explain the importance and role of cultural competence for health professionals

Key Words

Cultural competence	Diversity	Inclusion	Social justice
Culturally and Linguistically Appropriate Services (CLAS) standards	Food insecurity	Majority	Structural racism
	Health disparities	Minority	Upstream, midstream, and downstream health factors
	Health equality	Minority health	
	Health equity	Social determinants of health	
Discrimination	Implicit bias		

Today's American Culture and Population Health

What do you think? Is American culture a salad bowl, a melting pot, or a stir-fry (Civic Issues, 2019)? Regardless of which cooking analogy you selected; we can all agree that diversity exists within the United States, and our culture will continue to transform in the future. America's culture profile has a significant impact on population health. Let's begin with the concept of **diversity**, a term that means "an appreciation and respect for differences and similarities in the workplace (and beyond), including the varied perspectives, approaches, and competencies of coworkers and populations served" (Dicent Taillepierre, 2016).

Chapter Six Social Determinants of Health | 107

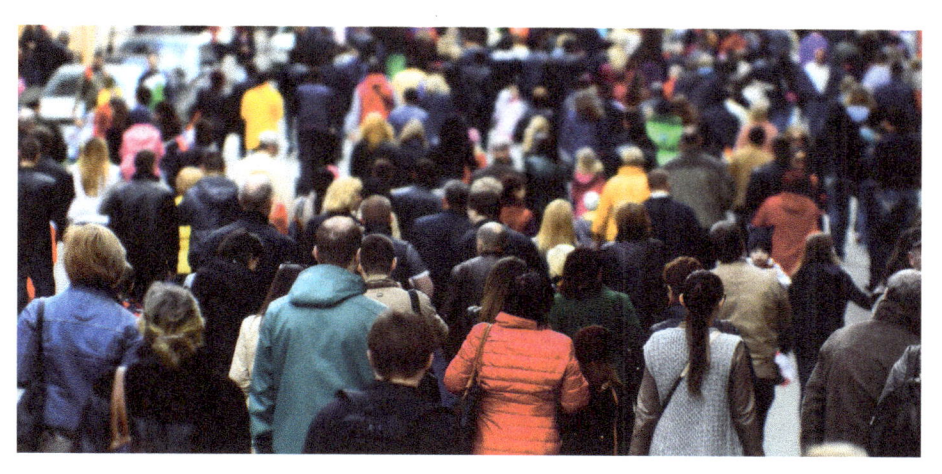

FIGURE 6.2 Culturally Diverse America

Diversity also means applying our skills to recognize individual differences whether they be on dimensions of race, ethnicity, gender, sexual orientation, socio-economic status, age, physical abilities, religious beliefs, political beliefs, or other ideologies (Queensborough Community College, n.d.).

Both appreciation and respect are expected and necessary character traits when we discuss cultural concepts. Cultures combine both ***majority*** (when characteristics are found in more than 50% of a population), and ***minority***

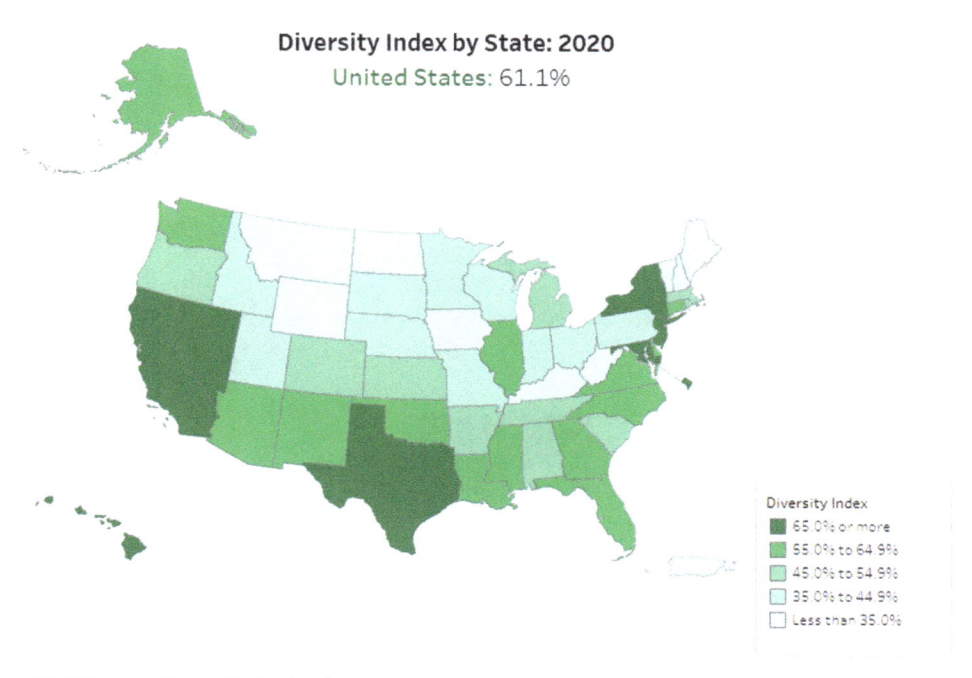

FIGURE 6.3 Diversity Index by State 2020

(which refers to a subgroup with fewer than 50% of the population) components. In the United States, **minority health** refers to the following groups: American Indians/Alaska Natives, Asian Americans, Native Hawaiians and other Pacific Islanders, African Americans, and Hispanics in our country (Seabert et al. 2022). In fact, the 2020 census revealed that the U.S. population is more racially and ethnically diverse than measured in 2010 (Jensen et al., 2021).

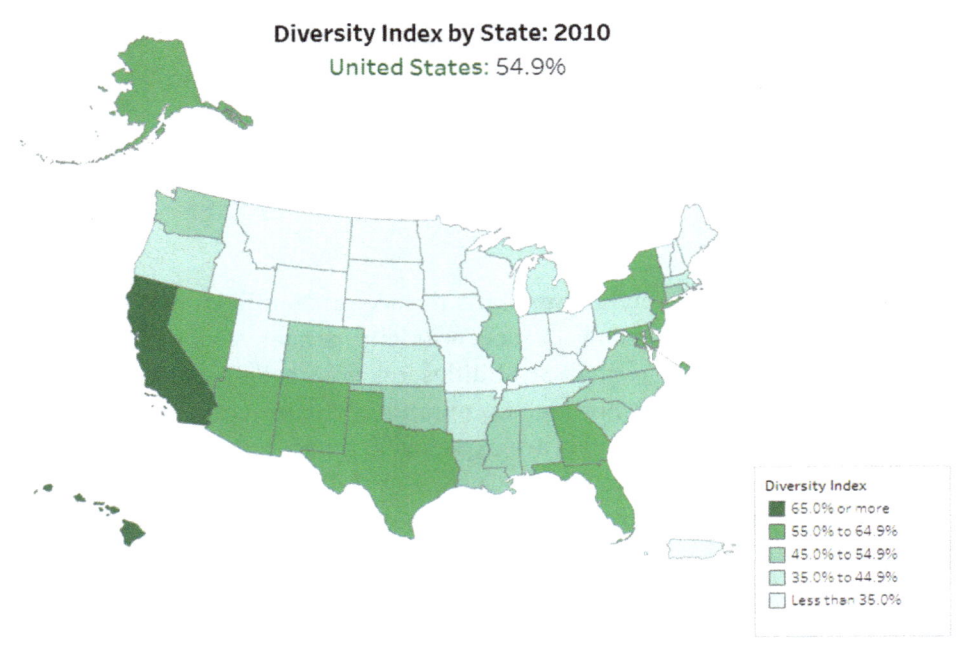

FIGURE 6.4 Diversity Index by State 2010

Practical Skill: Census Data and You

Use the following link to access the interactive U.S. Census Bureau maps: https://tinyurl.com/29f6rhft. Access your state. What did you discover about racial and ethnic diversity there?

Establishing a culture of health and positive population health outcomes requires both a recognition of diversity and a realization that **inclusion** is the essential process for accepting the variation and differences among all of us.

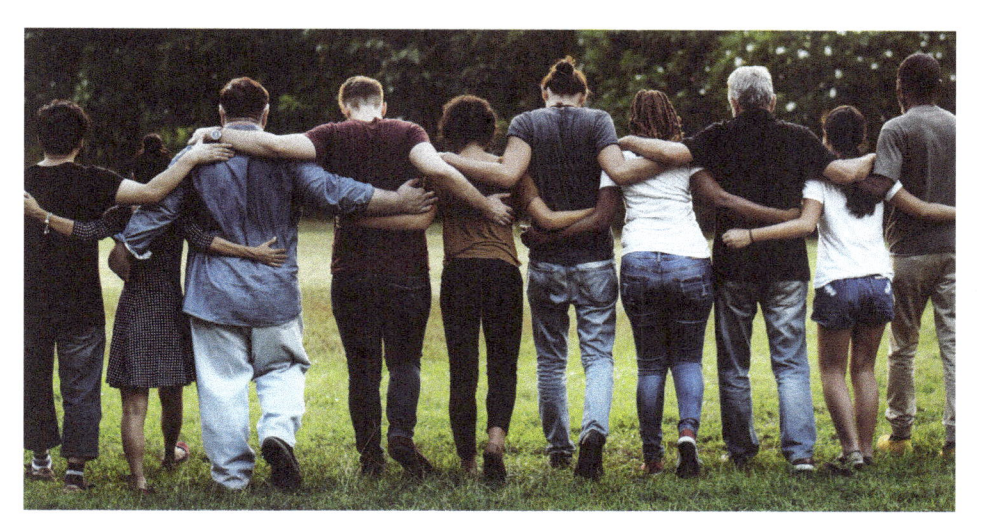

FIGURE 6.5   Inclusion

The core foundation for inclusion includes respect, support, and a sense of being valued. Inclusion also involves focusing on the needs of every individual and ensuring the right health conditions are available for each person to achieve their potential (U.S. Department of Housing and Urban Development, n.d.). Population health seeks to ensure and align all health efforts and activities to be inclusive regardless of the priority population.

Social Determinants of Health

Although public health has acknowledged the importance of the SDOH for many years, the most pressing health care sector issue today is the impact of these widespread and harmful factors on population health outcomes (Commission on the Social Determinants of Health, 2008). The exceptionally negative outcomes of higher COVID-19 mortality rates and excessive hospitalizations for minority populations, including both patients and health care workers, increased national awareness of health care disparities for at-risk groups (Birk, 2022; Getachew et al., 2020; Magesh et al., 2021, Ray, 2020). **Health disparities**, which include the burden of disease, injury, violence, or opportunities to achieve optimal health, continue to be experienced by socially disadvantaged populations (Centers for

Disease Control and Prevention [CDC], 2008). We also know that minority groups experience various levels of health disparities (National Academy of Sciences, 2017). For example, the Hispanic immigrant minority group has better health outcomes than do White Americans (Lara et al., 2005). And yet, infants born to African American mothers experience the highest rates of infant mortality (11.11 infant deaths per 1,000 births) as compared to infants born to Asian or Pacific Islander mothers, who experience the lowest rates (3.90 infant deaths per 1,000 births; National Center for Health Statistics, 2016).

For all Americans, the SDOH have powerful influences on overall health status. Experts have identified seven major areas of minority outcomes that are affected by the SDOH (see Figure 6.6).

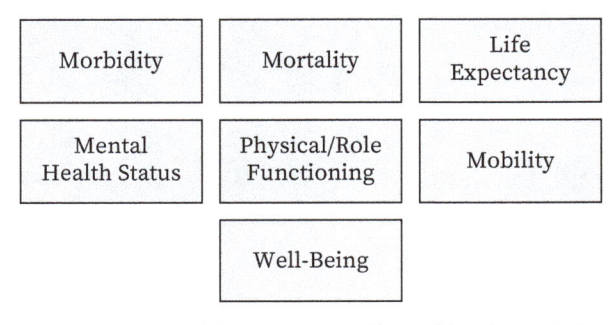

FIGURE 6.6 Health Outcomes Affected by the SDOH

Why are the SDOH such powerful predictors of health outcomes? **SDOH** refers to a group of major factors that have both direct and indirect impacts on the health status of any population. Experts define *SDOH* as "the places where people live, learn, work and play (U.S. Department of Health and Human Services, n.d.). Table 6.1 outlines the five recognized categories of SDOH and provides specific examples within each group (Braveman & Gottlieb, 2014; Artiga & Hinton, 2018).

TABLE 6.1 Social Determinants of Health Categories

Economic Factors	Access to Education	Health Care Access	Built Environment Neighborhood Safety	Social/Community Context
Employment Housing Instability Poverty	Quality schooling Access to early childhood education	Access to health care Access to preventive care and screenings	Quality housing Transportation Public safety Access to healthy foods	Civic engagement Structural racism/discrimination Social cohesion

Adapted from Braveman & Gottlieb, 2014; Brown et al., 2022; and CDC, 2020.

As you read the impact examples within each of the SDOH categories, imagine planning health care for a population who is unemployed, never graduated from high school because they needed to work to feed their family, always lacked access to health insurance or a primary care doctor, didn't have a safe and secure home with daily meals, and faced social prejudice everywhere they went. Now imagine that there are thousands of individuals in this population. These conditions are real and exist in the United States today.

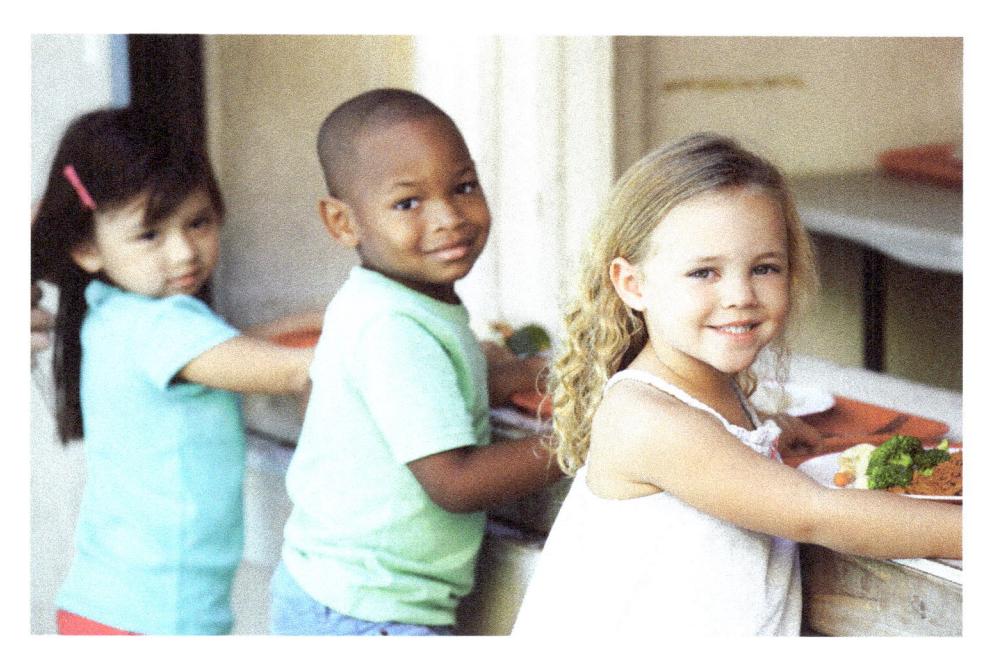

FIGURE 6.7   Preschool and School Lunch

Practical Skill: Food Insecurity

Food insecurity refers to an economic and social condition characterized by limited or uncertain access to adequate food (White-Williams, 2022; White-Williams et al., 2020). It was projected that one in eight Americans, including 13 million children, may have experienced food insecurity in 2021 (Feeding America, 2021). Before the impact of COVID-19, 30% of college students suffered from food insecurity with health consequences that included lower grade point averages, stress and depression, and reduced college completion rates (McCoy, 2022).

Select a local or regional college or university. Search their website and/or call to assess the availability of a food pantry for college students.

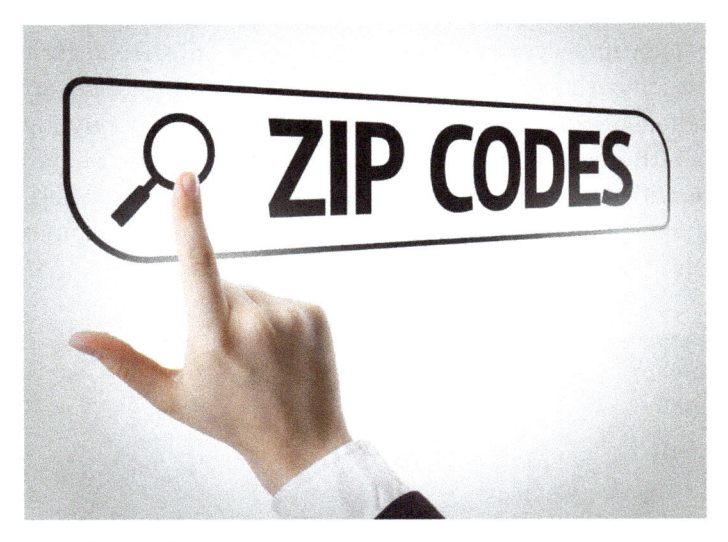

FIGURE 6.8 Zip code

The Relationship of SDOH to Population Health Outcomes

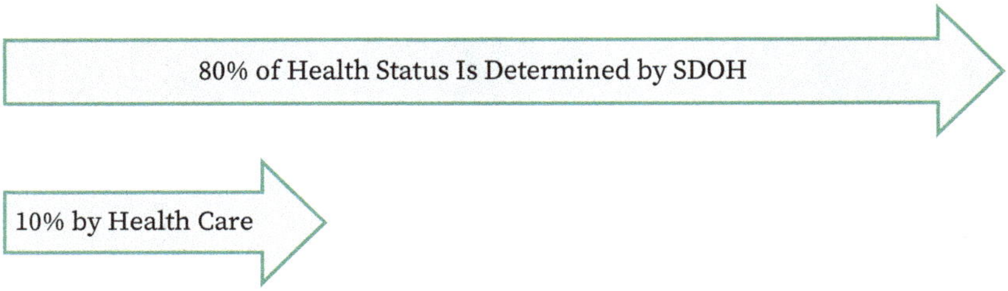

80% of Health Status Is Determined by SDOH

10% by Health Care

FIGURE 6.9 Percentage of Individual Health Status Determined by the SDOH

Population health research has established that the SDOH directly determines 80% of all individual health outcomes (Manatt Health & Phelps & Phillips, LLP, 2019) compared to only 10% attributed to health care. What difference does it make if you live two blocks from the best hospital in the country if you cannot afford health insurance or your family has food insecurity and is not sure if they have enough money for the next meal? Individuals affected by the SDOH **over a lifetime** face even lower life expectancy rates and higher incidences of chronic disease (Noonan et al. 2016). How does population health address these life-altering health impacts?

Population Health Strategies for SDOH

One useful SDOH strategy can easily be explained through a parable, which is a lesson illustrated in a story. A well-known public health parable focuses on the SDOH.

The Upstream/Downstream Parable

A group of college students were picnicking near a river and noticed a person in the water struggling against the river current. They quickly mobilized and saved the person, only to discover that another person needing help immediately appeared, followed by another. They discovered a rope and started tying people together to save them. One of the students decided to go upstream and figure out why this was happening. People were falling into the river and needed to be rescued. When they arrived upstream, they found a scenic bridge with a desirable view. However, to enjoy the view, you had to risk falling in the river. The group of college students worked with the community to build a barrier so that no one would fall in the river again. This public health parable has been modified over the years and shared with many students since it first appeared, but the main point remains clear. **How do you address upstream issues to avoid downstream problems?**

According to the upstream/downstream parable, the SDOH are an upstream problem. **Upstream health factors** are the conditions, situations, and environment that lead to health inequities and disparity. *Upstream* simply means that they are the causes (Manchanda, 2019: Merck, 2018). **Midstream factors** are often everyday individual lifestyle choices and risky behaviors. **Downstream factors** are the costs of treating any resulting condition or other consequences related to the SDOH impact.

Now let's examine this story from a population health's perspective on solving the problem. The upstream health factor is a SDOH, the built environment/environmental concern of an unsafe bridge, which would require installing a barrier, and safety boats along the river with trained personnel. The population health midstream response would be health promotion and disease prevention activities related to individual behaviors such as providing swimming lessons and water safety classes. The downstream factor population health activities would include treatment of chronic and relapsing conditions related to the near-drowning health crisis and/or the development of alternative and safer community activities. A population health expert sums up the situation with the quote "Shut off the faucet and stop mopping the floor" (Nash, 2018), meaning that if we do not address these upstream issues, we will continue to invest more resources in downstream interventions that tax our health care system.

114 | Population Health: Practical Skills for Future Health Professionals

Practical Skill: Student Activity

Take the time to watch the following YouTube video discussing upstream and downstream health issues.

Source: Upstream. (2013, September 25). Introduction to Upstream. *YouTube. https://tinyurl.com/2krc4vn9*

Using the textbook example, what type of upstream population health initiatives would be needed?

Population Health Outcomes and Health Equity

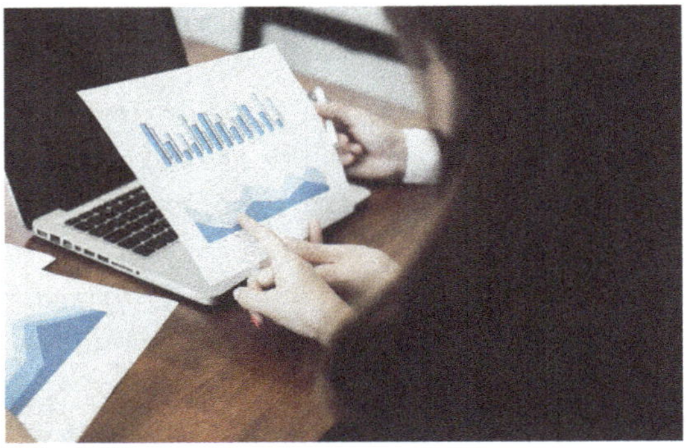

FIGURE 6.10   Population Health Outcomes and Health Equity

Although the SDOH can explain many of the causes of health disparities and poor health outcomes for vulnerable populations, population health also recognizes that health equality and equity are essential for ensuring positive outcomes for all. Healthy People 2030 strongly emphasizes the elimination of health disparities and the achievement of health equity as a primary goal (CDC, 2020). Eliminating bias and discrimination continues to remain a primary imperative for all health organizations and professionals as they seek to provide inclusive programs, opportunities, and interventions for better health status (American Public Health Association, n.d.). **Discrimination**, harmful beliefs, and behaviors come in many forms such as "isms" or phobias. These include ageism, tokenism, colorism, sexism, antisemitism, heterosexism, elitism, and others (College of Engineering, 2022). Recently racism was declared a public health issue (Ahmad, 2022), with more than 250 declarations across the United States (Late, 2022).

Chapter Six Social Determinants of Health | 115

Practical Skill: Discrimination

Discrimination against individuals can take several unique forms. Read the following article discussing a recent Massachusetts law and provide a summary of the issue: https://tinyurl.com/4fu3f8sx. Be sure to include a paragraph describing your own perspective. Note that Massachusetts is the 18th state to adopt what is known as the CROWN Act (Cornell, 2022).

Can you identify any other examples of discrimination that might be like this situation?

In addition to the negative issue of discrimination, population health is also concerned with both health equality and health equity. See Figure 6.11 for definitions of both terms.

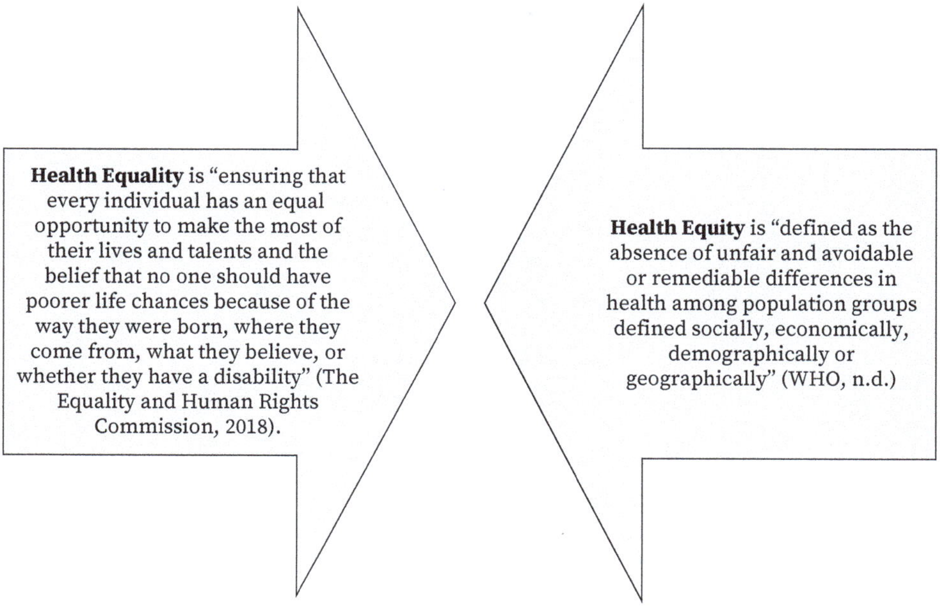

Health Equality is "ensuring that every individual has an equal opportunity to make the most of their lives and talents and the belief that no one should have poorer life chances because of the way they were born, where they come from, what they believe, or whether they have a disability" (The Equality and Human Rights Commission, 2018).

Health Equity is "defined as the absence of unfair and avoidable or remediable differences in health among population groups defined socially, economically, demographically or geographically" (WHO, n.d.)

FIGURE 6.11   Definitions of Health Equality and Health Equity

Review these definitions closely. Can you clearly explain the differences between these two key terms? Now review Figure 6.12. Does this visual help your understanding of health equality and equity?

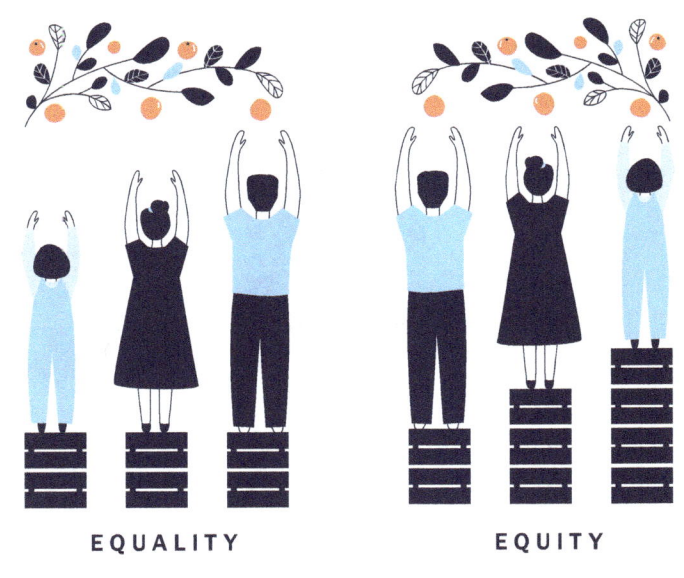

EQUALITY   **EQUITY**

FIGURE 6.12   Comparing Health Equality and Health Equity

Practical Skill: The AHA Health Equity Roadmap

The American Hospital Association (AHA) recently announced an initiative to improve health care outcomes and health equity, diversity, and inclusion. The framework, the Health Equity Roadmap, enables hospitals and health care systems to chart their own paths to become more equitable and inclusive organizations (AHA, 2021). After completing an assessment process, the roadmap provides step-by-step direction for building vision, strategy, and leadership to work internally and collaborative with community partners to advance health equity. View a short video on the AHA's Health Equity Roadmap using the following link: https://tinyurl.com/yc6ywd76.

Be sure to note the six levels of health equity transformation. The AHA also developed a document titled *Community Partnerships: Strategies to Accelerate Health Equity* to encourage strong collaborations with other health sector and non health sector organizations within the community to partner in equity-focused initiatives.

Several examples of cultural competence recommendations, roadmaps, and pathways are available to help health organizations and professionals ensure health equity in their work and the local community. A valuable framework for health organizations is Paving the Road to Health Equity, which was developed by the CDC and the Office of Minority Health and Equity (2020). This framework offers programs and evaluation measures and provides examples and recommendations for health policies.

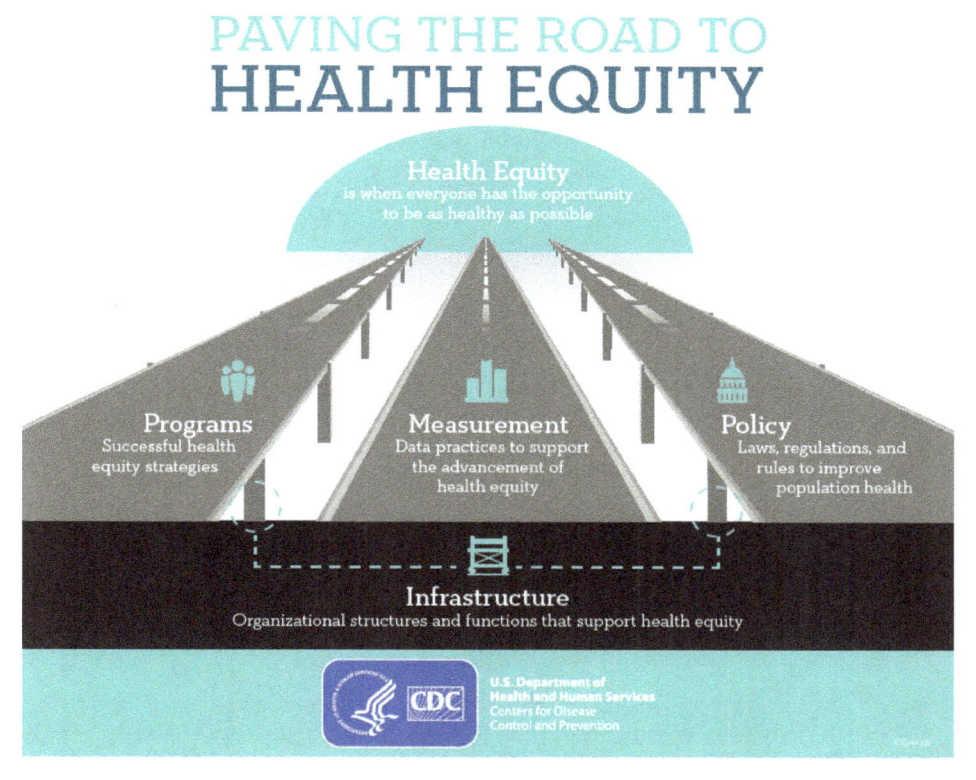

FIGURE 6.13   Paving the Road for Health Equity Framework

The National **Culturally and Linguistically Appropriate Services** (CLAS) standards are a blueprint to not only eliminate health disparities and advance health equity, but also improve service quality of care (Office of Minority Health, n.d.).

As you read the CLAS standards, did you notice that they focused on personal, professional, and organizational actions? Without leadership, training, and teamwork, any organization will not succeed in establishing a CLAS-oriented culture.

National CLAS Standards

The National CLAS standards are intended to advance health equity, improve quality, and help eliminate health care disparities by establishing a blueprint for health and health care organizations to achieve the following:

Principal Standard

1. Provide effective, equitable, understandable, and respectful quality care and services that are responsive to diverse cultural health beliefs and practices, preferred languages, health literacy, and other communication needs.

Governance, Leadership, and Workforce

2. Advance and sustain organizational governance and leadership that promotes CLAS and health equity through policy, practices, and allocated resources.
3. Recruit, promote, and support a culturally and linguistically diverse governance, leadership, and workforce that are responsive to the population in the service area.
4. Educate and train governance, leadership, and workforce in culturally and linguistically appropriate policies and practices on an ongoing basis.

Communication and Language Assistance

5. Offer language assistance to individuals who have limited English proficiency and/or other communication needs, at no cost to them, to facilitate timely access to all health care and services.
6. Inform all individuals of the availability of language assistance services clearly and in their preferred language, verbally, and in writing.
7. Ensure the competence of individuals providing language assistance, recognizing that the use of untrained individuals and/or minors as interpreters should be avoided.
8. Provide easy-to-understand print and multimedia materials and signage in the languages commonly used by the populations in the service area.

Engagement, Continuous Improvement, and Accountability

9. Establish culturally and linguistically appropriate goals, policies, and management accountability and infuse them throughout the organization's planning and operations.
10. Conduct ongoing assessments of the organization's CLAS-related activities and integrate CLAS-related measures into measurement and continuous quality improvement activities.
11. Collect and maintain accurate and reliable demographic data to monitor and evaluate the impact of CLAS on health equity and outcomes and to inform service delivery.

12. Conduct regular assessments of community health assets and needs and use the results to plan and implement services that respond to the cultural and linguistic diversity of populations in the service area.

13. Partner with the community to design, implement, and evaluate policies, practices, and services to ensure cultural and linguistic appropriateness.

14. Create conflict and grievance resolution processes that are culturally and linguistically appropriate to identify, prevent, and resolve conflicts or complaints.

15. Communicate the organization's progress in implementing and sustaining CLAS to all stakeholders, constituents, and the public.

Source: U.S. Department of Health and Human Services. (n.d.). National CLAS standards. *https://thinkculturalhealth.hhs.gov/clas/standards*

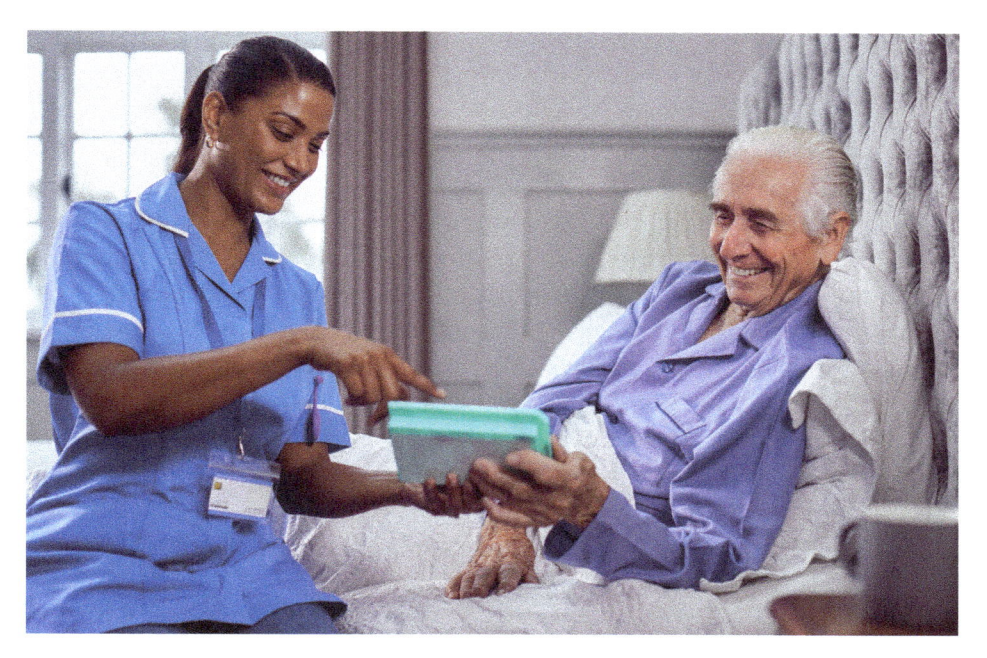

FIGURE 6.14   Ensuring CLAS standards for Population Health

The health sector can ensure health equality by increasing access and availability of all health services, but that step alone is not enough. A local health provider may accept a minority individual's health insurance, but if they do not offer office hours that are convenient in an office that is within easy transportation reach or recognize that language and health literacy can be barriers to care, then health equity will not be achieved. Discrimination affects more than just individuals and major subpopulations and is related to the construct of structural racism. **Structural racism** is defined as "the macrolevel systems, social forces, institutions, ideologies, and processes that interact with one another to generate and reinforce inequities among racial and ethnic groups" (Powell, 2008). At this level, discrimination is often embedded in policies that reinforce unequal treatment of individuals. The health sector and population health organizations can serve as advocates for policy changes to address structural racism. Population health can also focus on assessing health equity measures to better guide both health delivery and advocacy decision-making (Bailit & Kanneganti, 2022). We all know that you cannot change what you do not measure, and for population health, assessing the impact of structural racism is essential. (Onduo, 2022). Health advocacy and policy initiatives represent efforts to ensure social justice and health equity for all. **Social justice** is a cultural view that "everyone deserves equal economic, political, and social rights and opportunities" (San Diego Foundation, 2016). When social justice and health equity are aligned, all populations experience better health status.

Cultural Competence in Population Health

Health professionals and practitioners are required to practice cultural competence in health care by "providing high-quality respectful care, while decreasing inequities" (Molinari et al., 2020). **Culture competence** is a set of congruent behaviors, attitudes, and policies that come together in a system, agency, or among professionals that enables effective work in cross-cultural situations (National Prevention Information Network, 2021). As future health professionals, it is important to complete cultural competence training and reflect on "personal health biases—both explicit and implicit" (Ogden & Erwin, 2023). **Implicit bias** refers to a type of unconscious bias that occurs automatically and unintentionally and affects our judgments, decisions, and behaviors (National Institute of Health, 2022).

Summary

The health sector is not alone in recognizing the enormous challenges of reducing the negative impact of the SDOH on vulnerable populations. The SDOH are commonly grouped into five target areas for change: economic stability, educational access/quality, social and community context, health care access/quality, and neighborhood-built environment. Population health, along with other industry sectors, seeks to mitigate and eliminate negative health outcomes by focusing on upstream activities such as tailoring health promotion and care strategies specifically to vulnerable populations. The additional challenge of health disparities, which are often results of health inequality and inequities, was dramatically highlighted when Black, Latino, and Asian groups were disproportionately more likely to receive a positive diagnosis and to be admitted to intensive care units for COVID-19 than were other populations. Integrating proactive social justice policies can help eliminate discrimination and address the impact of structural racism for all populations.

Discussion Questions

1. The *social determinants of health* (SDOH) refer to a group of major factors that have both direct and indirect impacts on the health status of any population. They have also been defined as the places where people live, learn, work, and play. Why is the SDOH such a powerful influence on health status? The CDC classifies SDOHs into five distinct groups: economic factors, access to education, health care access, built environment, neighborhood safety, and social/community context. Select one of the impact factors with a particular group from Table 6.1. Locate a recent news article or video that demonstrates the impact of that specific SDOH factor on health status. Write a summary of the video and your assessment of the impact.

SDOH Factor:
Article Title: (URL)
Summary:

2. The upstream/downstream parable highlights the complexity of addressing SDOHs. Complete the grid below and assume that the SDOH of concern is housing.

Housing	Impact Factors
A. Upstream—conditions, situations and environment that lead to health inequities and disparity	
B. Midstream—everyday lifestyle choices and risk behaviors	
C. Downstream—cost of treating any resulting condition or other consequences related to the SDOH impact	

3. Research shows that SDOHs negatively affect diverse populations in the United States with minority groups experiencing significant health disparities in outcomes. To eliminate these variations in health care, the health care sector strongly supports the concept of inclusion which emphasizes respect, support, and a sense of being valued. How does population health emphasize inclusion? Provide three examples.
4. Population health focuses on at-risk populations and the delivery of health care. One goal is to eliminate all discrimination for every population. First, identify two areas where discrimination in health care can occur. Second, discuss the implications of health equity as compared to equality.
5. Common discrimination issues appear throughout the health sector and the healthcare delivery process. The National CLAS standards are intended to advance health equity, improve quality, and help eliminate health care disparities by establishing a blueprint for health and health care organizations. The framework focuses on three potential areas for improvement: governance, leadership and workforce, communication and language assistance, and engagement, continuous improvement, and accountability (see Figure 6.12). Review the standards for the communication and language assistance section. Can you provide any examples of industry efforts to improve this area? Have you ever experienced a need for a translator? Have you ever experienced not understanding care directions from a health care provider?

References

Ahmad, N. (2022, January 4). *Uprooting racism to advance health equity.* Robert Wood Johnson Foundation Blog. https://www.rwjf.org/en/blog/2022/01/uprooting-racism-to-advance-health-equity.html?rid=0034400001rm5zSAAQ&et_cid=2531808

American Hospital Association. (2021, November 4). *The AHA health equity roadmap.* https://www.youtube.com/watch?v=HRxP_y0-dBA

American Public Health Association. (n.d.). *Health equity.* https://www.apha.org/topics-and issues/health-equity

Artiga, S., & Hinton, E. (2018, May 10). *Beyond health care: The role of social determinants in promoting health and health equity.* https://www.kff.org/disparities-policy/issue-brief/beyond-health-care-the-role-of-social-determinants-in-promoting-health-and-health-equity/

Bailit, M., & Kanneganti, D. (2022, March 22). A typology for health equity measures. *Health Affairs.* https://www.healthaffairs.org/do/10.1377/forefront.20220318.155498?utm_medium=email&utm_source=newsletter&utm_campaign=hat&utm_content=-march+2022&utm_term=bailit&vgo_ee=7zjVhjEBDJ9hKDOcqHBj%2F7TV8qsFU-fI%2F1ISxnX2Ui4c%3D

Birk, S. (2022, June/August). Opening more doors: Increasing access to care. *Healthcare Executive, 37*(4), 8–14.

Braveman, P., & Gottlieb, L. (2014). The social determinants of health: It's time to consider the causes of the causes. *Public Health Reports, 129*(Suppl 2), 19–31. https://doi.org/10.1177/00333549141291S206

Brown, C., Jefcoat, C., & Barlow, J. (2022, June 29). Addressing *social determinants of health with companion* care. https://www.ecgmc.com/thought-leadership/blog/addressing-social-determinants-of-health-with-companion-care

Carlson, L. M. (2020). Health is where we live, work and play—and in our ZIP. codes: Tackling social determinants of health. *The Nation's Health, 50*(1), 3. http://www.thenationshealth.org/content/50/1/3.1

Centers for Disease Control and Prevention. (2008). *Community health and program services (CHAPS): Health disparities among racial/ethnic populations.* U.S. Department of Health and Human Services.

Centers for Disease Control and Prevention. (2020). *Sources for data on social determinants of health.* https://www.cdc.gov/socialdeterminants/data/index.htm Atlanta: U.S. Department of Health and Human Services.

Civic Issues. (2019, January 1). *Melting pot or salad bowl?* Penn State University. https://sites.psu.edu/ajwcivicissues/2019/01/21/melting-pot-or-salad-bowl/

College of Engineering. (2022). *A quick guide to the -isms and -phobias.* Ohio State University. https://engineering.osu.edu/quick-guide-isms-and-phobias

Commission on the Social Determinants of Health. (2008). *Closing the gap in a generation: Health equity through action on the social determinants of health; Final report of the Commission on Social Determinants of Health.* World Health Organization. https://www.who.int/social_determinants/final_report/csdh_finalreport_2008.pdf

Cornell, H. (2022, July 26). *The bill banning hairstyle bias signed into MA law.* Patch. https://patch.com/massachusetts/lexington/s/icbd3/bill-banning-hairstyle-bias-signed-into-ma-law?utm_term=article-slot-1&utm_source=newsletter-daily&utm_medium=email&utm_campaign=newsletter

Dicent Taillepierre, J. (2016). *Why diversity and inclusion matters in public health.* https://www.cdc.gov/minorityhealth/internships/2016/whydiversityinclusionmatterspublichealth.pdf

Equality and Human Rights Commission (2018). *Understanding equality: What is equality?* https://www.equalityhumanrights.com/en/secondary-education-resources/useful-information/understanding-equality

Feeding America. (2021, March). *The impact of the coronavirus on food insecurity in 2020–2021.* https://www.feedingamerica.org/sites/default/files/2021-03/National%20Projections%20Brief_3.9.2021_0.pdf

Getachew, Y., Zephyrin, L., Abrams, M., Shah, A., Lewis, C., & Doty, M. (2020, December 10). *Beyond the case count: The wide-ranging disparities of COVID-19 in the United States.* https://www.commonwealthfund.org/publications/2020/sep/beyond-case-count-disparities-covid-19-united-states?gclid=EAIaIQobChMI9JCo0L-Pu-AIV1v6zCh1Q6Qu8EAAYAyAAEgLdgvD_BwE

Jensen, E., Jones, N., Rabe, M., Pratt, B., Medina, L., Orozco, K., & Spell, L. (2021, August 12). *The chance that two people chosen at random are of different race or ethnicity groups has increased since 2010.* https://www.census.gov/library/stories/2021/08/2020-united-states-population-more-racially-ethnically-diverse-than-2010.html

Lara, M., Health, R., & Rand, C. (2005). *Acculturation and Latino health in the United States: A review of the literature and its sociopolitical context.* RAND Corporation.

Late, M. (2022, July 25). *Racism declarations pass new milestone.* Public Health News. http://www.publichealthnewswire.org/Articles/2022/07/25/Racism-Public-Health

Magesh, S., John, D., Li, W., Li, Y., Mattingly, A., Jain, S., Chang, E., & Ongkeko, W. (2021, November 11). Disparities in COVID-19 outcomes by race, ethnicity, and socioeconomic status: A systematic review and meta-analysis. *Journal of the American Medical Association Network Open, 4*(11), e2134147. https://jamanetwork.com/journals/jamanetworkopen/fullarticle/2785980

Manatt Health and Phelps & Phillips, LLP. (2019, February 1). *Medicaid's role in addressing social determinants of health.* Robert Wood Johnson Foundation. https://www.rwjf.org/en/library/research/2019/02/medicaid-s-role-in-addressing-social-determinants-of-health.html

Manchanda, R. (2019, January 17). *Making sense of the social determinants of health.* http://www.ihi.org/communities/blogs/making-sense-of-the-social-determinants-of-health

McCoy, M., Martinelli, S., Reddy, S., Don, R., Thompson, A., Speer, M., Bravo, R., Yudell, M., Darira, & S. (2022, January 31). Food insecurity on college campuses: The invisible epidemic. *Health Affairs.* https://www.healthaffairs.org/do/10.1377/forefront.20220127.264905

Merck, A. (2018, October 8). *The upstream-downstream parable for health equity.* Salud America. https://salud-america.org/the-upstream-downstream-parable-for-health-equity/

Molinari, C., Lundahl, S., & Shanderson, L. (2020). The culturally competent and inclusive leader. In L. G. Rubino, S. J. Esparza, & Y. Chassiakos (Eds.), *New Leadership for Today's Health Care Professionals: Concepts and Cases* (2nd ed.; pp. 49–67). Jones & Bartlett Learning.

Nash, D. B. (2018). Shut off the faucet and stop mopping the floor. *American Health & Drug Benefits*, *11*(9), 447–448. https://www.ncbi.nlm.nih.gov/pmc/articles/PMC6322593/

National Academy of Sciences. (2017). 2, The state of health disparities in the United States. In A. Baciu, Y. Negussie, A. Geller, et al. (Eds.), *Communities in Action: Pathways to Health Equity*. National Academies Press. https://www.ncbi.nlm.nih.gov/books/NBK425844/

National Center for Health Statistics. (2016). *Health, United States, 2015: With a special feature on racial and ethnic health disparities*. National Center for Health Statistics.

National Institutes of Health. (2022, June 3). Implicit Bias. https://diversity.nih.gov/sociocultural-factors/implicit-bias

National Prevention Information Network. (2021, September 21). *Cultural competence in health and human services*. Centers for Disease Control and Prevention. https://npin.cdc.gov/pages/cultural-competence

Noonan, A., Velasco-Mondragon, H., & Wagner, F. (2016). Improving the health of African Americans in the USA: An overdue opportunity for social justice. *Public Health Review*, *37*, 12. https://doi.org/10.1186/s40985-016-0025-4.

Office of Disease Prevention and Health Promotion (n.d.). *Social determinants of health: Interventions and resources*. Healthy People 2020. U.S. Department of Health and Human Services. https://www.healthypeople.gov/2020/topics-objectives/topic/social-determinants-health/interventions-resources

Office of Minority Health. (n.d.). *The case for national CLAS standards*. U.S. Department of Health and Human Services. https://thinkculturalhealth.hhs.gov/assets/pdfs/EnhancedNationalCLASStandards.pdf

Office of Minority Health and Health Equity. (2020, November 30). *Paving the road to health equity*. Centers for Disease Control and Prevention. https://www.cdc.gov/minorityhealth/publications/health_equity/index.html

Ogden, P., & Erwin, C. (2023). Professionalism and communication. In *Management of healthcare organizations* (4th ed.). Health Administration Press.

Onduo. (2022, April 27). *Onduo by Verily tackles social determinants of health in new commitment to the conversation series on health equity*. https://verily.com/blog/onduo-by-verily-tackles-social-determinants-of-health-in-new-commitment-to-the-conversation-series-on-health-equity/

Powell, J. A. (2008). Structural racism: Building upon the insights of John Calmore. *North Carolina Law Review*, *86*, 791–816.

Queensborough Community College. (n.d.) *Definition for diversity*. https://www.qcc.cuny.edu/diversity/definition.html

Raths, D. (2022, March 30). *Research explores patients' desire for assistance with unmet social needs*. https://www.hcinnovationgroup.com/population-health-management/social-determinants-of-health/news/21262318/research-explores-patients-desire-for-assistance-with-unmet-social-needs?utm_source=HI+Daily+NL&utm_medium=email&utm_campaign=CPS220331120&o_eid=6978A6266356F5Z&rdx.ident%5Bpull%5D=omeda%7C6978A6266356F5Z&oly_enc_id=6978A6266356F5Z

Ray, R. (2020, April 9). *Why are Blacks dying at higher rates from COVID-19?* Brookings Institution. https://www.brookings.edu/blog/fixgov/2020/04/09/why-are-blacks-dying-at-higher-rates-from-covid-19/

San Diego Foundation. (2016, March 24). *What is social justice?* https://www.sdfoundation.org/news-events/sdf-news/what-is-social-justice/

Seabert, D., McKenzie, J., & Pinger, R. (2022). Disparate populations and community and population health. In *McKenzie's, an introduction to community and public health* (10th ed.; pp. 252–284). Jones & Bartlett Learning.

U.S. Census Bureau. (2021, August 12). *Racial and ethnic diversity in the United States: 2010 census and 2020 census*. https://www.census.gov/library/visualizations/interactive/racial-and-ethnic-diversity-in-the-united-states-2010-and-2020-census.html

U.S. Department of Health and Human Services. (n.d.). *National CLAS standards*. https://thinkculturalhealth.hhs.gov/clas/standards

U.S. Department of Housing and Urban Development. (n.d.). *Diversity and inclusion definitions*. https://www.hud.gov/program_offices/administration/admabout/diversity_inclusion/definitions

White-Williams, C. (2022, March 31). *Social determinants of health and heart failure. The Art of person-centered care*. PowerPoint presentation. American Heart Association.

White-Williams, C., Rossi, L. P., Bittner, V. A., Driscoll, A., Durant, R. W., Granger, B. B., Graven, L. J., Kitko, L., Newlin, K., Shirey, M.; on behalf of the American Heart Association Council on Cardiovascular and Stroke Nursing; Council on Clinical Cardiology; and Council on Epidemiology and Prevention. (2020, April 30). Addressing social determinants of health in the care of patients with heart failure: a scientific statement from the American heart association. *Circulation, 141*, e841–e863. https://www.ahajournals.org/doi/10.1161/CIR.0000000000000767

World Health Organization. (n.d.). *Social determinants of health: Health equity*. https://www.who.int/health-topics/social-determinants-of-health#tab=tab_3

Credits

Fig. 6.1: Generated with FreeWordCloudGenerator.com.

Fig. 6.2: Copyright © 2015 Depositphotos/nikolaev.

Fig. 6.3: Source: https://www.census.gov/library/visualizations/interactive/racial-and-ethnic-diversity-in-the-united-states-2010-and-2020-census.html.

Fig. 6.4: Source: https://www.census.gov/library/visualizations/interactive/racial-and-ethnic-diversity-in-the-united-states-2010-and-2020-census.html.

Fig. 6.5: Copyright © 2017 Depositphotos/Rawpixel.
Fig. 6.7: Copyright © 2013 Depositphotos/monkeybusiness.
Fig. 6.8: Copyright © 2015 Depositphotos/gustavofrazao.
Fig. 6.10: Copyright © 2018 Depositphotos/psisaa.
Fig. 6.12: Copyright © 2020 Depositphotos/Vectorbox.
Fig. 6.13: Source: https://www.cdc.gov/minorityhealth/publications/health_equity/index.html.
Fig. 6.14: Copyright © 2022 Depositphotos/monkeybusiness.

CHAPTER SEVEN

Health for All Populations

Focus on Health Behaviors and Consumerism

Chapter Description

This chapter transitions from identifying the impact of the social determinants of health (SDOH) on higher-risk populations to concentrate on two strategies that can improve health outcomes. Patients are individuals with personal lifestyles and health behaviors that directly impact their health status. Health education and health behavior change form the foundation of health promotion activities targeting vulnerable groups. Patients are also consumers as they can select who will be their health provider and when to seek care. This chapter describes two useful health behavior models and explains basic behavior economic concepts to increase our understanding of why and how people make their health decisions. Changing negative health decisions and behaviors to positive ones can improve the quality of life and life expectancy for all.

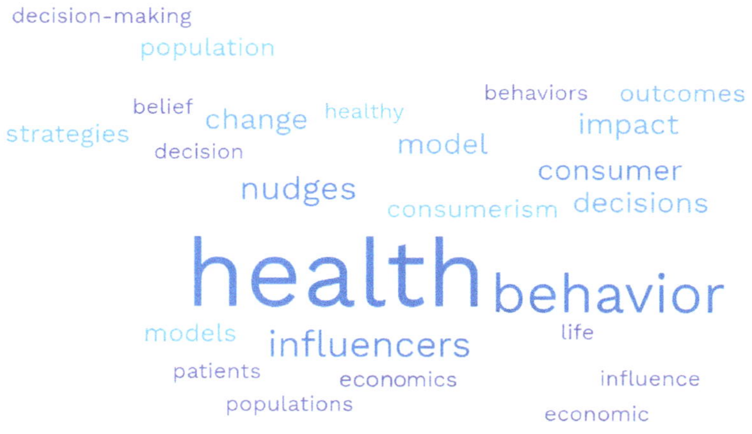

FIGURE 7.1 Chapter Word Cloud

Chapter Objectives

After completing this chapter, students will be able to:

1. Discuss the relationship between health behavior and health outcomes
2. Describe two common health behavior change models
3. Explain the role of consumerism and its impact on health decision-making
4. Identify ways behavioral economic concepts influence individuals' health decision-making processes
5. Provide examples of the two behavior change strategies called "nudges" and "influencers"

Key Words

Behavior economics	Health belief model	Mental accounting	Transtheoretical (stages of change) model
Consumer	Heuristics	Nudges	
Consumerism	Influencers	Self-efficacy	
Health behavior	Loss aversion		

Changing Health Behaviors: A Population Health Challenge

80 is the new 60

FIGURE 7.2   Living Longer

Most of us would like to live forever. In ancient times, Herodotus, who was an historian and geographer, first mentioned a mystical fountain of youth, and for centuries after, explorers searched in vain for a water of life that prevented aging (Greek Boston, n.d.). Unfortunately, it has not yet been discovered. What we do know about longevity and life expectancy is that our everyday health behavior choices can increase or decrease how long we live and our quality of life.

Why is this important to population health? First, the health care industry has long known that seniors are the largest consumers of health care. At least 80% of American seniors have been diagnosed with at least one chronic disease, and more than 50% are being treated for two conditions (American's Health Rankings, n.d.). Second, the senior population is expected to increase faster than any other age group. Figure 7.3 presents the projected world population by broad age groups.

World: Population by Broad Age Groups

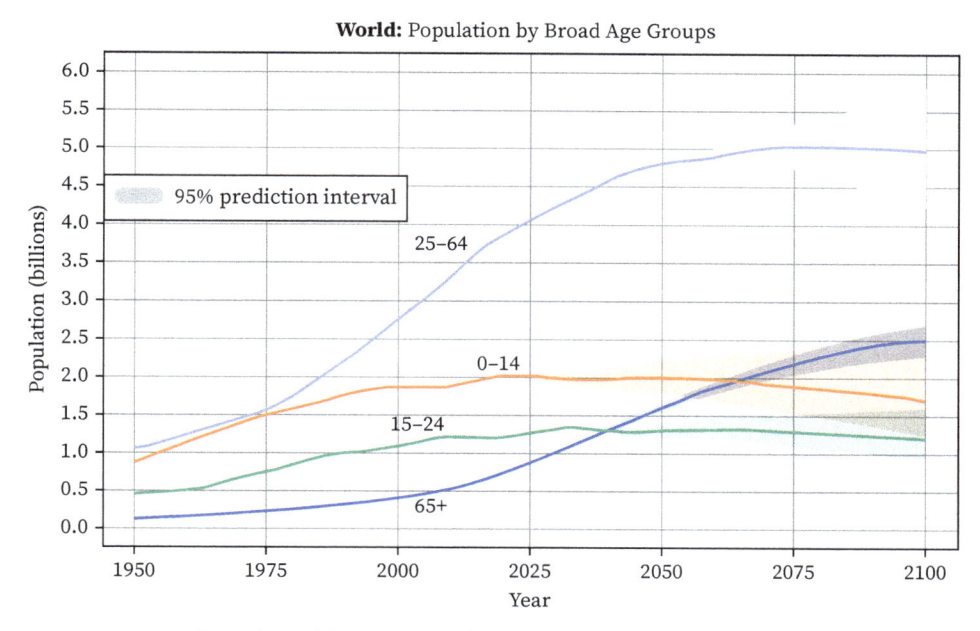

FIGURE 7.3 Projected World Population by Broad Age Groups

What did you notice about the projected age of future world populations? Of course, the senior age group is the fastest growing, and the same can be said for the United States. Because seniors often become part of higher-risk populations due to chronic diseases such as diabetes, heart disease, arthritis, and other conditions, population health remains focused on identifying and reducing these major risk factors (see Figure 7.4).

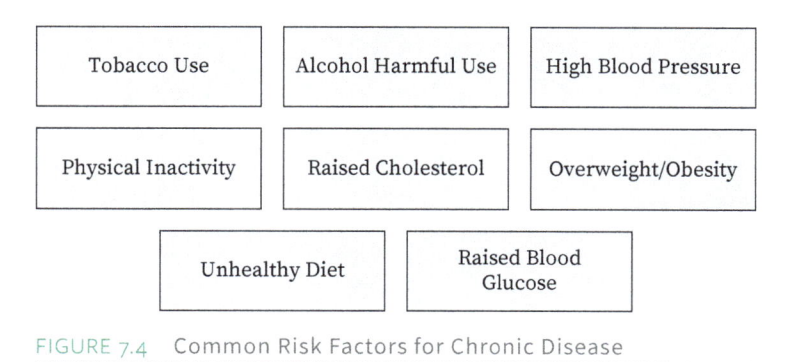

- Tobacco Use
- Alcohol Harmful Use
- High Blood Pressure
- Physical Inactivity
- Raised Cholesterol
- Overweight/Obesity
- Unhealthy Diet
- Raised Blood Glucose

FIGURE 7.4 Common Risk Factors for Chronic Disease

Health Behavior Population Health Strategies

Given the projected growth of the senior population and knowing that health behaviors can directly influence chronic disease risk factors, positive health

132 | Population Health: Practical Skills for Future Health Professionals

behavior change has become a major health promotion strategy. **Health behaviors** are any actions and activities individuals undertake that affect their health (County Health Rankings & Roadmaps, 2022). Everyone's lifestyle reflects a collection of daily health behavior choices.

Practical Skill: Your Health Behaviors

What did you eat for breakfast this morning? Did you plan any exercise for today? Do you feel stressed out over upcoming courses or assignments? Were you able to spend time with family or friends over the weekend? These are all common daily situations that require health behavior decisions, and over time their impact can have a considerable influence on health status.

But how does population health change someone's negative health behavior? How do we encourage seniors to get their annual checkups? What can we do to prevent obesity in preschool and elementary school children? Which population health strategies will encourage people of all ages that activity and exercise are beneficial for both the mind and the body? The answers to these questions will aid in furthering the population health goals of preventing future chronic diseases and reducing the cost of health care for all.

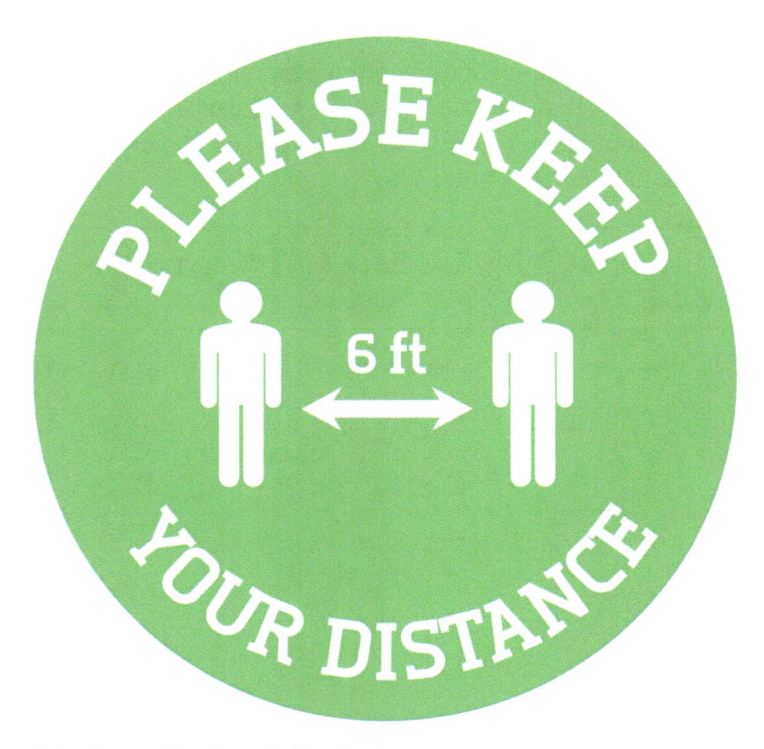

FIGURE 7.5   For Your Safety Poster

Health Behavior Models

Health behaviors, which can be both positive and negative, involve personal preferences and habits, as well as external factors that are also important influences (Glanz & Kahan, 2014). For example, during the COVID-19 pandemic, some individuals chose not to follow distancing guidelines or wear masks. Although numerous models and frameworks for changing health behaviors exist, population health programs rely on health behavior change models that represent best practices and have been proven successful. Three of the most common frameworks are presented in Figure 7.6.

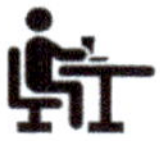

Intra-Personal Health Behavior Change
- Health Belief Model
- Transtheoretical Model (Stages of Change)

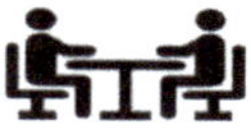

Interpersonal Health Behavior Change
- Social Cognitive Theory

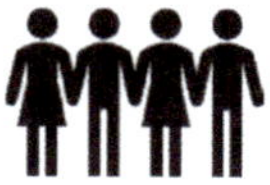

Population Health Behavior Changes
- Social Ecological Model
- Diffusion of an Innovation
- Social Marketing
- Media Advocacy

FIGURE 7.6   Health Behavior Change Frameworks

Health behavior change frameworks such as the health belief model and the transtheoretical/stages of change model are most effective when changes within the individual are needed. The social cognitive theory focuses on interpersonal relationships with others and the environment. For major health behavior changes that affect society, the social-ecological model includes all levels of influence, including worksites, communities, and society, via the use of public health policy. Large national health campaigns that often involve social media and health promotion advocacy are included at this level.

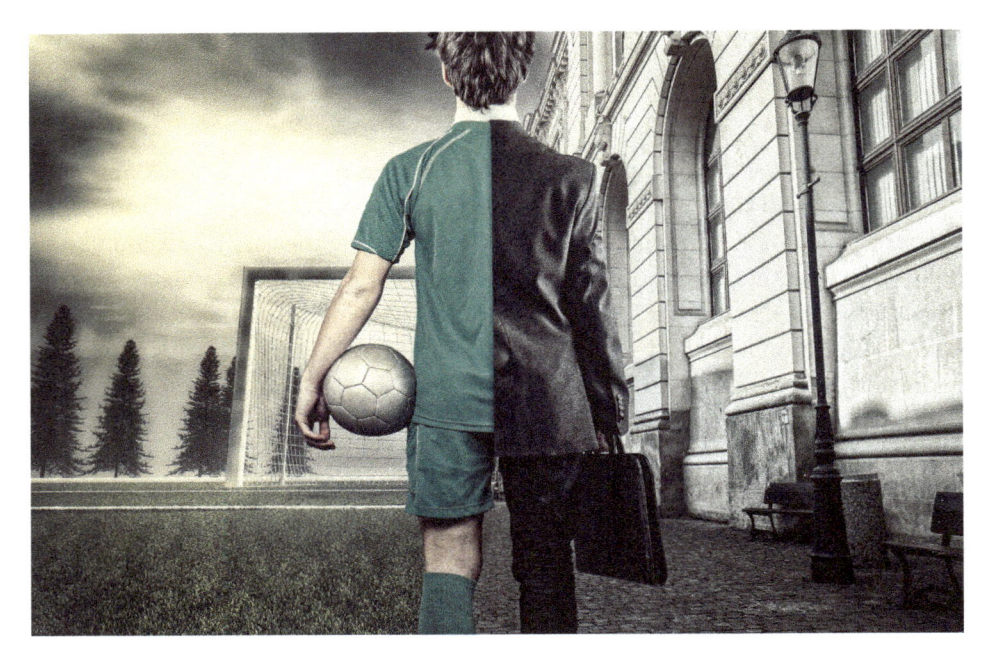

FIGURE 7.7   Self-Efficacy

Health Belief Model

The U.S. Public Health Service developed the **health belief model (HBM)** more than 50 years ago with the purpose of trying to explain human health behavior (Champion & Skinner, 2008). This model suggests that an individual's health behavior choices are influenced by their expectations, threats, and cues to action (Rosenstock et al., 1988). The model includes one of the essential psychological components for change: self-efficacy. *Self-efficacy* refers to an individual's perception of their capabilities for changing a behavior (American Psychological Association, 2009). Here is a quick example of how this theory would work for an individual who is overeating and may have prediabetes. Review Table 7.1 to see how the HBM concepts are applied.

Asking someone to change a health behavior takes time because many actions are ingrained habits and personal attitudes may have been formed early in life. Although this example is at the intrapersonal level, within any given population, many individuals would benefit from this behavior change model. The HBM will increase the individual's likelihood of positive behavior change, but this intervention can even be shared with large at-risk populations.

Negative health behaviors are not the same and some have stronger negative consequences than others. What if the risky health behavior that needs to be altered is a severe addiction?

TABLE 7.1   Application of the Health Behavior Model Theory

HBM Theory Components	COVID-19 Example
Expectations	
Perceived benefits of action	If I quit overeating, I may not develop diabetes, and my family will be happy.
Perceived barriers to action	It's so hard when everybody else can eat everything they want. I hate being different when I go out with friends.
Perceived self-efficacy	My aunt lost 50 pounds. I can do it, too.
Threats	
Perceived susceptibility	Not everybody who overeats get diabetes, but some do.
Perceived severity	I know obesity is linked to heart disease and that kills a lot of people.
Cues to action	
Media	I keep seeing this message at work about a walking group and a weight-loss program that's even virtual.
Personal influences	I know my friends and family would support me and help me reach my weight goal.
Reminders	I'll keep a bottle of water or some fruit in the car so that the next time I think about eating fast food, I can do something else.

The Transtheoretical Model

The **transtheoretical model (TTM)**, an individual-level model of behavior change, addresses the cycle of addictive lifestyle behavior issues. The stages of change include precontemplation, contemplation, preparation, action, maintenance, and termination (Prochaska et al., 2008). We know that often individuals pass through a series of stages as they seek to change their habits and, in fact, that many individuals relapse. See Figure 7.8 for the TTM cycle of health behavior change.

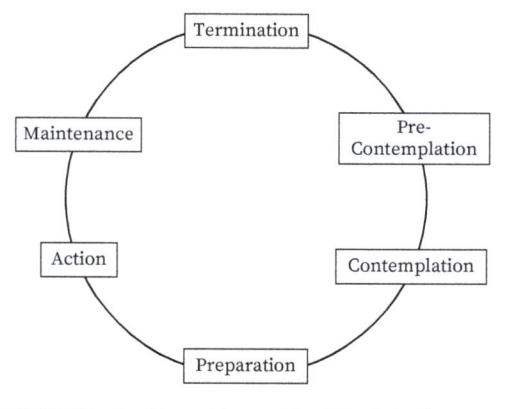

FIGURE 7.8   Transtheoretical Model of Health Behavior Change

This model helps the individual to recognize their current stage and supports them with stage designed communications and key reminders for sustained behavior change. Each person and their addiction are different, and individuals can skip over stages or need to cycle through one of them again (LaMorte, 2019). Review Table 7.2 to view a TTM example in which a person became addicted to pain medication (opioids) following a severe car accident.

TABLE 7.2   Application of the Transtheoretical Model (Stages of Change)

Precontemplation: Individual may be unaware of problem behavior or devalue the need to change	"I'm fine. Everybody takes pills when they have pain."
Contemplation: Awareness and thinking about the near future—6 months	"What if I cut down on these pills? They are supposed to be addictive. Should I?"
Preparation: Individuals may start to take small positive action steps in the next 30 days	"OK, I am ready to change. I know there are safer ways to manage my pain, and my doctor has outlined a plan of action for me."
Action: Behavior change has begun with intention to continue	"It has been 6 months since I stopped taking those pills. It wasn't easy, but I do feel better, and the coaching and extra activities with my family have really helped."
Maintenance: Evidence of positive behavior change for at least 6 months; however, chance of relapse	"I pulled my back, and it wasn't easy not to reach for those pills, but I'm not going to start using them again."
Termination: A possible stage of no relapse indications; however, rarely achieved	"I know how powerful those drugs can be, but I don't intend to go back to that again."

Health behavior changes can extend one person's life for years and, for population health, can prevent thousands of chronic diseases in the future. These two health frameworks are examples of population health strategies for health promotion and disease prevention. Other models, such as the social cognitive theory and the social-ecological model, are appropriate options for groups, subpopulations, and societal health initiatives. As you can imagine, these models

Practical Skill: Personal Application of the Health Belief Model

All of us struggle with negative health habits, and every day we have an opportunity to change our health behaviors. Review the HBM again and think about one negative health habit you would like to change. Answer each of the following questions:

- If I change, what will be the benefit?
- If I change, what will be the main barriers?
- Do I think I can change?
- If I don't change, do I know what will happen?
- Even if I don't change, how dangerous will the consequences be?
- Would setting a goal be a great cue to action for me?
- I know other friends who have started a support group. Could I just use a health app on my phone?

What was the outcome of this exercise? Do you think you can make a positive health behavior change now?

are more sophisticated and require health educators trained in developing appropriate interventions and programs.

The Impact of Consumerism

Health behavior change theories are most valuable with patients recognizing the need for changing negative lifestyle choices. However, we also need to reach individuals and populations who are not yet patients. Improving population health outcomes requires a relationship between the patient and the health system before initiating health behavior change. The first step is making a connection, and that depends on the patient's decision to participate in health care. Accepting that patients are also consumers has been a challenge for the health sector (Gusmano et al., 2019), but the COVID-19 pandemic dramatically increased the impact of consumerism on the American health system (Martin & Gundling, 2022).

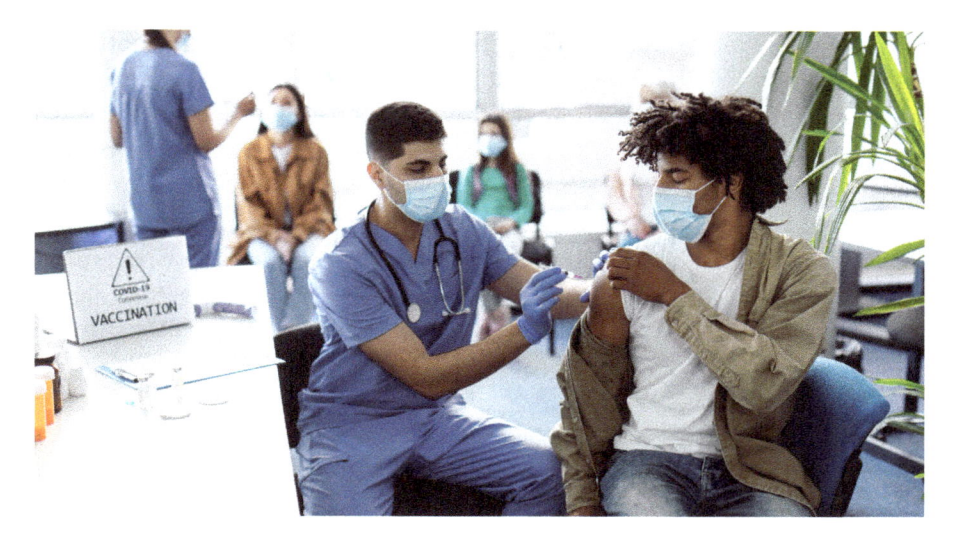

FIGURE 7.9   COVID-19 Vaccination at Nontraditional Health Care Sites

For almost two years, COVID-19 disrupted the traditional relationships between primary care and other health system components and their patients. Most hospitals reduced the number of elective services they provided, and primary care facilities also closed temporarily (Technical Resources, Assistance Center, and Information Exchange, n.d.). Older adults delayed treatments, children did not receive vaccines, and important clinical trials were interrupted. COVID-19 vaccines were offered by state and local public health departments, local community clinics, and participating pharmacies (Michaud & Kates, 2020).

The trusted and continuous relationship with a single health provider was disrupted for a significant length of time. Patients quickly became **consumers** as they recognized they had a choice in where and when to seek health care. Recent technology has made decisions to switch health providers even more convenient with the result that today's patients think of themselves as consumers.

Practical Skill: On Consumerism Activity

Where did you receive your COVID-19 vaccinations? Did you go somewhere different from your normal care provider? Did that change make any difference in where you will seek care in the future? Briefly describe your vaccination circumstances and situation. Did it change your perspective as a consumer of health care?

Health care consumerism refers to "people proactively using trustworthy, relevant information and appropriate technology to make better-informed decisions about their health care options" (Carman et al., 2019). Consumers have the right to make choices, and with the number of increasing options for health care from primary care visits, urgi-centers, pharmacies, and even large retail stores (Walmart, 2022; MinuteClinic, n.d.), consumers now are faced with multiple and diverse choices. Today, the consumer experience is the primary concern for health care organizations, as health consumers expect to find the same convenient service for health care as they do for banking or ordering take-out food. For health care, the shift has been from simply offering a service to recognizing the consumer may or may not choose your service (Morehouse,

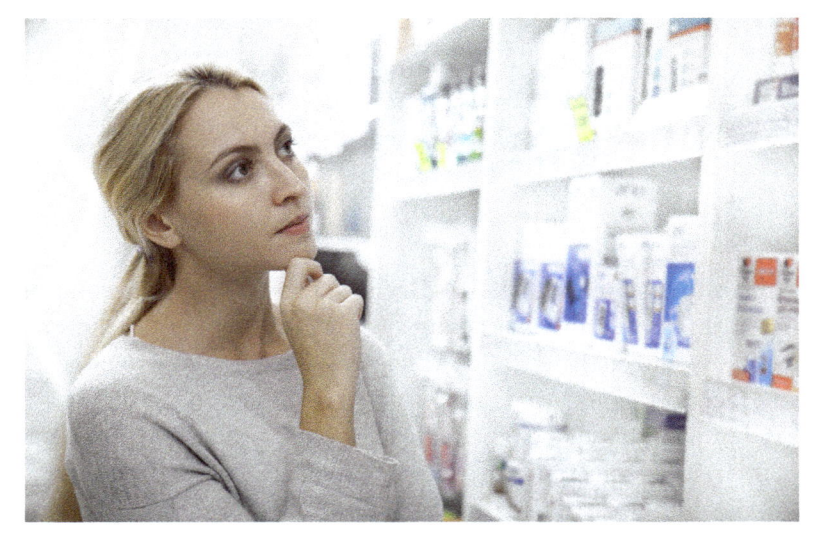

FIGURE 7.10   Consumer Decision-Making

2021). The focus is now on the entire customer experience, beginning with the first virtual encounter and including all interactions along the pathway, not only with health practitioners, but with staff as well. Today's consumers have definite expectations, are comfortable with mobile encounters and virtual experiences, and expect the same from their health care providers (Rubenfire, 2022).

A primary commonality among all potential health consumers is the health care decision-making process. Behavior economics can explain how individuals make those health care decisions. However, once a consumer selects a health care provider or organization, tailored activities must begin to ensure positive health outcomes.

Behavior Economics

The public health system has ensured that each one of us is aware of potential health hazards and risks, such as excessive or misuse of substances including drugs, alcohol, and nicotine. And yet, there are Americans every day who do not buckle up their seat belts or avoid harmful sun exposure. It has been said that people are illogical when they make health decisions and that they often put themselves at health risk (Gutman & Kawachi, 2013).

Consumers follow a decision-making pathway when they make choices, but their behavior still may not be economical, rational, or even predictable. **Behavioral economics** is a field of study that describes the how and why health consumers and patients make important health decisions. This concept blends both the economics of choice (cost) with social psychology (motivation) to help explain individuals' decision-making (Lin, 2016). Outlined below are three basic health economics concepts that help population health professionals understand how patients and consumers make their decisions.

1. A ***heuristic*** refers to decision-making based on using a "rule of thumb" (Lin, 2016). We often make choices based on short-cut thinking from past experiences. Individuals often equate situations that are not similar and may choose the tried and true without thinking about new or better options.

    o **Consumer example:** "The last time I had a headache, I took xyz medication, and it worked. So, I'm trying it again with my stomachache."

2. Did you ever use a pro and con decision-making process? Based on how a decision is presented and described, patients often use a **mental accounting** (pro-and-con) system to make a choice. Their intent in doing so is to determine the "probability" of an outcome so that they can make the best decision. Health care providers receive requests asking about the likelihood

of success for a potential recommended treatment or medication. The patient can then apply that information to their own situation.

- **Consumer example:** "Do I really need to get a mammogram every year? I don't. But my grandmother got breast cancer, so the probability of my getting the disease could be higher. My doctor said it could be higher. I'd better schedule the mammogram."

3. **Loss aversion** means that an individual has a personal preference for loss avoidance as compared to acquiring gains. Therefore, their choice is directed more toward changes that avoid perceived losses and less toward those that will make gains in the future (Decision Lab, 2022).

    - **Consumer example:** "My doctor wants me to lose weight, but it means giving up some of the foods that I really like or going on a diet. I'm not sure that going on this diet is worth it now."

Practical Skill: Student Activity

Think back to your health decisions this past week. Can you find any examples that fit into the three behavior economic concepts discussed? Now, imagine that there are 10,000 other college students who made the same type of decision. How does this affect population health over time?

Population Health Strategies to Improve Decision-Making

Health behavior similarities occur among various at-risk and priority populations and are related to how choices are made regardless of the decision-making process. For example, people may choose to remain obese rather than to adopt a healthy diet, and even though 70% of smokers say they want to quit, only 2%–3% of smokers effectively quit each year (Volp & Lowenstein, 2014). What type of population health strategies can we use to mitigate negative health behavior choices based on common decision errors? **Nudges** and **influencers** are two familiar patient impact strategies that can be highly effective with at-risk populations.

Nudges + Influencers = Health Behavior Choices

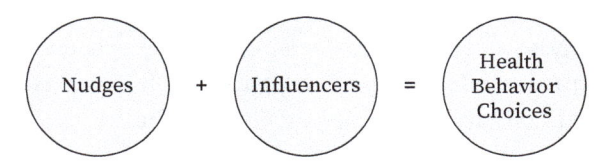

FIGURE 7.11 Strategies for Improving Population Health Behaviors

Based on proven health behavior theories and models, we know that reinforcement has a strengthening effect and can be beneficial in helping patients change their behavior (McKenzie et al., 2017). **Nudges** are targeted and tailored information that can be used as reinforcement to encourage consumers' and patients' participation in healthy actions and activities. Nudges should be relatively simple and not difficult to complete (Hansen, 2016). For example, in addition to an individual receiving a yearly postcard reminding them that it has been a year since their last mammogram exam, they might receive a follow-up email or text reminder 2 weeks later asking whether they have already made an appointment or would like assistance.

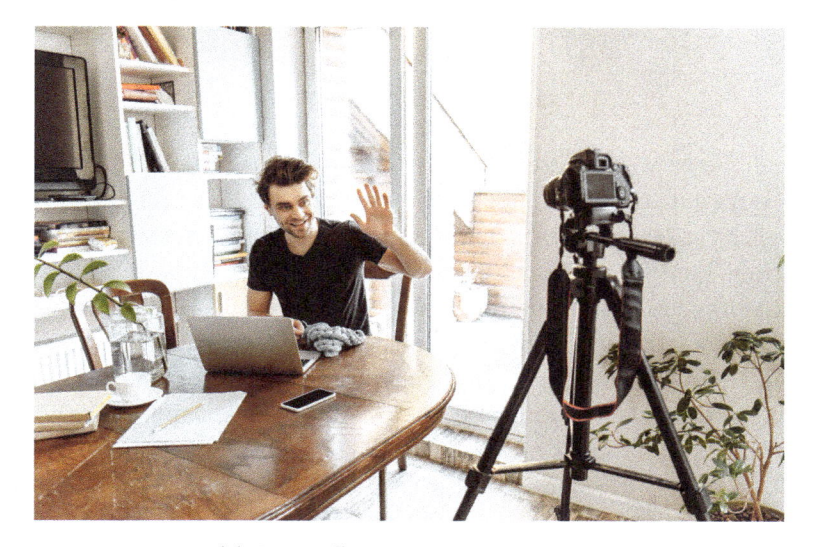

FIGURE 7.12   Health Care Influencers

Another type of behavior change strategy to improve consumer health decisions is the use of an **influencer**. An *influencer* is someone with the power to influence the perception of others or get them to behave in a different way (Dada, 2017). In terms of behavior change, the influencer role is a trusted individual to promote a health idea (lose weight) or a cause, such as wellness. Influencers encourage populations of followers to adopt suggested preferences with the purpose of shaping behaviors (Coughlin & Felts, 2021).

Summary

To meet the challenge of improving health and quality of life for all, population health relies on identifying at-risk populations and implementing behavior change intervention strategies. Health promotion programs that encourage positive behavior change use of health behavior models such as the HBM and the TTM to affect individuals' attitudes and daily activities. Population health also recognizes the increasing impact of consumerism on the choice of health care practitioners and providers. The primary criterion is convenience. Behavior economics concepts such as heuristics, mental accounting, and loss aversion can explain patients' decision-making processes. To reinforce positive behavior change, disease prevention approaches include the use of nudges and influencers to encourage at-risk populations to start and maintain necessary health changes. Understanding the impact of consumerism and patient-choice options involves guiding decision-making processes for both individuals and vulnerable populations.

Discussion Questions

1. Describe why the increase in chronic diseases in the United States has encouraged population health to focus on lifestyle and health behaviors.
2. Over the years, health experts have designed, implemented, and assessed various health behavior theories developed to help individuals change unhealthy habits. Population health recognizes the need for using various theories at the intrapersonal, interpersonal, group, organizational, and social levels. Identify a health behavior theory appropriate for each level.
3. Changing negative health behaviors and habits, especially those with chronic conditions, is not easy. People often lack the skills to help themselves make important and positive health changes. Which aspect (expectations, threats, cues to action) of the HBM do you believe would be most effective for this population?
4. Although it is not often listed as a chronic disease even though it is just as destructive over time, substance abuse or misuse requires significant lifestyle changes to prevent negative impacts on an individual's health status. Which aspects of the TTM make it a common population health–recommended choice for helping this at-risk population?
5. Today's consumers expect convenience whether it is banking on their smartphone, having their dinners delivered, or buying a new car online. Why should health care be any different? Outline expectations that today's consumers have for their health care.
6. *Behavior economics* refers to the field of study that describes the how and why health consumers and patients make important health decisions. In the grid below, three basic health concepts are listed. Please provide a personal example of how you have used these strategies when making decisions in your life.

Behavior Economic Concept	Student Example
1. Heuristic—a rule-of-thumb decision.	
2. Mental accounting—keeping a pro/con system for a choice	
3. Loss aversion—choosing another option perceiving a loss	

References

America's Health Rankings. (n.d.). About the senior report. *America's Health Rankings® senior report: A call to action for individuals and their communities*. https://www.americashealthrankings.org/about/page/about-the-senior-report

American Psychological Association. (n.d.). *Teaching tip sheet: Self-efficacy*. https://www.apa.org/pi/aids/resources/education/self-efficacy

Carman, K., Lawrence, W., & Siegel, J. (2019, March 5). The 'new' health care consumerism. *Health Affairs*. https://www.healthaffairs.org/do/10.1377/hblog20190304.69786/full/

Champion, V. L., & Skinner, C. S. (2008). The health belief model. In K. Glanz, B. K. Rimer, & K. Viswanath (Eds.), *Health behavior and health education: Theory, research, and practice* (4th ed.; pp. 45–66). Jossey Bass.

Coughlin, J., & Felts, A. (2021). Consumer engagement and technology. In D. B. Nash, R. J. Fabius, A. Skoufalos, & J. L. Clarke (Eds.), *Population health: Creating a culture of wellness* (pp. 181–193). Jones & Bartlett Learning.

County Health Rankings & Roadmaps. (2022). *Health behaviors*. https://www.countyhealthrankings.org/explore-health-rankings/measures-data-sources/county-health-rankings-model/health-factors/health-behaviors#:~:text=Health%20behaviors%20are%20actions%20individuals,intake%2C%20and%20risky%20sexual%20behavior

Dada, G. A. (2017, November 14). What is influencer marketing and how can marketers use it effectively? *Forbes*. https://www.forbes.com/sites/forbescommunicationscouncil/2017/11/14/what-is-influencer-marketing-and-how-can-marketers-use-it-effectively/?sh=1567c48f23d1

Decision Lab. (2022). *What is loss aversion?* https://thedecisionlab.com/biases/loss-aversion

Glanz, K. (n.d.). *Social and behavioral theories*. https://obssr.od.nih.gov/sites/obssr/files/Social-and-Behavioral-Theories.pdf

Glanz, K., & Kahan, S. (2014). Conceptual framework for behavior change. In S. Kahan, A. C. Gielen, P. J. Fagan, & L. W. Green (Eds.), *Health behavior change in populations* (pp. 9–25). John Hopkins.

Greek Boston. (n.d.). *All about the fountain of youth in Greek mythology.* https://www.greekboston.com/culture/mythology/fountain-of-youth/

Gusmano, M., Maschke, K., & Solomon, M. (2019, March). Patient-centered care, yes; patients as consumers, No. *Health Affairs, 38*(3). https://doi.org/10.1377/hlthaff.2018.05019

Gutman, A., & Kawachi, I. (2013, Spring). *Q&A: The science of irrationality.* https://www.hsph.harvard.edu/news/magazine/qa-the-science-of-irrationality/

Hansen, P. G. (2016, August 16). *What is nudging?* https://behavioralpolicy.org/what-is-nudging/

LaMorte, W. (2019). *Transtheoretical model of change/stages of change.* Boston University School of Public Health. https://sphweb.bumc.bu.edu/otlt/mph-modules/sb/behavioralchangetheories/BehavioralChangeTheories6.html

Lin, J. (2016). Chapter 8: Behavioral economics. In D. B. Nash, R. J. Fabius, A. Skoufalos, & J. L. Clarke (Eds.), *Population health management: Creating a culture of wellness* (2nd ed.; pp. 153–165). Jones & Bartlett Learning.

Martin, S., & Gundling, R. (2022, May 24). Episode 230: *How COVID-19 impacted consumerism and how healthcare organizations can adapt.* Oracle/Cerner Podcast. https://www.cerner.com/perspectives/how-covid-19-impacted-consumerism-and-how-healthcare-organizations-can-adapt

McKenzie, J., Neiger, B., & Thackeray, R. (2017). *Planning, implementing & evaluating health promotion programs: A primer* (7th ed.). Pearson.

Michaud, J., & Kates, J. (2020, October 20). *Distributing a COVID-19 vaccine across the U.S.—A look at key issues.* Kaiser Family Foundation. https://www.kff.org/report-section/distributing-a-covid-19-vaccine-across-the-u-s-a-look-at-key-issues-issue-brief/

MinuteClinic. (n.d.). *How can a MinuteClinic® provider work with my PCP (primary care physician)?* CVS Pharmacy. https://www.cvs.com/minuteclinic/why-choose-us/primary-care-physician

Morehouse, A. (2021, July/August). Building the branding experience. *Healthcare Executive,* 30–31.

Painter, J., Borba, C., Hynes, M., Mays, D., & Glanz, K. (2008). The use of theory in health behavior research from 2000–2005: A systematic review. *Annals of Behavioral Medicine, 35,* 358–362.

Prochaska, J. O., Redding, C. A., & Evers, K. E. (2008). The transtheoretical model and stages of change. In K. Glanz, B. K. Rimer, & K. Viswanath (eds.), *Health behavior and health education: Theory, research, and practice* (4th ed.; pp. 97–121). Jossey Bass.

Public Health Agency of Canada. (2015). *Chronic disease risk factors: What are the primary risk factors?* https://www.canada.ca/en/public-health/services/chronic-diseases/chronic-disease-risk-factors.html

Rosenstock, J. M., Strecher, V. J., & Becker, M. H. (1988). Social learning theory and the Health Belief Model. *Health Education Quarterly, 15,* 175–183.

Rubenfire, A. (2022, April 22). *5 ways consumer expectations have changed and how to align your organization for success.* https://www.phreesia.com/2022/04/22/5-ways-consumer-expectations-have-changed-and-how-to-align-your-organization-for-success/

Technical Resources, Assistance Center, and Information Exchange. (n.d.). *COVID-19 healthcare delivery impacts.* Office of the Assistant Secretary for Preparedness and Response. https://files.asprtracie.hhs.gov/documents/covid-19-healthcare-delivery-impacts-quick-sheet.pdf

United Nations. (2022). *World population health prospects 2022.* https://population.un.org/wpp/Graphs/DemographicProfiles/Line/900

Volp, K., & Loewenstein, G. (2014). Behavioral economics and incentives to promote health behavior change. In S. Kahan, A. C. Gielen, P. J. Fagan, & L. W. Green (Eds.), *Health behavior change in populations* (pp. 417–434). Johns Hopkins University Press.

Walmart. (2022). *Walmart health.* https://corporate.walmart.com/purpose/health-wellness#:~:text=The%20patient%20is%20at%20the,door%20to%20the%20Walmart%20Supercenter

Credits

Fig. 7.1: Generated with FreeWordCloudGenerator.com.

Fig. 7.2: Source: https://www.ubs.com/us/en/investor-watch/2018/living-longer.html.

Fig. 7.3: Copyright © by United Nations, DESA, Population Division (CC BY 3.0 IGO) at http://population.un.org/wpp/.

Fig. 7.5: Copyright © 2020 Depositphotos/tupungato.

Fig. 7.6a: Copyright © by Microsoft.

Fig. 7.6b: Copyright © by Microsoft.

Fig. 7.6c: Copyright © by Microsoft.

Fig. 7.7: Copyright © 2016 Depositphotos/ALLVISIONN.

Fig. 7.8: James O. Prochaska, Colleen A. Redding, and Kerry E. Evers; , "The Transtheoretical Model and Stages of Change," *Health Behavior and Health Education: Theory, Research, and Practice*, ed. Karen Glanz, Barbara K. Rimer, K. Viswanath. Copyright © 2008 by John Wiley & Sons, Inc.

Fig. 7.9: Copyright © 2021 Depositphotos/Milkos.

Fig. 7.10: Copyright © 2019 Depositphotos/bjjenzor@gmail.com.

Fig. 7.12: Copyright © 2020 Depositphotos/AlexShadyuk.

PART III

Management

The chapters included in Part III challenge students to develop management skills in the areas of health data analytics, risk management, and financial and quality accountability. Chapter 8 provides a base for understanding data aggregation, analytics, and reporting, and available tools such as electronic health records (EHRs) and artificial intelligence applications. Students learn to identify which data sources will provide the best information for decision-making, whether it be clinical, public, industry, or patient-generated data. Chapter 9 outlines a real-world population risk assessment process, including identification of risk factors, segmentation, stratification, and care management. Another major population health management function is accountability, which requires financial, quality, and safety competencies. Chapter 10 provides financial examples such as completing the volume-to-value transition, quality process basics using the Plan, Do, Check, Act (PDCA) model, and patient safety standards. Chapter 11 frames the process of population health management decision-making needed to select the best strategies for improving chronic care and facilitate care coordination. The specific aims and delivery process of two care models, accountable care organizations and patient-centered medical homes, illustrate the current processes of population healthcare delivery today. The chapters in Part III emphasize the data skills, accountability competencies, and model strategies necessary for future population health professionals.

CHAPTER EIGHT

Measuring and Assessing Population Health

Chapter Description

Chapter 8 describes data strategies, skills, and tools needed to ensure effective population health service delivery and positive health outcomes. This chapter explains the importance and relevance of health technology advances and innovations. These include essential population health management tools such as health information systems, electronic health records, and health data analytic processes. Other chapter topics include interoperability capabilities, predictive modeling, and artificial intelligence. The rapid adoption of data analysis and integrated technology systems has increased health sectors' ability to assess population health risks with a greater degree of certainty and aggregate patient health data and other database information to improve decision-making.

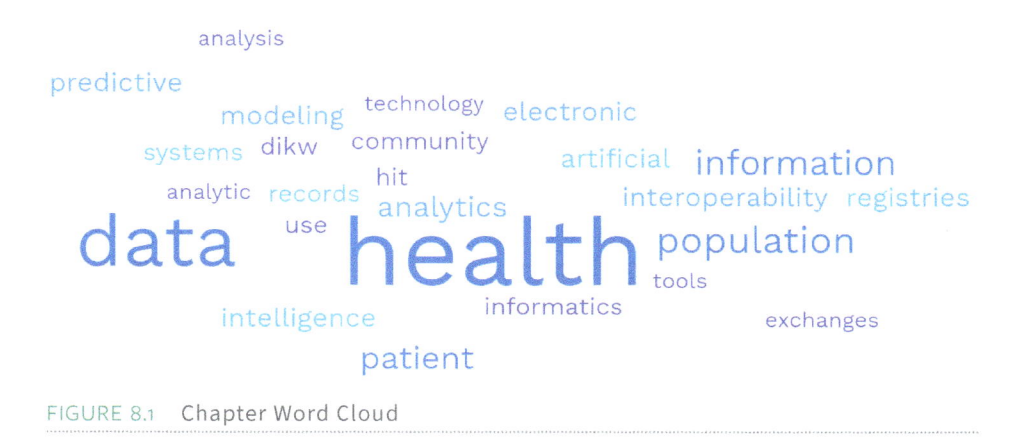

FIGURE 8.1   Chapter Word Cloud

149

Chapter Objectives

After completing this chapter, students will be able to:

1. Discuss the Data, Information, Knowledge, and Wisdom (DIKW) continuum and the role of health information technology
2. Describe the importance of electronic health records
3. Compare health information exchanges and patient registries
4. Define and discuss the role of health data analytics
5. Clarify the concept of interoperability and advantages of real-time data
6. Identify the potential benefits of artificial intelligence
7. Summarize the issue and impact of health data inequality and data bias
8. Explain the data benefits from community health needs assessments

Key Words

Algorithm	Data justice	exchange	Health (HITECH) Act
Artificial intelligence	Electronic health records	Health Insurance Portability and Accountability Act of 1996 (HIPAA)	Interoperability
Big data			Meaningful use
Data, Information, Knowledge, and Wisdom (DIKW) continuum	Health data analytics		Patient registries
	Health informatics	Health Information Technology for Economic and Clinical	Predictive modeling
	Health information		

The Role of Data and Population Health

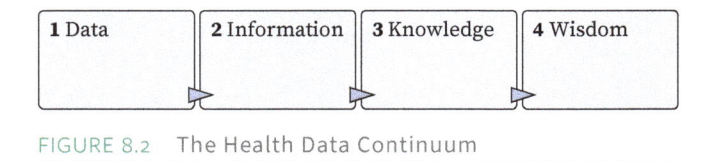

1 Data → 2 Information → 3 Knowledge → 4 Wisdom

FIGURE 8.2   The Health Data Continuum

Data → Information → Knowledge → Wisdom

Population health relies on constant and reliable data, and without the technology innovations of the past 20 years, population health management would not function as efficiently as it does currently. The **Data, Information, Knowledge, and Wisdom (DIKW) continuum** is a framework to explain the four data levels (data, information, knowledge, wisdom) and their relationships leading to higher-order thinking (i.e., decision-making). Data are in real time, which means they surround us, so we know precisely when a patient procedure has been completed and what the outcome is. For population health, those data need to be collected and aggregated, as the goal is to manage priority populations and not just individuals, and at-risk groups can have 10,000, 100,000, or even 1 million members. However, basic data tell us nothing until they are connected to yield information. Information needs to be analyzed and interpreted into meaningful content before it can become knowledge (Brahmachary, 2019). Additionally, knowledge needs to be conceptualized and examined before it becomes useful wisdom and aids decision-making. For instance, we know that certain priority groups are at risk for the social determinants of health (SDOH), which can result in negative health outcomes. Without health information systems (HIS), these vulnerable populations can be overlooked or missed entirely. The digitization of health data has long been considered the foundation for patient safety, operational efficiency, and quality of care (Abernathy et al., 2022).

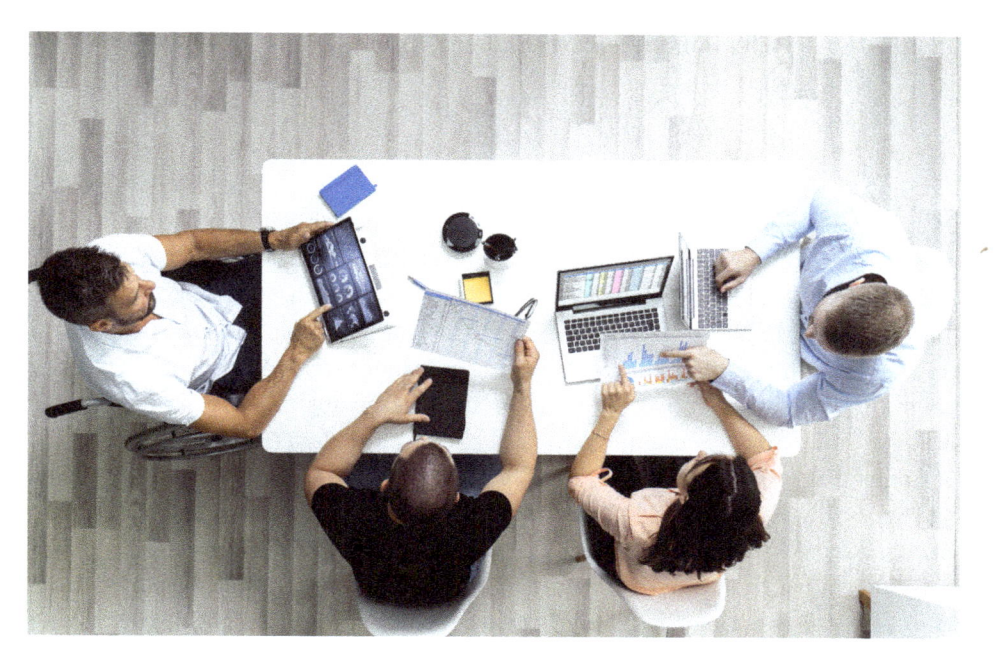

FIGURE 8.3   Computer Systems for Population Health

An enormous industry built on the development, maintenance, and implementation of HIS exists today. **Health informatics** is the term used to describe "the science of information management in health care" (Mastrian & McGonigle, 2017). It seems almost unbelievable that it took monetary incentives, as part of a national health mandate, to force health systems, hospitals, and health providers away from patient paper file folders into the digital era (Brown et al.,

2019). The **Health Information Technology for Economic and Clinical Health (HITECH) Act**, passed in 2009, required health care entities to install computerized systems and demonstrate their meaningful use (HIPAA Journal, 2020) *Meaningful use* is a term used to describe the requirement for providers to demonstrate performance on defined metrics and measures from their electronic health record. The goal was to ensure national data to improve quality of care. A second act, the **Health Insurance Portability and Accountability Act of 1996 (HIPAA)**, established privacy and security requirements for health care providers and organizations (U.S. Department of Health and Human Services, n.d.). The HIPAA Security Rule standards continue to protect personal health data and require specific administrative, physical, and technical safeguards to ensure confidentiality, integrity, and security of health information. Over time, national legislation that initially encouraged the adoption and integration of HIS has produced significant and positive impacts on the American's health status by ensuring real-time availability and reliability of data that assists in identifying priority populations with unmet needs.

Major Health Informatic Tools for Population Health

Population health professionals should recognize major health informatic tools, beginning with the **electronic health record (EHR)**, also known as an *electronic medical record* (EMR), which serves as a universal repository of a patient's information. The EHR is a digital platform and database that includes an individual's relevant health data, personal profile, and administrative information. Over the years, EHRs have been expanded to include items designed to capture SDOH information to provide complete patient background data (National Association of Community Health Centers, 2019). One of these additional EHR additions is known as *PRAPARE*, which is an acronym for *Protocol for Responding to Assessing Patient Assets, Risks, and Experiences*. This helps collect SDOH data.

EHR use improves patient safety compared to using paper records and increases access to patient records and conditions in real time. By providing aggregate priority **population health data**, EHRs have become instrumental in identifying elevated risk populations (Scherpbier et al., 2021). Today, the EHR is the cornerstone for population HIS.

Several major companies offer EMR software, and recently other non-health sector entrants such as Amazon and Google have developed competitive options. As you can imagine, these HIS and software often cost millions of dollars and require additional investments for training and support. Health professionals both in clinical and administrative positions rely on data collected in real time from EMRs. As technology has advanced, the complexity and utility of EMRs

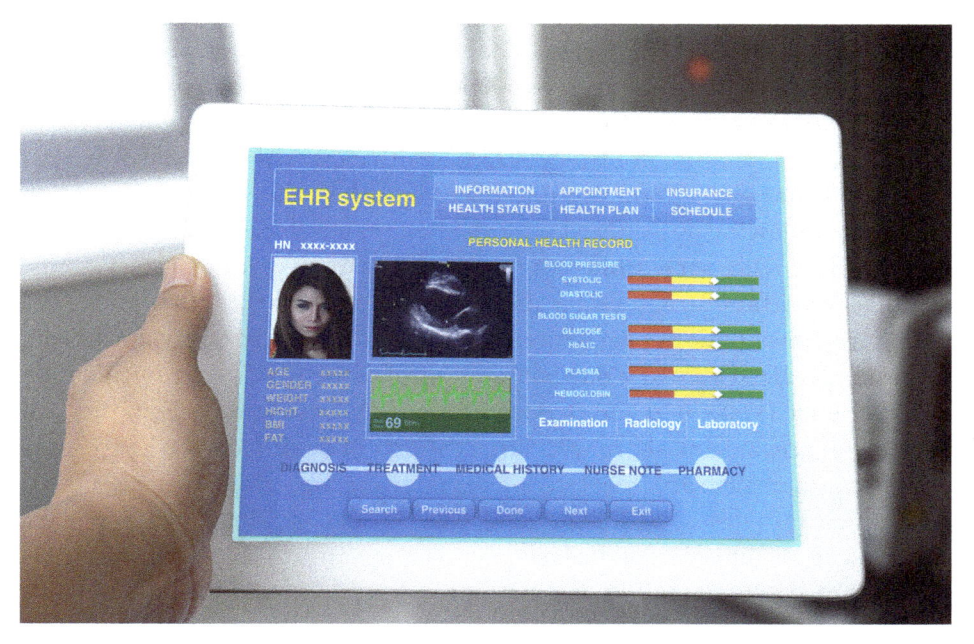

Chapter Eight Measuring and Assessing Population Health | 153

FIGURE 8.4   Major EHR Vendors

have improved as well. Experts recently outlined six major EMR trends for 2022 (Dugar, 2022). These six trends can be divided into two major categories: external pressures and technological advancements. External pressures include both clinical and environmental with the impact of COVID-19 on individual practitioners and policy requirements for standardization among various platform elements. Technology advancements include the collection and integration of patient wearable data, increased use of IoT (Internet of Things) and **artificial intelligence (AI)** within decision-making protocols, 5G networking capability for better connectivity, and increased security measures. However, many physicians are waiting for EMRs to have voice-recognition capabilities. The impact of that technology would certainly be to free the clinicians and other health care providers from all the manual data entry.

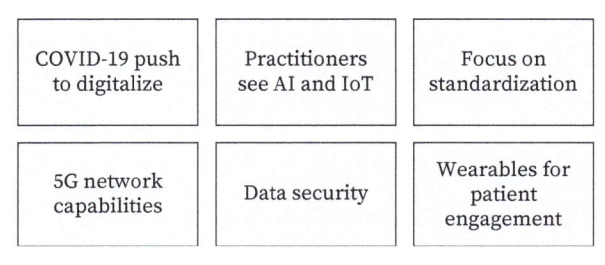

COVID-19 push to digitalize	Practitioners see AI and IoT	Focus on standardization
5G network capabilities	Data security	Wearables for patient engagement

FIGURE 8.5   Six Major EHR Future Trends

The data revolution continues to benefit population health based on the ability to aggregate data for unique purposes, and a data tool for creating and sharing data is a **health information exchange (HIE)**. HIEs permit access to patient data and treatment history across health care providers and organizations (HealthIT.gov, 2020). As a database repository of patient information developed following universal standards, HIEs can be local, state, or national and easily provide accessible patient data to hospitals and health systems. Another important data tool that specifically benefits at-risk populations is a patient registry. **Patient registries** are patient information repositories that store standardized information about a group of patients who share a condition or experience (Workman, 2013). Because the data are standardized, they are easier to aggregate and share with large cohorts of qualified health providers and researchers who are interested in researching and treating a specific disease. In certain cases, patients and or patient advocacy organizations have encouraged the creation of disease registries specific to their own concerns (Gliklich et al., 2014). Well-known national registries include the Alzheimer's Prevention Registry and the population-based Surveillance, Epidemiology, and End Results (SEER) program registries of the National Cancer Institute (National Institute of Health, 2022). Algorithms aid in the database search processes for both HIEs and patient registries.

Practical Skill: Population Health Algorithms

Algorithm has become a familiar term to all Americans. An **algorithm** is a machine process used for solving a problem or performing a technical computation (Gillis, 2022). Algorithms can be a coded list of instructions that identify step-by-step desired digital actions. Many types of algorithms perform complex tasks, such as those that function as search engines, sorting processes, and encryption tools. Algorithms enable smartphones and watches and Wi-Fi and can select our online shopping choices, but they also provide positive enhancements for population health. They can enable consumers to find local health providers and participate in their health care via patient portals. Other population health benefits can be classified as clinical, such as completing clinical trial outcomes, comparing two treatments over time for selecting evidence-based programs or medications, and enhanced medical imaging. Algorithm advancements also enable other types of health activities, such as telemedicine via the Internet, encryption for patient record safety, determination of disease probabilities, and human genome explorations (Stewart, n.d.). Even Google searches with page rankings can be attributed to algorithms along with determining health scores such as the Apgar score, which is used to assess a newborn's condition at birth. The value of algorithms for population health decision-making is their ability to complete varied data analytical tasks for priority groups regardless of the size of the at-risk population.

Health Data Analytics

Health data and information can be overwhelming, but the capacity and capability to move to the knowledge level and then on to wisdom requires the use of data analysis. Transforming population health data into knowledge requires sophisticated levels of data analysis. **Health data analytics** "focuses on the technologies and processes that measure, manage, and analyze healthcare data" (Looker Data Sciences, Inc., 2020). Notice that this definition emphasizes a data pathway of measurement, management, and analysis for quality purposes. This is the framework for implementing population health. Previously, the health sector depended on hospital data and insurance claim data and included information from public health sources for population health issues. Health data analytics has enabled more advanced analysis beyond basic aggregation and algorithms. New HIS technologies based on the incredible power of data analytics include **predictive modeling**, artificial learning, and machine learning (see Figure 8.6).

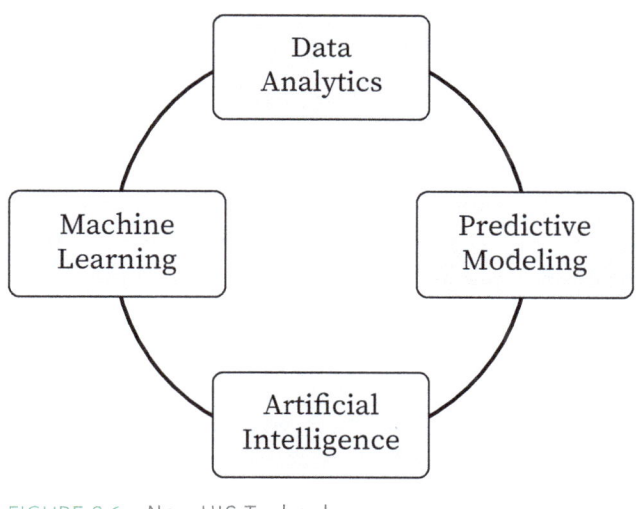

FIGURE 8.6   New HIS Technology

The original role of data analytical activities included data aggregation, analytics and reporting, and visualization (Johri, 2021). Other advanced health analytics tasks now use data for sophisticated techniques valuable to innovative decision-making. A recent study reported that COVID-19 hospitalizations could accurately be predicted using Google searches (Gonzalez, 2022). Table 8.1 provides definitions and population health examples for predictive modeling, AI, and machine learning.

TABLE 8.1   Health Data Analytical Tools

Data Analysis Process Tool	Population Health Example
Predictive modeling uses databases to forecast future needs, costs, and other outcomes.	Example: Predictive modeling uses large databases to determine characteristics of at-risk populations who may be at risk for infectious or chronic diseases, such as identifying teens at risk for not getting important vaccines such as human papillomavirus (Raths, 2020). Google can now predict COVID-19 hospitalizations (Gonzalez, 2022).
AI relies on technologies capable of capturing the complex process of human thought and intelligence (McGonigle & Mastrian, 2017, p. 65).	Example: When implemented in an HIS, AI can coordinate basic health care tasks, such as monitoring patients' vital signs and sending to appropriate providers or alerting attending health professionals of a clinical need for intervention.
Machine learning, a subset of AI, repeatedly learns from large data sets and improves the identification of patterns of health status and outcomes (Johri, 2021). It uses inductive machine learning (a process of reasoning) for generalizing from huge data sets (**big data**), and deductive reasoning assumes that premises made are assumed to be true and conclusions are true based on these premises (McGonigle et al., 2017).	Example: The randomized controlled trial (RCT) is the best-known deductive reasoning analysis for health care. The most recent RCT example is the positive findings for remdesivir, the Food and Drug Administration–approved drug for emergency use in severely ill hospitalized COVID-19 patients (Ellen, 2020).

AI is a tech-savvy process that allows computerized machines to align with human thinking and complete decision-making tasks by collecting and analyzing enormous amounts of data at unimaginable speeds. Chatbots, predictive and targeted content, content creation, and image recognition technology are already in use (Gupta, 2023). Although AI has been adopted throughout the health sector, a generative AI platform known as ChatGPT is now available to the public (Gupta, 2023). ChatGPT, an AI chatbot, can be used to focus on content creation such as imitating human writing and generating text to respond to an unimaginable list of potential questions or prompts (Tirth et al., 2023). The implications for use in the health care sector are substantial opportunities for reimagining workflow, documenting health interactions, maintaining patient records, and assessing consumer preferences for treatments and health professionals. Two issues of concern with the use of AI have emerged. The first focuses on the intent of use of data and is being addressed by the Blueprint for an AI Bill of Rights, which identifies five nonbinding guidelines for use of the technology to protect data privacy and avoid bias in algorithms (Burky, 2022). Privacy concerns also are considered a threat to the use of AI, and health institutions will need to guarantee safety and privacy to ensure trust among stakeholders and consumers (Gupta, 2023).

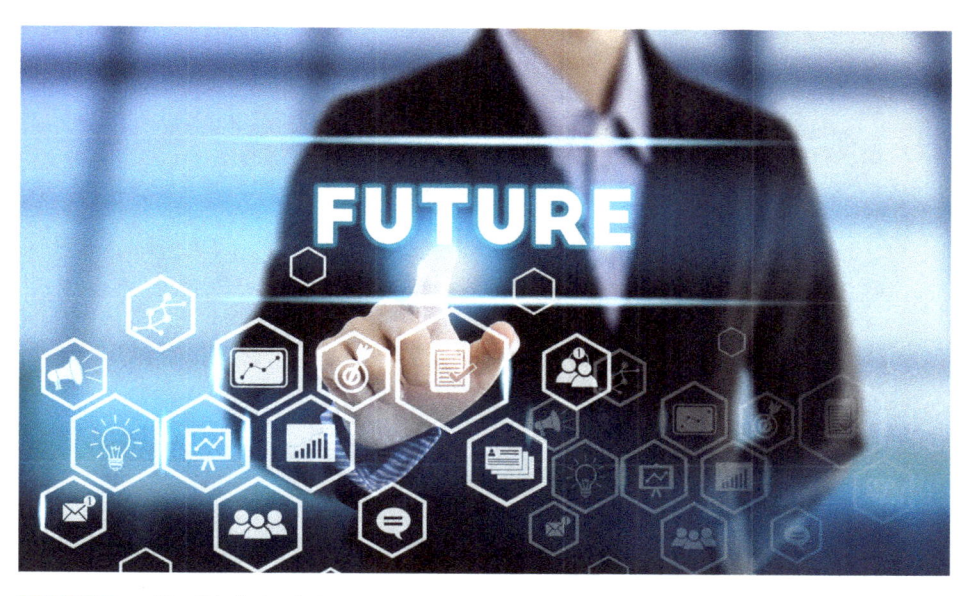

FIGURE 8.7   Health Data Future

Each of the three advanced data analytics processes described above benefits enormously from the HIS capability known as *interoperability*. **Interoperability** permits the process of data integration and the ability to interface with multiple databases (Roberts, 2017). Interoperability moves beyond data integration and allows access between various data sets (e.g., between medical treatment, patient outcomes, and diverse health care providers). Health care professionals can now make sophisticated clinical and administrative interpretations to ensure better health care planning for individuals and vulnerable populations.

Population Health Data Sources

Why are we collecting all this data? Population health needs to assess everyone's health status within a priority population to design the best system of care and monitor and ensure positive outcomes. To harness the power of health data analytics, health care organizations have transitioned beyond basic clinical and administrative data to include additional information to make better informed choices (Bresnick, 2019). Public health sources, primary care providers, ambulatory care, proprietary insurance and companies, pharmacies and the pharmaceutical industry, and other major health payers all provide additional and useful data. As covered in Chapter 3, public health data provide detailed mortality and morbidity reports and continually track incidence and prevalence of disease. The Google Flu Trends Estimate, which aggregates search

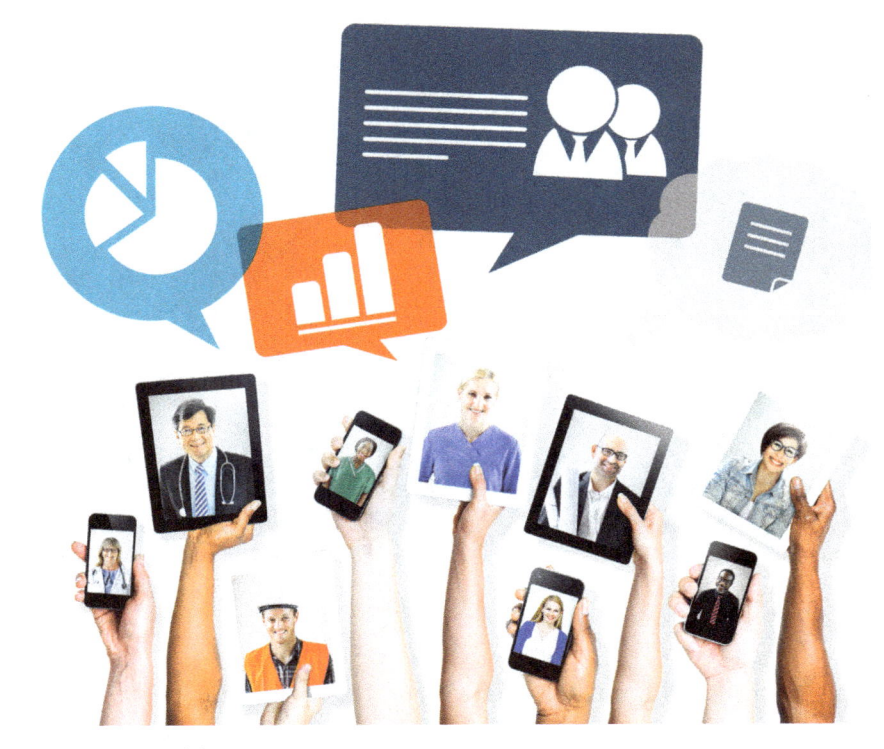

FIGURE 8.8   Health Care Data Sources

query data across regions, can reliably identify common flu trends (Google Inc., 2014). Table 8.2 identifies the types of data available when assessing a specific priority population.

As population health is concerned with more than medical treatment, all these data sources are required to develop appropriate and cost-effective population health plans of action for at-risk groups. Population health also focuses on the SDOH to facilitate designs for health promotion and disease prevention efforts to prevent chronic diseases that can affect quality of life. No longer can a physician prescribe a medication without assessing a patient's capabilities for receiving the medication and enabling the follow-up protocols. Data analytics compiles and helps interpret comprehensive data to frame the complete health care context and healthscape for vulnerable groups.

Challenges

As the health care sector becomes more cognizant of health disparities and inequities, population health also recognizes the critical issue of data equity and data bias. Inherent biases can be found in all aspects of data analysis and

TABLE 8.2 Types of Health Data Available for Population Health Decision-Making

Data Type/Source	Example
Clinical outcomes	Data such as patient history and basic demographics, vital signs, medications, lab results admissions, discharges, etc., from electronic health records
Patient-generated data	Data provided by the patient/consumer from personal health devices, trackers, and other wearable technologies or home devices and/or provided via mobile portal or applications; patient-reported outcomes from surveys and interviews (Fisher, 2022)
Administrative and analytic data	Utilization and hospital admission rates, with financial and claims data, including attribution data that connects the patient to the provider
Public health data	Community health assessments and disease surveillance, epidemiological information
SDOH indicators	Hospital's community health needs assessments and County Health Rankings & Roadmaps data, data from local and national nonprofit health organizations that identify common issues such as lifestyle behaviors, safe housing, transportations, food insecurity, and access to care
Community data	Community health needs assessment reports: municipal surveys and reports, including economic, educational, access to care, built environment, and social/community context factors from other organizations and coalitions
Private databases	Google, Amazon, proprietary health insurance companies, pharmacies, and pharmaceutical companies
Other/Industry groups	Health information exchanges, disease registries, census data research

Sources: Johri. N. (2021). Health data analytics for population health management. In A. Hewitt, J. Mascari, & S. Wagner (Eds.), Population health management: Strategies, tools, applications, and outcomes *(pp. 79–101). Springer Publishing Company; Scherpbier, H., Walsh, K., Skoufalos. (2021). Population health data and analytics. In D. B. Nash, R. J. Fabius, A. Skoufalos, & J. L. Clarke (Eds.),* Population health: Creating a culture of wellness *(3rd ed.; pp. 114–135). Jones & Bartlett Learning.*

are even apparent in commonly used algorithms (Obermeyer et al., 2019). **Data justice** has been proposed as a potential strategy to apply ethics and equity in data. These strategies may include the use of open-source data (Jorgenson, 2022) and participant-centered algorithms for big data (Norori et al., 2021). Data justice is a proactive strategy necessary for all components of the health sector with a goal to remediate and eliminate the possibility of prejudiced or unfair data design, collection, interpretation, or use (Parker, 2022). The purpose is not just to treat the disease, but also to ensure quality of life for all populations and the best possible outcomes. Health data analytics must include data justice to truly impact the continuum of care (Surendrank, n.d.).

Summary

The 21st-century health sector digital technology transition produced one of the most valuable tools for health care today: the EMR. Other advances in health care technology include the application of interoperability to access multiple population health databases, including those from health administration systems, community health reports, public health epidemiological rates, SDOH, and various other valuable resources from nonhealth sector industries. Using sophisticated data analytics techniques has allowed population health professionals to develop predictive models, learn from big data information, implement large-scale health programs, and improve decision-making to produce better health outcomes at lower costs. Despite the persistence of disparities in health care, population health will continue to be responsive using techniques such as data justice to ensure elimination of bias to obtain data that is already easily available, accurate, timely, and trustworthy. The key issue is the creation of integrated technology to produce affordable health care for all populations.

Discussion Questions

1. Why is it so critical that the pathway from data to information to knowledge and, finally, to wisdom is completed?
2. What role do EHRs play in population health?
3. In the context of health data analytics, what is *interoperability*, why is it needed, and how will it be used?
4. Machine learning, AI, and predictive analytics are technologies that will define the workflow process of population health in the future. Although Table 8.1 depicts the definitions of these technologies and current examples, the adoption of these technologies is escalating at a rapid rate in health. Provide a recent example of each application in the health care sector and include a URL.
5. Despite the pledges of some ransomware gangs in 2020 to refrain from attacking medical facilities, the health care sector continues to be targeted by hackers who demand huge ransoms to secure the privacy of patients' data. Read the article titled "No Relief in Sight for Ransomware Attacks on Hospitals" and identify why health care data are so vulnerable. Provide at least three solutions to this dilemma.

Source: Zacharakos, A. (February 2023). *No relief in sight for ransomware attacks on hospitals. https://tinyurl.com/39xycswy*

References

Abernethy, A., Adams, L., Barrett, M., Bechtel, C., Brennan, P., Butte, A., Faulkner, J., Fontaine, E., Friedhoff, S., Halamka, J., Howell, M., Johnson, K., Long, P., McGraw, D., Miller, R., Lee, P., Perlin, J., Rucker, D., Sandy, L., ... Valdes, K. (2022). The promise of digital health: Then, now, and the future. *NAM Perspectives.* Discussion paper, National Academy of Medicine. https://doi.org/10.31478/202206e

American Hospital Association. (2020, July 15). *IRS extends deadline for hospitals to complete community health needs assessments.* https://www.aha.org/news/headline/2020-07-15-irs-extends-deadline-hospitals-complete-community-health-needs-assessments

Brahmachary, A. (2019, May 4). *DIKW model: Explaining the DIKW pyramid or DIKW hierarchy.* https://www.certguidance.com/explaining-dikw-hierarchy/

Bresnick, J. (2019, April 30). *Data analytics in widespread use, but not for population health.* HealthITAnalytics. https://healthitanalytics.com/news/data-analytics-in-widespread-use-but-not-for-population-health

Brown, G. D., Pasupathy, K. S., & Patrick, T. B. (2019). *Health informatics: A systems perspective* (2nd ed.). Health Administration Press; Association of University Programs in Health Administration.

Burky, A. (2022, October 5). *Biden administration unveils AI bill of rights laying out voluntary guidelines to avoid AI misuse.* Fierce Healthcare. https://www.fiercehealthcare.com/ai-and-machine-learning/biden-administrations-blueprint-ai-bill-rights-lays-out-voluntary

ChatGPT. (n.d.). *Optimizing language models for dialogue.* OpenAI. ChatGPT: Optimizing Language Models for Dialogue (openai.com)

Dugar, D. (2022). *Future of electronic medical records: Experts predict EMR trends in 2022.* https://www.selecthub.com/medical-software/emr/electronic-medical-records-future-emr-trends/

Ellen, J. (2020, May 7). *You can observe a lot just by watching: Inductive reasoning is the key to medical science.* https://www.city-journal.org/inductive-reasoning-medical-science#:~:text=Perhaps%20the%20best%20known%20and,ill%20hospitalized%20Covid%2D19%20patients

Fisher, J. (2022, April 18). *The power of patient-reported outcomes: Helping patients tell their stories.* Phreesia. https://www.phreesia.com/2022/04/18/power-of-patient-reported-outcomes/?utm_source=marketo&utm_medium=snl_email&utm_destinationmedium=blog&utm_campaign=pro&utm_vendor=phreesia&utm_audience1=cross_market&utm_content=patient_reported_outcomes_blog_post&utm_date=apr_20_22&mkt_tok=NTA4LUFITS00MzcAAAGD64r5gKG7NhN-fPqr91Nj55JfwB1dLzdWGN2x_ywlms3Y4aC2InFFUBLk9U8IXFsfPkm3zV0y5O1X-QFC47sFWHMuO0FT4FgYPfsu392xIYP5P-

Gillis, A. (2022, May). *What is an algorithm?* TechTarget. https://www.techtarget.com/whatis/definition/algorithm

Gliklich, R. E., Dreyer, N. A., Leavy, M. B. (2014). *Registries for evaluating patient outcomes: A user's guide [Internet]* (3rd ed.). Agency for Healthcare Research and Quality. https://www.ncbi.nlm.nih.gov/books/NBK208628/

Goldstein, F., Shephard, V., & Duda, S. (2016). Policy implications for population health: Health promotion and wellness. In D. B. Nash, R. J. Fabius, A. Skoufalos, & J. L. Clarke (Eds,). *Population health: Creating a culture of wellness* (pp. 43–58). Jones & Bartlett Publishing.

Gonzalez, G. (2022, June 30). *COVID-19 hospitalizations can be predicted through Google searches.* https://www.beckershospitalreview.com/healthcare-information-technology/covid-19-hospitalizations-can-be-predicted-through-google-searches.html?origin=CIOE&utm_source=CIOE&utm_medium=email&utm_content=newsletter&oly_enc_id=1450I5993723C6U

Google Inc. (2014). *Google flu trend estimates.* https://www.google.com/publicdata/explore?ds=z3bsqef7ki44ac_

Gupta, S. (2023, February 26). *How startups are leveraging AI to scale their digital marketing efforts.* https://inc42.com/resources/how-startups-are-leveraging-ai-to-scale-their-digital-marketing-efforts/

Hagland, M. (2022, February). *Healthcare associations call on congress to spur APM adoption.* HC Innovation. https://www.hcinnovationgroup.com/policy-value-based-care/alternative-payment-models/news/21255759/healthcare-associations-call-on-congress-to-spur-apm-adoption

HealthIT.gov. (2020, July 4). *What is a HIE?* https://www.healthit.gov/topic/health-it-and-health-information-exchange-basics/what-hie

HIPAA Journal. (2020). *What is the HITECH act?* https://www.hipaajournal.com/what-is-the-hitech-act/

Internal Revenue Service. (2020). *Community health needs assessment for charitable hospital organizations—Section 501(r)(3).* https://www.irs.gov/charities-non-profits/community-health-needs-assessment-for-charitable-hospital-organizations-section-501r3

Johri, N. (2021). Health data analytics for population health management. In A. Hewitt, J. Mascari, & S. Wagner (Eds.), *Population health management: Strategies, tools, applications, and outcomes* (pp. 79–101). Springer Publishing Company.

Jorgenson, J. (2022, March 15). *The importance of equitable data science*. CGI. https://www.cgi.com/us/en-us/blog/technology-innovation/equitable-data-science

Looker Data Sciences, Inc. (2020). *Healthcare analytics.* Looker. https://looker.com/definitions/healthcare-analytics

Mastrian, K., & McGonigle, D. (2017). Informatics, disciplinary science, and the foundation of knowledge tools. In K. Mastrian & D. McGonigle, (Eds.), *Informatics for health professionals*. Jones & Bartlett Learning.

McGonigle, D., & Mastrian, K. (2017). Introduction to cognitive science and cognitive informatics. In K. Mastrian & D. McGonigle (Eds.), *Informatics for health professionals* (p. 65). Jones & Bartlett Learning.

McGonigle, D., Mastrian, K., & McGonigle, C. (2017). Data mining as a research tool. In K. Mastrian & D. McGonigle (Eds.), *Informatics for health professionals* (p. 318). Jones & Bartlett Learning.

Monegain, B. (2018, April 20). *Black book: Epic, Cerner, Meditech take top scores in new EHR survey but Amazon and Google pose a threat to market*. HealthcareITNews. https://www.healthcareitnews.com/news/black-book-epic-cerner-meditech-take-top-scores-new-ehr-survey-amazon-and-google-pose-threat

National Association of Community Health Centers. (2019). *Chapter 1: Understand the PRAPARE project.* http://www.nachc.org/wp content/uploads/2019/04/NACHC_PRAPARE_Chpt1.pdf

National Institute of Health. (2022). *List of registries.* https://www.nih.gov/health-information/nih-clinical-research-trials-you/list-registries

Norori, N., Hu, Q., Aellen, F., Dalia Faraci, F., & Tzovara, A. (2021, October 8). Addressing bias in big data and AI for health care: A call for open science. *Patterns, 2*(10). https://www.sciencedirect.com/science/article/pii/S2666389921002026#:~:text=Bias%20in%20AI%20algorithms%20for,existing%20datasets%2C%20further%20amplifying%20inequalities

Obermeyer, Z., Powers, B., Vogeli, C., & Mullainathan, S. (2019). Dissecting racial bias in an algorithm used to manage the health of populations. *Science, 366*(6464), 447–453. doi: 10.1126/science.aax2342

Parker, R. P. (2022, June 6). *Want to achieve health equity? Start by eliminating data*. https://www.cgi.com/us/en-us/blog/health/health-equity-eliminating-data-bias

Raths, D. (2020, September 25). *The predictive analytics journey at Texas Children's Hospital*. Healthcare Innovation. https://www.hcinnovationgroup.com/analytics-ai/artifical-intelligence-machine-learning/article/21155910/the-predictive-analytics-journey-at-texas-childrens-hospital

Roberts, B. (2017). *Integration vs. interoperability: What's the difference?* SIS BLOG. https://blog.sisfirst.com/integration-v-interoperability-what-is-the-difference.

Saidy, N. T. (2021, November 18) *Artificial intelligence in healthcare: opportunities and challenges*. TEDxQUT. YouTube. https://www.youtube.com/watch?v=uvqDTbusdUU

Scherpbier, H., Walsh, K., & Skoufalos, A. (2021). Population health data and analytics. In D. B. Nash, R. J. Fabius, A. Skoufalos, & J. L. Clarke (Eds.), *Population health: Creating a culture of wellness* (3rd ed.; pp. 114–135). Jones & Bartlett Learning.

Stewart, K. (n.d.). *10 algorithms that are changing health care—Algorithms for innovation*. University of Utah Health Sciences. https://uofuhealth.utah.edu/innovation/blog/2015/10/10AlgorithmsChangingHealthCare.php#:~:text=Medical%20algorithms%20remove%20some%20of,%2Dbased%20and%20data%2Dddriven

Surendrank, B. (n.d.). *Use of data analytics to improve Continuum of Care*. KP INSIGHT (Data & Analytics Group). Kaiser Permanente. http://or.himsschapter.org/sites/himsschapter/files/ChapterContent/or/OR19_Use_of_Data_Analytics_to_Improve_Continuum_of-Care.pdf

Tirth, D., Athaluri, S.A., & Singh, S. (2023). ChatGPT in medicine: an overview of its applications, advantages, limitations, future prospects, and ethical considerations. Front. Artif. Intell., 04 May 2023.https://www.frontiersin.org/articles/10.3389/frai.2023.1169595/full#:~:text=ChatGPT%20is%20a%20state%2Dof,patient%20monitoring%2C%20and%20medical%20education.

U.S. Department of Health and Human Services. (n.d.). *Health information privacy*. https://www.hhs.gov/hipaa/index.html

Workman, T. A. (2013). *Engaging patients in information sharing and data collection: The role of patient-powered registries and research networks [Internet]*. Agency for Healthcare Research and Quality. https://www.ncbi.nlm.nih.gov/books/NBK164514/

Credits

Fig. 8.1: Generated with FreeWordCloudGenerator.com.

Fig. 8.3: Copyright © 2020 Depositphotos/AndreyPopov.

Fig. 8.4: Copyright © 2016 Depositphotos/pandpstock001.

Fig. 8.5: Adapted from Kashish Arora, "Future of EHR/EMR: Experts Predict Trends in 2023," https://www.selecthub.com/medical-software/emr/electronic-medical-records-future-emr-trends/. Copyright © by SelectHub.

Fig. 8.7: Copyright © 2017 Depositphotos/baramee2017.

Fig. 8.8: Copyright © 2014 Depositphotos/Rawpixel.

CHAPTER NINE

Risk Management

Population Health's Challenge

Chapter Description

Chapter 9 examines the importance of individual health decision-making and the role of population health in finding solutions to prevent unhealthy decisions and behaviors. Human beings are not logical and often do not make the best health decisions, which, over time, can result in chronic diseases such as diabetes, cancer, and addiction. Managing health risks by identifying, monitoring, and intervening appropriately remains a primary population health goal. Risky behaviors indicated by aggregating diverse databases can produce sub-population risk factors. These can be mitigated through tailored plans of action for specific higher-risk populations. This chapter presents a step-by-step risk management process, which includes determining an individual risk score,

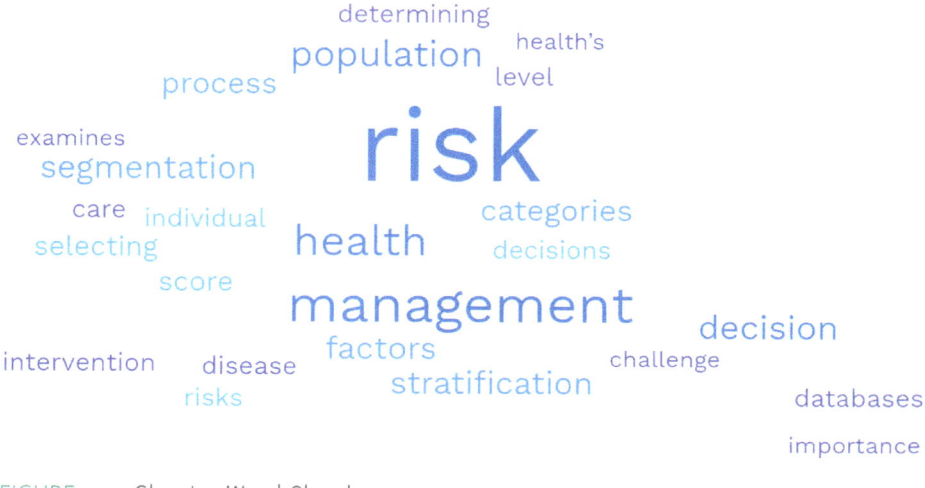

FIGURE 9.1   Chapter Word Cloud

completing a risk segmentation selection process, and performing a detailed risk stratification analysis. The final stage in the decision-making process is selecting the health care intervention components (i.e., who, what, where, when, and how) for each level of population risk.

Chapter Objectives

After completing this chapter, students will be able to:

1. Define *risk, risk score, segmentation,* and *stratification*
2. Discuss which databases should be selected to obtain a valid risk factor score
3. Describe and provide an example for each step in the risk management process
4. Differentiate between the risk levels of low, medium, rising, and high risk
5. Segment a population into population health risk management categories
6. Develop a visual that depicts a contemporary continuum of care

Key Words

| Risk | Risk management | Risk stratification |
| Risk factor | Risk segmentation | |

Introduction to Risk Management

What Is a Health Risk?

Review the pictures at the beginning of this chapter. Do you consider any of these activities to be evidence of risky behavior? Of course, what *you* may consider to be a risky behavior another person may view as a regular activity. For population health, **risk** is a probability or a chance that a health event or condition may occur. Determining a health risk requires both analytical and clinical expertise to select characteristics that determine the likelihood (probability) of impacting a priority population's health status. The health risk selection process leads to the identification of **risk factors**, which indicates an exposure that is associated with a disease or condition, without certainty.

For population health, identification of risk factors is necessary for designing appropriate programs and interventions that will be offered and tailored for at-risk populations. The process is known as **risk management**, and it represents

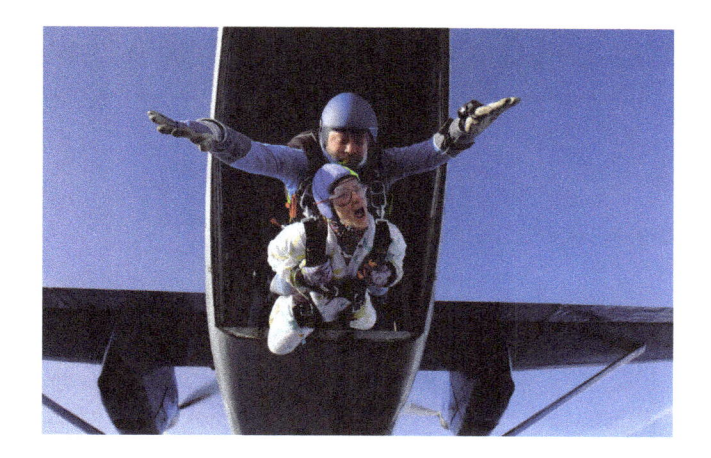

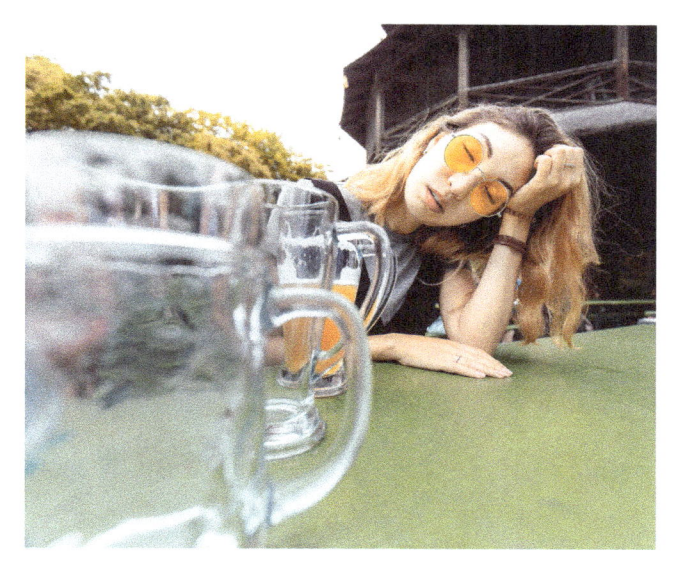

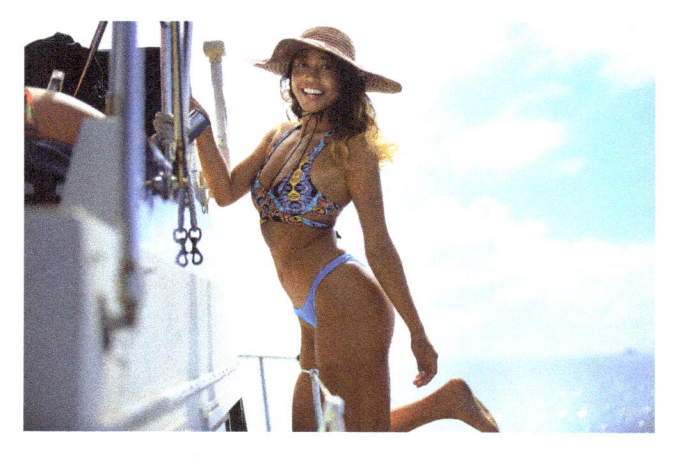

FIGURE 9.2 Risky Health Lifestyle Behaviors

one of the primary decision-making activities for population health. To understand the risk analysis step by step, let's follow a fictitious patient through the process.

Risk Management Case Study

Meet Jennifer, a married, 55-year-old woman living in a suburban area in Florida. She recently attended her office health fair, where the nurse reported that she had elevated blood pressure. Since Jennifer had not seen her primary care physician (PCP) in more than 5 years, the nurse advised her to schedule an appointment. Jennifer agreed and completed a virtual health assessment before meeting face to face with the health care provider.

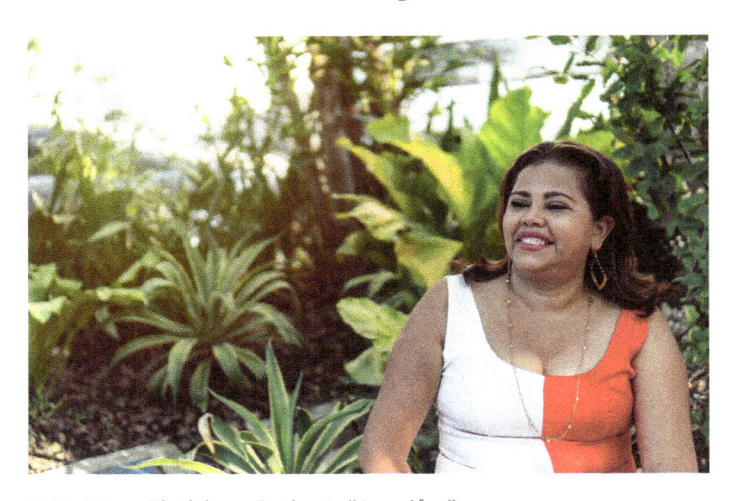

FIGURE 9.3 Fictitious Patient: "Jennifer"

Practical Skill: Risk Management Decision Point 1

Which health-related data should be selected to determine Jennifer's health risks based on her elevated blood pressure? Which data will be relevant to the health care provider? Which data will be important for the population health analyst? What information will the patient, Jennifer, want to know?

- First, consider all the databases and categories of health information available for Jennifer and discussed in Chapter 8. Which databases would you select?
- Second, identify which health risk factors you think will affect Jennifer's health status. How would you prioritize her disease risk?
- Now, let's review Jennifer's results.

Although Jennifer appears healthy, the checkup identified results linked to specific health risks.

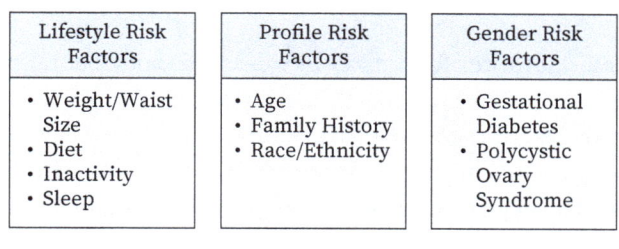

Lifestyle Risk Factors	Profile Risk Factors	Gender Risk Factors
• Weight/Waist Size • Diet • Inactivity • Sleep	• Age • Family History • Race/Ethnicity	• Gestational Diabetes • Polycystic Ovary Syndrome

FIGURE 9.4   Risk Factors for Prediabetes

Jennifer's risk factors include being overweight with a large waist size. She has reported not being an active person and lacks any regular exercise habits. She shared with her PCP that her family eats few fresh fruits and vegetables due to their busy work schedules. Jennifer has a Hispanic heritage and a family history of diabetes. She believes that she had gestational diabetes during her only pregnancy but is not sure.

Practical Skill: Risk Management Decision Point 2

What should be the next step in Jennifer's health plan? Do we know her primary health risks and risk factors? What should her health care plan options be going forward?

Jennifer's primary health risk is a condition known as *prediabetes*. Individuals with this condition have a higher-than-normal blood sugar level, but with lifestyle changes, adults with prediabetes can prevent type 2 diabetes (Mayo Clinic, n.d.). Health promotion and disease prevention efforts are needed immediately to delay any long-term diabetic damage to the heart, blood vessels, and kidneys.

Risk factors (an exposure that is associated with a disease or condition, without certainty) are combined to develop a risk score (Mascari & Hewitt, 2022). The *risk score* refers to the likelihood of an event occurring within a short time frame, such as 6 months. This risk score forms the basis for the selection for appropriate health interventions. The higher the risk score is, the more intensive the health promotion and disease prevention activities will be needed at a higher cost.

Based on her risk score, Jennifer's risk management strategy begins when her health care provider arranges a consultation meeting with a dietitian or coach. She also receives detailed health education materials and links to health motivation videos for exercise and improving sleep patterns. As a follow-up, Jennifer gets regular monthly phone calls and/or text messages checking on her progress.

Five years later, Jennifer feels dizzy at work and passes out. She is rushed to the nearest emergency department (ED) and held for observation and additional testing. She shares with the health care providers that she has noticed having a dry mouth and being thirsty more often. She states that she has been tired recently but suggests it is because of her age. Jennifer is surprised her weight has decreased compared to 5 years ago, and she also mentions frequent urination. Her clinical symptoms show a slightly elevated glucose level.

What do we know? Jennifer exhibits the classic signs of prediabetes. The clinical signs of prediabetes and potentially type 2 diabetes include increased urination, thirst and hunger, weight loss, fatigue, blurred vision, frequent infections, slow-healing sores, and numbness or tingling in the feet or hands (Arrigo, 2021).

Practical Skill: Risk Management Decision Point 3

Based on this recent acute care episode, Jennifer's risk score for diabetes has increased significantly. Her population health management strategy needs to reflect her current condition. The evidence is clear that she potentially meets the criteria for inclusion in a rising risk (prediabetes) population. Jennifer represents one example of many thousands of patients with similar symptoms.

How do population health managers decide which patients are most at risk and which types of interventions should be chosen to produce positive outcomes? Risk scores form the basis for the selection of a subpopulation appropriate for health interventions, but specific risk factors are used optimally to identify a distinct vulnerable population. This process is known as *risk segmentation*. Table 9.1 shows a fictitious risk segmentation grid for a generic disease.

TABLE 9.1 Segmentation of Risk Factors for a Generic Disease

Diagnosis	Age	Gender	Comorbidities	PCP Visits	Medications	ED Visits	Lifestyle Behaviors	Social Determinants of Health (SDOH) Factor	Hospital Length of Stay

These risk segmentation factors represent diverse types of data as they use current and prospective health status, medical costs based on health utilization, patient attitudes and lifestyles, and levels of health care engagement to identify an at-risk priority population. Note that a risk segmentation grid will change based on the condition or the disease. Review a fictitious risk segmentation example for patients such as Jennifer who have symptoms of prediabetes or type 2 diabetes in Table 9.2.

TABLE 9.2   Fictitious Risk Segmentation Factors for Prediabetes

Prediabetes Condition	Age	Gender	Family History	Lifestyle Behaviors	SDOH Factors	Clinical Indicator (Elevated Glucose)	Increase in Symptoms	Comorbidities	Medical Cost

Jennifer is about to be released from the hospital. Her health care provider has discussed her clinical conditions. She and her family are frightened and unsure of the next steps.

Practical Skill: Risk Management Decision Point 4

Jennifer's risk for prediabetes clearly places her in a rising risk or high-risk subpopulation. Which treatments, interventions, and activities should be provided? What are the action steps needed to ensure that any further increase in symptoms or relapse for prediabetes or type 2 diabetes doesn't occur?

Not all prediabetes patients are like Jennifer. To ensure that each subgroup receives the optimal guidance and support, the next risk analysis step is **risk stratification**. Once the major risk factors are identified, the next step would be to complete a patient risk stratification grid based on the selected risk factors and scores. Since the risk factors are known, the grid identifies the level of risk for each factor either low, medium, rising, or high risk. Table 9.3 shows a generic example of a risk stratification matrix.

Assumptions: The patient has a family history of diabetes.

Jennifer has been placed in the rising-risk category based on her recent ED visit and overnight stay in the hospital. It is important to note that patients often transition from one category to another depending on their symptoms and health outcomes. Jennifer's disease prevention care plan will be aligned with her risk segmentation category.

TABLE 9.3 Prediabetes to Type 2 Diabetes Risk Stratification Matrix (Fictitious Example)

Risk Factor	Low	Medium	Rising	High
Age	<50 years	50–55 years	56–65 years	65+ years
Exercise	Consistent exercise	Occasional/Some weekends	Primarily sedentary/ Few walks	Sedentary
Blood pressure	Normal	Elevated	Medium/Medication	High/Medication
Blood glucose	None	Single medication		Severe/Requires oxygen
Weight	Normal weight	Overweight (Weight problem)	Obese (Weight problem)	Morbidly obese (Excess weight)
Health care usage	PCP regular visits	• Intermittent visits with PCP • Recommended care plan	• Specialist visits/ low patient engagement • Care plan inconsistent	• Intermittent visits/ uncoordinated care • Use of emergency room/overnight stay

Practical Skill: Risk Management Decision Point 5

Which types of health interventions will produce a positive health outcome for Jennifer? Does she need a single care visit or daily check-in? Who will provide the care? Which type of health care practitioner is needed? Should it be a social worker, nurse, patient advocate, nurse practitioner, or physician? How will the care be delivered? Will it be offered via mobile, virtually, at home, or face to face in an office visit? How often should she be contacted? Each of these decisions will be made based on Jennifer's specific risk factors and identified contact preferences.

Jennifer's disease prevention plan includes an initial face-to-face meeting with a care manager, followed by weekly check-ins, a prescribed change in medications, a virtual assistant for planning a healthy diet, and a health coach visit for exercise options. She also receives regular mobile app reminders with an option to chat with a health care professional when questions or issues arise. Six months later, Jennifer reports losing weight and following her Medicaid regimen, and her family is now practicing several of Jennifer's new positive health behavior changes.

Practical Skill: Risk Management Decision Point 6

Jennifer shows progress maintaining her disease management plan. What types of adjustments should be made to ensure that she maintains these healthy behaviors? How often should Jennifer be monitored? The risk management process and strategies appear to have successfully helped Jennifer and prevented chronic disease.

Chapter Nine Risk Management | 173

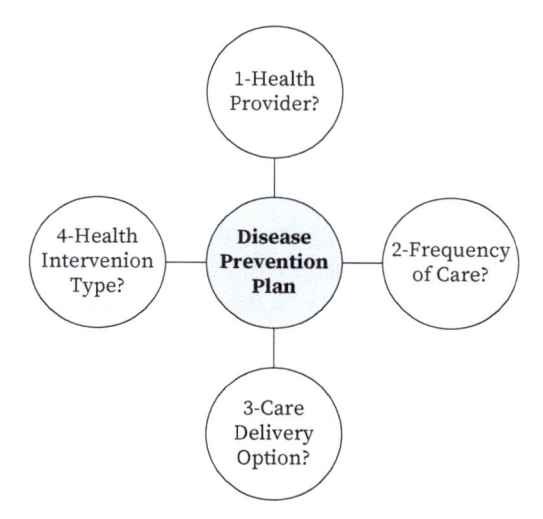

1 = Patient navigator, social worker, licensed practical nurse, nurse, nurse practitioner, physician assistant, physician; allied health practitioners (dietitian, pharmacist, physical therapist, occupational therapist, speech/language pathologist)
2 = Daily, weekly, monthly, quarterly, bi-annually, annual
3 = Home, office visit, virtual care
4 = Face-to-face office visits, specialty clinic visit, virtual visit, smartphone messages, phone calls, mobile unit house calls, traditional house visit

FIGURE 9.5   Disease Prevention Intervention—Population Decisions

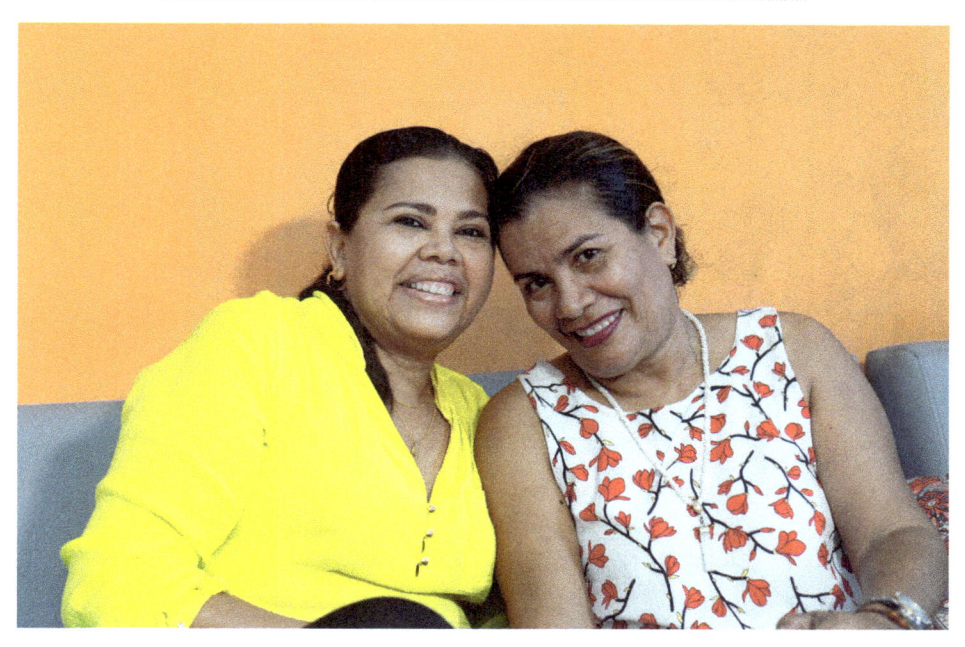

FIGURE 9.6   Risk Management Improves Population Health Outcomes

Risk Management and Personalized Care

Population health's goal is to manage risk for all priority populations. The example above represents a protocol for only one disease and for patients in a particular risk category. We need to imagine a system that includes hundreds of thousands of individuals, all with diverse health care needs.

One of the first available systems of risk categories was published in early 2000s and included five continuum of care categories (McAlearney, 2003).

Each of these original risk management categories was overly broad and lacked a complete range of options for diverse patients, conditions, and alternatives for individuals who might need to transition from one stage to another along a continuum of care. The *Continuum of Care* refers to care provided over time (Health Information Management System Society, 2014; National Cancer Institute, n.d.).

Lifestyle
- Offers a collection of health promotion and disease prevention strategies and approaches to facilitate health behavior change for decreased risk and improved populations' health habits

Demand
- Emphasizes remote directing consumers within specific populations toward appropriate utilization of medical care services

Disease
- Appropriate for populations with a particular disease and includes care coordination (medical and care management) tailored to the specific patients' needs with that condition

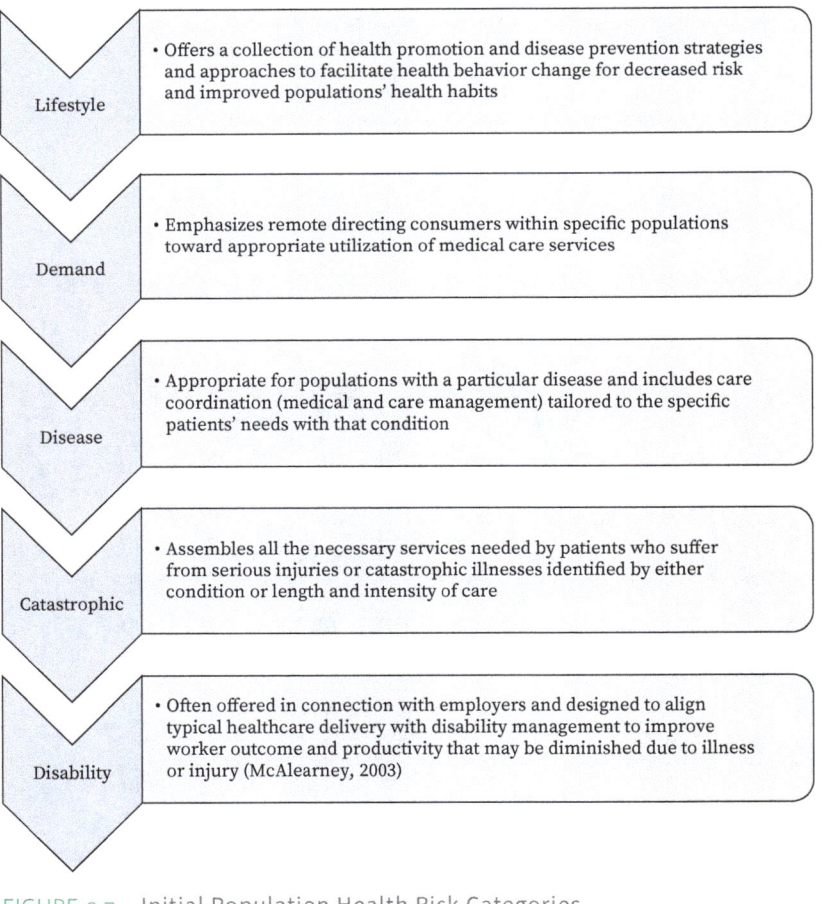

Catastrophic
- Assembles all the necessary services needed by patients who suffer from serious injuries or catastrophic illnesses identified by either condition or length and intensity of care

Disability
- Often offered in connection with employers and designed to align typical healthcare delivery with disability management to improve worker outcome and productivity that may be diminished due to illness or injury (McAlearney, 2003)

FIGURE 9.7 Initial Population Health Risk Categories

Practical Skill: Risk Management and Personalized Care

Unlike the limited five risk categories outlined above, population health benefits from the expanded continuum of care with numerous care modality options are now available for interactions with the consumer or patient. Patients complete initial surveys that ask, "Please indicate your preferred method of communication." The options include mobile (home/cell), virtual (video/audio), home visit, face-to-face office visit, or mobile van visit. These options provide additional flexibility to meet the needs of the patient and ensure follow-up and maintenance for their personalized health action plan. More than 80% of recently surveyed patients and consumers report they want their health providers to understand their lifestyle habits and their personal health goals (Minemyer, 2022). Personalized care coordination requires population health strategies capable of meeting the intimate needs of the individual and managing them across populations.

1. What is your preferred venue of communication with a health care professional?
2. Does it change based on your health status?
3. How important is it for you to know that the health care professional understands your personal health goals?

The Cost and Benefit of Population Health Risk Segmentation

After completing health risk segmentations, population health managers develop prediabetes intervention and care plans for patients such as Jennifer and thousands like her. Let's calculate the fictitious cost and benefit.

Practical Skill: Completing a Cost-Benefit Analysis (Fictitious Example)

- Step 1: Determine the unit cost of this disease prevention intervention. In this fictitious example, the cost is set at $1 per patient per month (PPPM). *COST*
- Step 2: Determine the cost-effectiveness for this intervention. Based on medication usage and cost for this fictitious disease condition, research suggests the risk segmentation process could reduce overall health costs by $12 PPPM. *BENEFIT*
- Step 3: Complete the cost equation: Benefit – Cost/PPPM.

There are 10,000 individuals who receive the fictitious disease prevention plan. If none of these individuals develops the disease, the cost equation shows a benefit or savings of $11,000.

- Step 4: If the intervention's actual cost exceeds more than $12 per person, the population health manager will have lost a significant amount, and the intervention may be unsustainable.

Linking risk management outcomes to cost-effectiveness relies on real-time, accurate data and tailored care coordination to be productive across populations. Fortunately, recent technological advances and the interoperability between data systems increase the ability of population health managers to make the best decisions on the use and outcomes of risk segmentation and stratification processes. The health benefits far outweigh the costs.

Summary

Risk management continues to dominate the role of population health as health planners seek improved and innovative options to improve outcomes for all populations. Understanding the primary steps involved in identifying risks, developing risk scores, and completing rigorous risk segmentation and stratification requires real-time, dependable, and sensitive data that includes both analytical and clinical information. Costs spent for medications, care treatment visits or hospital usage, and clinical symptoms or conditions data contribute only part of the individual's risk score. Other risk factors such as lifestyle behaviors and SDOH can provide guidance for developing an appropriate action plan that will ensure patients are engaged in their care and more likely to succeed. Today's multiple options for patient interactions and the use of preferred methods of communication can increase the success of personalized care interventions for all populations.

Discussion Questions

1. A *risk* refers to the probability or chance that a health event or condition may occur. Often a risk is dependent on exposure to a risk factor. Define *risk factors* and describe the process for identifying risk factors in a population. Then discuss the role of a risk score.
2. Population health focuses on large groups of people who may share risk factors and even risk scores for a particular condition or disease. Review tables 9.1 and 9.2. Identify the differences between the generic risk segmentation and the risk segmentation table for prediabetes. Why were these risk factors chosen?
3. Explain the ways risk segmentation and stratification differ.
4. Review the five basic risk categories that were previously used before population segmentation was developed as a tool. Why have they changed, and what additional options have emerged for the continuum of care?
5. Which data sources would you seek before developing a risk segmentation and risk stratification for a particular disease or condition?

References

Arrigo, T. (2021, June 22). *Early signs and symptoms of diabetes*. WebMD. https://www.webmd.com/diabetes/guide/understanding-diabetes-symptoms

Centers for Disease Control and Prevention. (2021). *Diabetes tests*. https://www.cdc.gov/diabetes/basics/getting-tested.html#:~:text=A%20fasting%20blood%20sugar%20level,higher%20indicates%20you%20have%20diabetes

Health Information Management System Society. (2014). *Definition: Continuum of care*. http://s3.amazonaws.com/rdcms-himss/files/production/public/2014-05-14-DefinitionContinuumofCare.pdf

Mascari, J., & Hewitt, A. (2022). Population health decision-making: Risk segmentation, stratification, and management. In A. Hewitt, Mascari, J., & Wagner, S. (Eds.), *Population health management: Strategies, tools, applications, and outcomes* (pp. 103–119). Springer Publishing.

Mayo Clinic. (n.d.). *Prediabetes risk factors*. https://www.mayoclinic.org/diseases-conditions/prediabetes/symptoms-causes/syc-20355278

McAlearney, A. (2003). *Population health management: Strategies to improve outcomes*. Health Administration Press/Association of University Programs in Health Administration.

Minemyer, P. (2022, July 13). *Consumers seeking personalized, integrated care post-COVID, CVS survey finds*. Fierce Healthcare, July 13, 2022. https://www.fiercehealthcare.com/providers/consumers-seeking-personalized-integrated-care-post-covid-cvs-survey-finds

National Association of Community Health Centers. (2019). *Population health management. Risk stratification*. https://www.nachc.org/wp-content/uploads/2019/03/Risk-Stratification-Action-Guide-Mar-2019.pdf

National Cancer Institute. (n.d.) *Continuum of care*. National Cancer Institute Dictionary. https://www.cancer.gov/publications/dictionaries/cancer-terms/def/continuum-of-care

Ranganathan, P., Aggarwal, R., & Pramesh, C. (2015). Common pitfalls in statistical analysis: Odds versus risk. *Perspectives in Clinical Research, 6*(4), 222–224. https://doi.org/10.4103%2F2229-3485.167092

Substance Abuse and Mental Health Services Administration. (n.d.). *Risk and protective factors*. https://www.samhsa.gov/sites/default/files/20190718-samhsa-risk-protective-factors.pdf

Credits

Fig. 9.1: Generated with FreeWordCloudGenerator.com.
Fig. 9.2a: Copyright © 2019 Depositphotos/skyantonio.
Fig. 9.2b: Copyright © 2019 Depositphotos/frantic00.
Fig. 9.2c: Copyright © 2018 Depositphotos/vitaliy_sokol.

Fig. 9.3: Copyright © 2021 Depositphotos/HectorPertuz.

Fig. 9.4: Source: Adapted from https://www.mayoclinic.org/diseases-conditions/prediabetes/symptoms-causes/syc-20355278.

Fig. 9.6: Copyright © 2021 Depositphotos/HectorPertuz.

CHAPTER TEN

Population Health Accountability

Financial and Quality Outcomes

Chapter Description

Chapter 10 covers key population health strategies that help health professionals align cost outcomes (fiscal responsibility) and quality of care. Financial accountability is affected by commercial, nonprofit, and government health plans and payers, including Medicare and Medicaid. Today, managing cost outcomes involves a major transition from a volume (quantity) to a value-based payer system. The basic financial equation of value equals outcome divided by cost is the foundation for new alternative payment systems that spread financial risk among all three major stakeholders: payers, providers, and patients/consumers. Population health accountability also includes an obligation to ensure quality of care with a special emphasis on safety and care equity for all. The National Center for Quality Assurance (NCQA) provides established guidelines for meeting quality standards and safety criteria. Quality benchmarks for

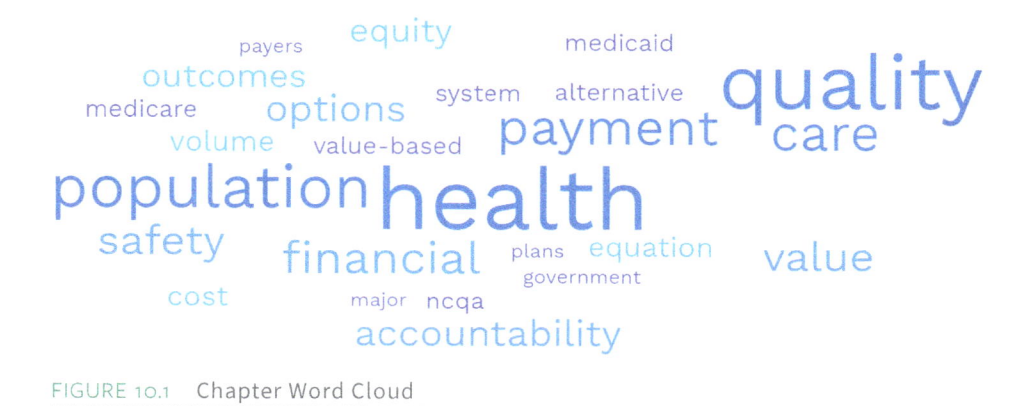

FIGURE 10.1   Chapter Word Cloud

population health organizations also mandate the identification and prevention efforts to reduce health disparities in care outcomes. Regardless of any priority population's health characteristics or type of insurance, financial and quality considerations are primary goals for population health.

Chapter Objectives

After completing this chapter, students will be able to:

1. Summarize the main responsibilities of population health accountability
2. Discuss population health's transition from a volume- to a value-based payment system
3. Identify the value equation
4. Examine and describe both current and emerging alternate payment system options
5. Define quality and its role as a key population health strategy
6. Explain why the concepts of safety and equity are integrated in quality outcomes
7. Review the role of the NCQA

Key Words

Alternative payment models	Episodes of care	NCQA	Quality improvement
Bundled payments	Managed care	Patient safety	Value equation
Dual eligibility	Medicaid	Performance measurement	Value over volume
	Medicare	Quality	

Population Health Accountability

One of the key distinctions between population health and previous health approaches is the direct link between quality of care and health care provider payments. As discussed in Chapter 1, the rising cost of health care has continued to spiral upward. Health insurance costs, for those lucky enough to be insured, rise annually placing undue stress on the American health consumer.

Millions of Americans enroll in the top five commercial health plans: UnitedHealth Group, Anthem, Aetna, Cigna, and Humana (Townsend, 2022). And millions more receive coverage from the U.S. government's major health plan programs such as Medicaid and Medicare (Guinan, 2022). Even with

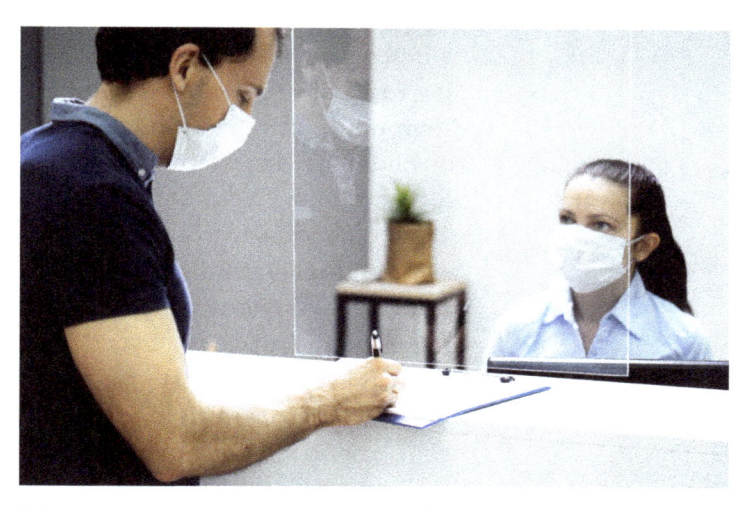

FIGURE 10.2 Population Health Fiscal Accountability

employer-sponsored health insurance, an estimated 23.6 million Americans will spend a large share of their income (10%) on health care premiums (monthly payments), out-of-pocket costs, or both (Hayes et al., 2019).

Practical Skill: Health Insurance—Student Activity

Check with your classmates to see if they are currently insured. Does your university require health insurance? If your colleagues have jobs, how many of them receive health insurance through their employers? Do any of your friends receive health insurance through spousal benefits? How many students in the class are younger than age 26 and eligible to receive care under their parents' insurance? The commercial health insurance industry is complex, and any health plan changes have an immediate impact on consumers and patients.

The Impact of Government Health Plans on Population Health

Medicare and **Medicaid** are two very well-known government-sponsored health care plans, although other major federal programs include the Children's Health Insurance Program (CHIP) and the Indian Health Service, which provides coverage for American Indian and Alaska Natives (Higbea et al., 2022). Medicare covers individuals older than age 65, people younger than age 65 with certain disabilities, and people of all ages with end-stage renal disease. Medicaid, considered health insurance, is a social protection program in which eligibility

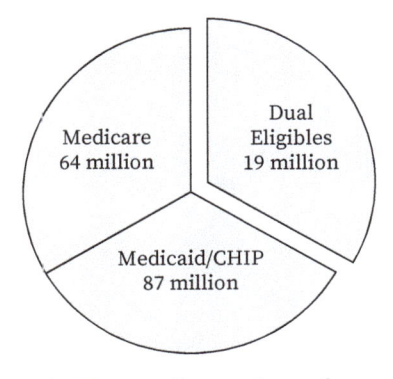

FIGURE 10.3 Comparison of Medicare, Medicaid/CHIP, and Dual-Eligible Enrollments

- Medicare: 64 million
- Dual Eligibles: 19 million
- Medicaid/CHIP: 87 million

is determined by income and designed for low-income Americans (UnitedHealthcare Community Plan, 2021). CHIP and Medicaid are both funded in part by the federal and state governments. These complex health plans require participants to meet all eligibility criteria. **Dual eligibility** is a term that refers to individuals whose living circumstances make them eligible for both Medicare and Medicaid coverage. This priority population often includes people with chronic diseases who use a maximum amount of care from the health system.

Americans with vulnerable health conditions often qualify as dual-eligible. To improve and coordinate services, recent proposed legislation suggests combining Medicare and Medicaid benefits to ensure less fragmented care and reduce duplication (Guinan, 2022). Because diverse at-risk populations are often insured by these government plans, population health financial affordability is a major concern.

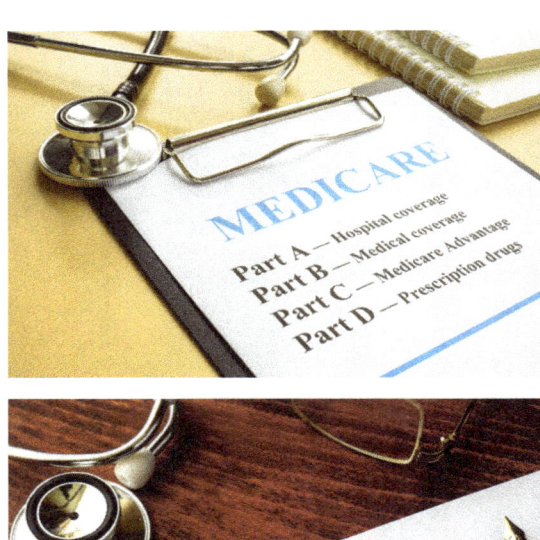

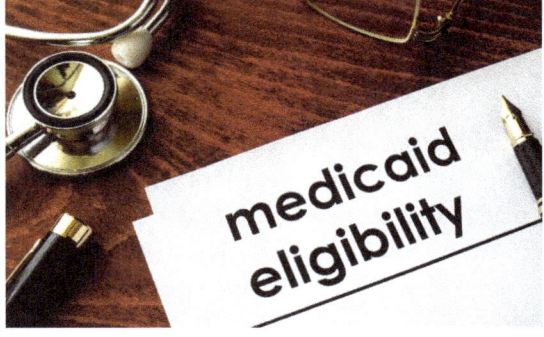

FIGURE 10.4 Medicare and Medicaid

Practical Skill: Medicare and Medicaid

Regardless of the type of insurance payer, health plan organizations seek to improve health outcomes for all their constituents by implementing population health strategies such as risk management (Chapter 9), health promotion and wellness (Chapter 5), and patient engagement activities (Chapter 12). Population health care gatekeepers also rely on health care outcome assessments (Chapter 8) to monitor vulnerable groups. Establishing accountability means assuming responsibility for doing what you say you are going to do or achieve (Johns, 2017), so it is not surprising that health care payers seek innovative options for improving health status and lowering costs.

Population Health and Cost of Care

Two important points underpin today's population health processes for financial accountability. The first is simply that the previous fee-for-service (see Chapter 1) health care financial model was unsustainable, as was emphasized by multiple reports over the years (Health Research & Educational Trust, 2014). Second, given that almost one-fifth of the entire nation's economy (gross domestic product) involves the health care sector, any major health payment reform change will need to be transformational. Transformation changes are often visionary or focused on the future and need to alter the current status quo (Johns, 2017). In the case of population health, the transformational financial change requires a shift from fee-for-service to value-over-volume payment policies (Buehler et al., 2018).

Value refers to an economic concept that states that the value or worth of any good or service is relative to what a person would be willing to pay for it either monetarily or by giving other resources, such as time or effort (Vocabulary.com, n.d.). **Value over volume** refers to a complex health care sector reimbursement process transformation that moves from volume-based care, in which the provider is paid by patient for the number of services, to pay for performance, in which payment is directly aligned with patient positive outcomes (Miller & Woodard, 2022). The **value equation** shows the relationship between value, outcome, and cost.

$$\text{Value} = \frac{\text{Outcome}}{\text{Cost}}$$

FIGURE 10.5 Value Equation

For population health, the value equation strategy places the emphasis on population outcomes versus an individual treatment focus and the alignment with cost. Figure 10.6 presents a contemporary and simplified version of key change components in the transition between volume and value approaches.

Volume

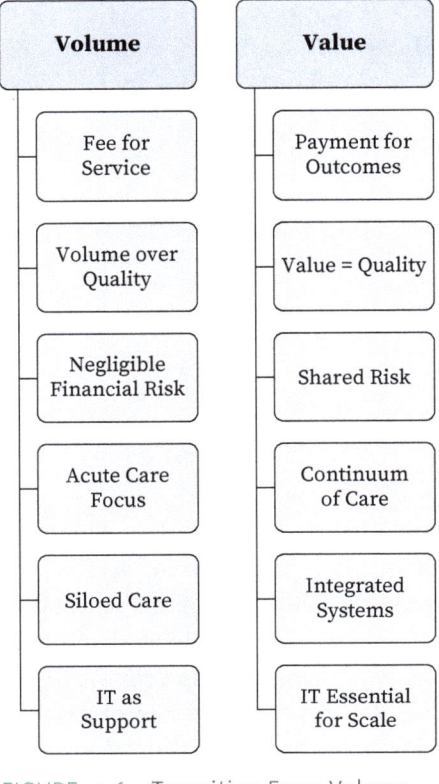

- Fee for Service
- Volume over Quality
- Negligible Financial Risk
- Acute Care Focus
- Siloed Care
- IT as Support

Value

- Payment for Outcomes
- Value = Quality
- Shared Risk
- Continuum of Care
- Integrated Systems
- IT Essential for Scale

FIGURE 10.6 Transition From Volume to Value Approaches

New Population Health Payment Models

Value-based financial arrangements are known as ***alternative payment systems***. Although various definitions exist for these emerging health financial compensation arrangements, the payment options divide financial risk between payers, providers, and patient/consumers.

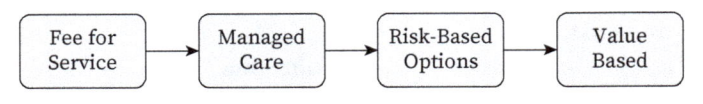

Fee for Service → Managed Care → Risk-Based Options → Value Based

FIGURE 10.7 New Population Health Payment Model Options

One technique for understanding value-based payment is to visualize a continuum. Each step shows a different type of alternative payment options from low to high risk. The farther you proceed on the continuum, the greater the financial risk for the payer, patient/consumer, and provider. As previously discussed, fee for service is a basic economic exchange system where the provider receives payment per episode of care (Fee for Service, n.d.). The first payment transition away from fee for service appeared in managed care health plans. This financial model sought to align and control administrative and service costs.

Practical Skill: What Is Managed Care?

Did you know that managed care was originally associated with the Health Maintenance Organization (HMO) Act of 1973 (U.S. Government Accountability Office, 1978)? **Managed care** refers to a type of health care delivery system organized to manage cost, utilization, and quality (Medicaid, n.d.). Managed care organizations (MCOs) have existed for almost 50 years and, during that time, have evolved into multiple and complex versions. The HMO Act represented the first attempt to collectively control health care costs. Managed care plans, also called *gatekeeper care plans*, as the plan assumes accountability for coordination of care (Niles, 2021). Today, the following four major managed care models are known by the public:

- The term *health maintenance organization* (HMO) refers to the most generic type of managed care health insurance plan. Consumers must select a primary care doctor who coordinates care and provides references for specialists. Primary care physicians may receive payment based on a capitation system by which the provider receives a fixed amount for each patient they agree to treat, regardless of whether the physician provides any care (Wagner, 2018). *Capitation* refers to contracted arrangements between state Medicaid agencies and MCOs that accept a set per-member-per-month (PMPM, or capitation) payment for these services (Medicaid, n.d.). Only care within a predetermined provider network coverage is part of the plan.
- Preferred provider organizations (PPO) usually pay for more care if you seek care within the network. However, the consumer pays part of the cost of care if the care is provided outside of the network. The plan may or may not require referrals.
- The most flexible managed care option is known as a *point-of-service (POS) plan*, which allows the consumer the opportunity to choose between an HMO or a PPO for each health care visit or care need (MedlinePlus, 2019).
- Physician hospital organizations (PHOs) combine physician hospitals, surgical centers, and other medical providers together, enabling the entire organization to contract with a managed care plan to provide numerous services (Niles, 2021).

Instructions: Create a grid featuring advantages and disadvantages by comparing the four managed care options described above. Which one would you select, and why?

The pathway for today's population health alternative payment systems began with the managed care approach. One point has remained fixed over time: The more flexible a managed care plan's options are, the greater the consumer cost.

Population Health and Shared Financial Risk

While managed care integrated cost containment options, previous health plans did not include the concept of financial risk among the three groups of stakeholders: payers, providers, and patients/consumers. Today, financial payment options for population health are increasingly moving toward the value-over-volume options and introducing shared risk. In 2017, health experts developed a sample model for Medicaid payments with four financial arrangements identified.

TABLE 10.1   Definitions for Population Health Financial Payment Options

Type of Population Health Financial Payment Option	Definition
Fee for service	Established system of volume-based payment with no risk (Fee for Service, n.d.)
Managed care	Based on a gatekeeper arrangement system to manage care, utilization, and cost outcomes
Risk-based options	Arrangements in which the degree of risk is spread between the payer, provider, and patient/consumer
Value-based	Payment system that requires quality services, positive health outcomes, and cost reduction and may use incentives as part of the alternative payment system

This financial risk continuum reflects the changing relationships between payers, providers, and, of course, patients/consumers. Although financial risk increases with each level, reimbursement opportunities for health providers also increase to offset risk *if* health outcomes reach established goals. Today, health payers recognize primary care incentives and performance-based payment contracts as among the first alternative payment options to integrate the concept of population health outcomes as a prerequisite for provider reimbursement. Positive population health outcomes create value for all health stakeholders.

Value-Based Payment Options for Health Systems and Providers

Transitioning to value-based payment options requires complex implementation strategies for delivering health care. Choices for the degree of care (**quality**), integration among diverse types of health providers, and accountability (varying share of risk) all factor into the cost of care. Population health managers face the challenge of developing health service contracts with health providers that satisfy all three major stakeholders: payers, patients, and providers. A health service contract explains the provider's reimbursement arrangement for delivering healthcare services to patients covered by a specific health plan (LaPointe, 2018). These binding and legal agreements hold both parties accountable. Figure 10.8 shows a comparison between fee-for-service and value-based alternative payment systems.

Fee-for-Service	Performance-Based Payments	Bundled/Episodes of Care Payments	Accountable Care Programs
• Volume-Based Payments	• Primary Care Incentives • Performance-Based Contracts	• Condition of Service Line Programs	• Shared Savings • Shared Risk • Capitation

FIGURE 10.8 Fee-for-Service and Value-Based Alternative Payment System Contract Components

Research suggests that health care systems are moving slowly away from fee-for-service payments toward performance-based payments (Lockner, 2018). Performance-based contracts rely on pay for performance arrangements in which providers receive payment based on meeting specific performance measures. Bundled payments pay for specified **episodes of care** and usually involve teams of diverse health providers. In 2022, 483 ACOs existed, serving more than 11 million beneficiaries (National Association of ACOs, n.d.).

Practical Skill: Bundled Payment Examples

A **bundled payment** for episodes of care is a viable reimbursement option for treatments that are more than just a single visit and often require lengthy post-acute follow-up. For example, these might be service lines such as chronic cardiac conditions or orthopedic replacement surgeries that required surgery followed by rehabilitation and physical therapy over time. Other types of episodes of care commonly involved in bundled payments are total joint replacements, diabetes, and breast cancer (Struijs et al., 2020).

Bundled refers to the payment system where a team of health providers receive a specified payment amount for both acute and post-acute expenditures for a predetermined episode of care. This type of alternative payment system expands the risk to multiple health providers and not just the health payer. For example, a bundled payment single fixed fee can cover costs of all health providers (physicians and other clinicians), medications and devices, facilities, and other necessary resources (Lockner, 2018). The challenge is defining the type of care and coordination needed for both acute and post-acute care and determining a target price.

Instructions: You own a physical therapy clinic that works frequently with a large orthopedic medical practice. Would you participate in a bundled payment contract? Why or why not?

Developing and implementing innovative financial health payments systems remains a priority task for the health sector. Innovation in payment types and arrangements will continue to affect all major stakeholders as population health financial payment systems transition to meet health policy mandates that seek lower health care costs and improve health outcomes. Seeking improved health outcomes also requires an emphasis on quality and equity of care for all.

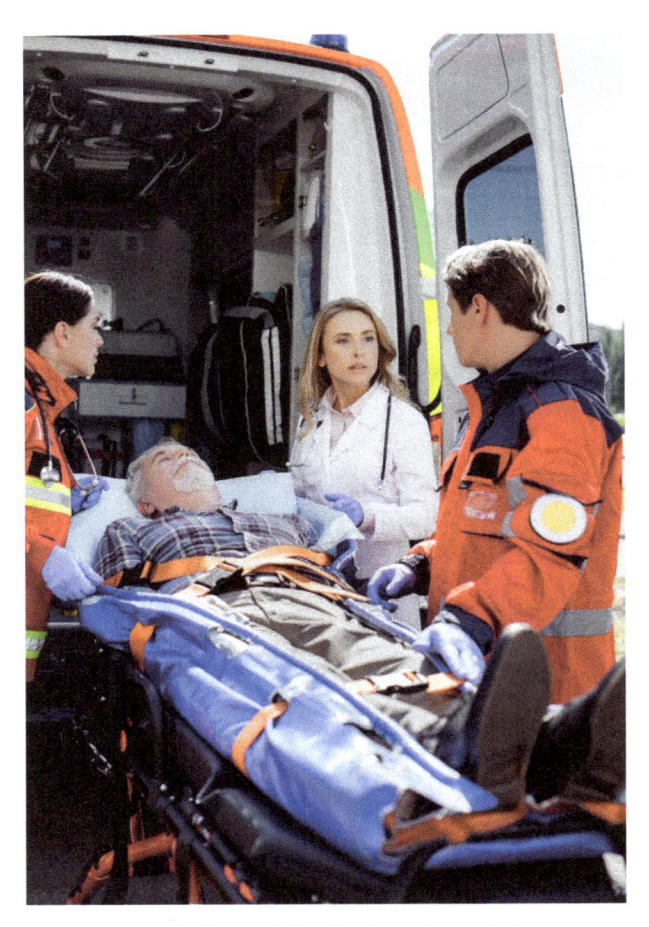

FIGURE 10.9 Patient at the Center of Population Health Accountability

Population Health's Accountability: Quality, Safety, and Equity of Care

Population health accountability involves four major components: financial outcomes, **patient safety**, health equity for all, and quality of care (see Figure 10.10). Although these outcomes appear as disparate parts of the health care delivery system, their interrelatedness is key to successful population health management.

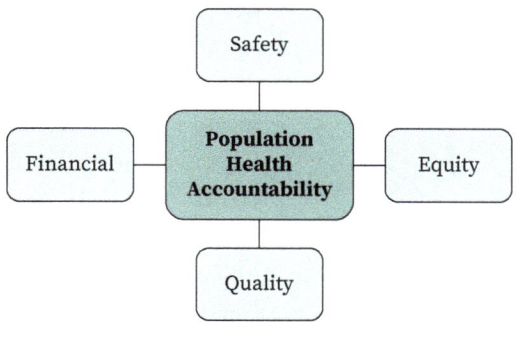

FIGURE 10.10 Four Major Components of Population Health Accountability

Providing quality care has always been essential for America's health sector. The National Committee on Quality Assurance (**NCQA**), established in 1990, focuses on lowering costs and maintaining quality for both Medicare and Medicaid patients (McIntire et al., 2001). In the early 2000s, two major Institute of Medicine (IOM; now known as the National Academy of Medicine) reports, *To Err Is Human* (IOM, 2000) and *Crossing the Quality Chasm* (IOM, 2001), became the catalysts for improving health care throughout the entire system. These national call-to-action documents urged health providers and systems to eliminate medical errors and preventable adverse events (Joshi, 2019). An adverse or temporary harm event occurs because of medical care in a health care setting (Office of Inspector General [OIG], 2022). Common harm event examples include medical errors, substandard care, known side effects, and unexpected complications that may not have been preventable.

Patient Safety and Equity

Take the time to review the following statistics, which highlight the continuing magnitude of our population health safety issue:

- In 2022, the Food and Drug Administration received more than 100,000 reports related to medication errors. It is estimated that 7,000 to 9,000 people die each year due to medication errors (SingleCare Administration, 2022).
- A 2018 report found that one-quarter of Medicare patients (25%) experienced adverse events and temporary harm events during their hospital stays (OIG, 2022).
- One state recently reported that its healthcare-associated infection (HAI) rates cost $124 million to $348 million each year in direct expenditures (North Carolina Department of Health and Human Services, 2022). Imagine the fiscal impact for all 50 states.

FIGURE 10.11 The Six Domains of Quality

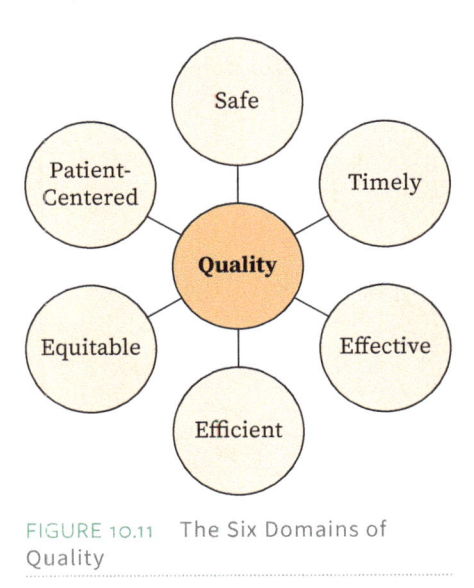

To provide the best quality, population health must address care equity for all populations. Over the years, reliable data repeatedly identified the inconsistency of health care treatment and outcomes for populations. Research identified both racial and ethnic populations as at greatest risk for health disparities, but as Chapter 5 highlights, health inequities can result from multiple social determinants of health and other characteristics such as age, gender identity and orientation, geography, language, disability status, and citizenship status (Ndugga & Artiga, 2021). The health sector continually seeks to eliminate this entrenched health disparity issues and remains committed to implementing and standardizing care that meets the six domains of quality.

The Relationship Between Quality and Performance

Quality care is related to performance issues whether it be (a) organizational such as availability of resources (b) processes that involve procedures and workflow or (c) outcomes that refer to the effectiveness of care (Donabedian, 2003). Contrary to public opinion, inferior quality is not always related to an individual practitioner. See the examples below that illustrate the three areas of performance—organizational, processes, and outcomes—that affect quality of care.

One of management's primary functions is controlling all aspects of the health organization to achieve desired quality standards. Health sector organizations can adopt this simple three-step control method process for improving quality (Olden, 2019). Figure 10.12 shows the three-step control quality performance process flow.

1 Setting performance standards	2 Measure actual performance and compare standards	3 Improve performance if it does not meet standard

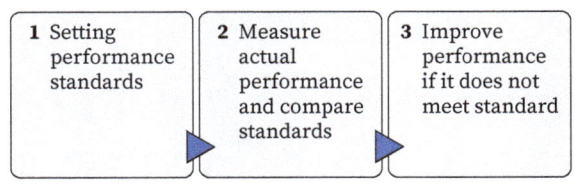

FIGURE 10.12 Three-Step Control Process for Quality Improvement

Population Health Practice Example

Follow the outlined steps below to understand the performance control process as applied in health care:

- **Step 1: Set the standards.** A population health manager receives performance standards from the organization's quality team for unnecessary hospitalization rates of three priority populations: Medicare, Medicaid, and dual-eligible.
- **Step 2: Measure and compare performance.** View the data analysis as presented in Figure 10.13. The sample control chart for the three priority groups shows the performance standard (gray line) and hospitalization rates for the most recent 3 months. A control chart simply visually depicts a comparison between data points in relationship to a performance standard, also called a *benchmark*. The orange bar represents the level for the dual-eligible group, and the blue and orange bars represent the Medicare and Medicaid hospitalizations.

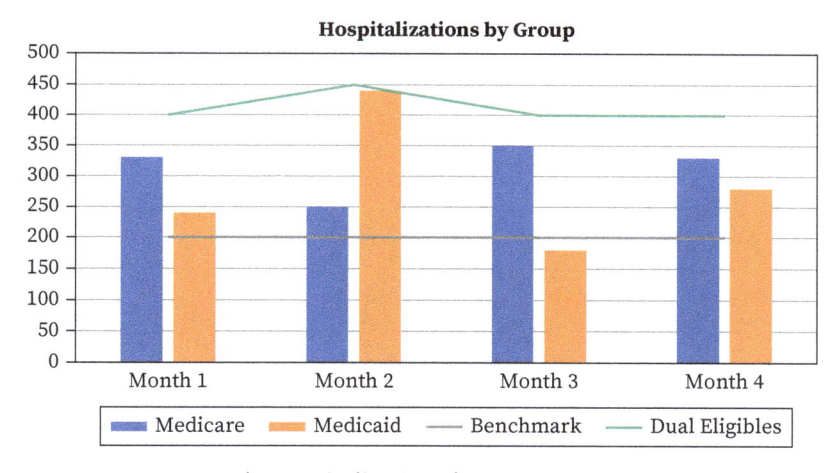

FIGURE 10.13   Sample Hospitalizations by Priority Group Control Chart

What did you notice? Which group had the least change in hospitalizations? Which group had the most variation? This information helped the population health managers make the decision to add outreach and coaching to the dual-eligible group to lower their unnecessary hospitalization rates.

- **Step 3: Improve performance and measure.** To improve quality of care and ensure the priority population (dual-eligible group) is receiving the appropriate care, the next step involves implementing additional outreach and coaching. A basic **quality improvement** four-step process, the Plan-Do-Check-Act (PDCA) model, is a framework used for the activities in Step 3 (American Society for Quality, 2022).

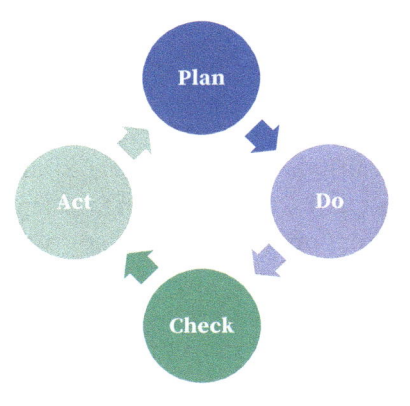

FIGURE 10.14 Plan-Do-Check-Act Model

The population health manager would develop and implement the outreaching and coaching activities in the first two steps. Then, managers would monitor, assess, and develop a control chart comparing the preintervention levels of hospitalization to the postintervention levels. The comparison between the preintervention and postintervention findings would determine whether the interventions were successful and should continue or additional efforts needed. The PDCA cycle ties the quality improvement intervention and monitoring together and assesses its value for improving care.

Practical Skill: Student Activity

To view up-to-date and publicly available hospital comparison data, go to Hospital Compare at https://tinyurl.com/5bvfyyx3.

Be sure to select at least three health organizations to review their data in a comparison chart. The NCQA developed the Health Plan Employer Data and Information Set (HEDIS), which is one of the most widely used performance improvement tools and has a data set with 90 measures (NCQA, n.d.).

Source: National Committee for Quality Assurance. (n.d.). HEDIS and performance measurements. https://www.ncqa.org/hedis/

Review the six domains that categorize the 90 different measures.

Population Health: Quality Improvement

Quality improvement tools continue to evolve and develop even more effective options for increasing positive outcomes. One primary example is the quality improvement tool Six Sigma, which expands the original PDCA cycle into five steps to integrate additional detail and statistical rigor (Ogden, 2019). Six Sigma, developed by Motorola in the 1980s, became one of the most popular quality improvement tools (Bhargav, 2021). Figure 10.15 shows a comparison between the basic PDCA model (Institute for Healthcare Improvement, 2020) and Six Sigma, which is known by the process step acronym *DMAIC*.

Population Health Performance Measures

Performance measures and quality improvement tools continue to advance as technology develops and supports even more advanced assessment systems. Basic performance measures include not only the standard control chart as illustrated in Figure 10.13 but also simple line and bar charts, histograms, and pie charts. More sophisticated analyses used include cause-and-effect diagrams and the Five Why's for solving problems and finding root causes. Based on Six Sigma, another quality improvement process is LEAN, which focuses on eliminating waste and emphasizing value (IHI, 2005). Basic process maps and more complex value-stream mapping are two additional quality improvement tools available to population health managers.

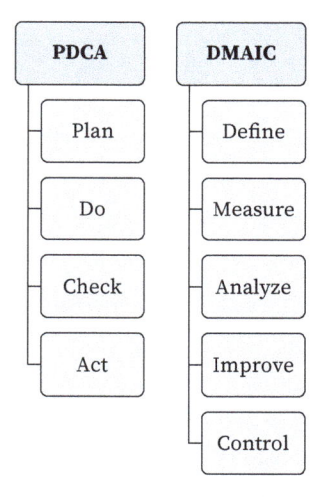

FIGURE 10.15 Comparison of PDCA and Six Sigma (DMAIC) Frameworks

Practical Skill: Understanding and Applying Quality Improvement

Additional information on quality improvement tools is available at the following well-known national organization websites:

Agency for Healthcare Research on Quality. (n.d.). Tools. https://tinyurl.com/4c34ycva

Center for Nursing Inquiry. (2022, March). *Quality improvement*. Johns Hopkins University School of Nursing. https://www.hopkinsmedicine.org/nursing/center-nursing-inquiry/nursing-inquiry/qualityimprovement.html#:~:text=As%20previously%20mentioned%2C%20the%20three,%2C%20Lean%2C%20and%20Six%20Sigma.

Institute for Healthcare Improvement. (n.d. https://tinyurl.com/ms9vsdkm

Summary

Population health accountability ensures continued progress on the overall goals of quality care, access for all and cost containment. Since the beginning of managed care, significant financial model transitions from volume to value-based care have culminated into today's alternative payment systems. These new and emerging financial payment options address risk and accountability for payers, patients, and providers. Both the continuum of alternative pay options (managed care and risk- and value-based) and the systems for payment (performance-based, bundled, ACO options) show innovation and stakeholder engagement based on shared risk and savings opportunities. Population health's accountability for quality and the inherent characteristics of safety and equity also document a similar progression of advancement. Safety initiatives based on performance measures have developed over the years to reduce unnecessary patient harm and preventable infections. Performance measures for health equity goals ensure that monitoring strategies inform initiative-taking, decision-making, and improvements. The diversity, scope, and complexity of emerging quality improvement tools provides increased opportunity to ensure all aspects of health care meet national quality standards such as those identified by the NCQA. Today's health sector integrates quality improvement processes within all aspects of population health delivery systems.

Discussion Questions

1. Both federal and state governments are major payers for health care through their sponsorship of Medicare and Medicaid. Briefly describe the eligibility requirements for each health insurance option and discuss the role of dual eligibility.
2. One of the key principles of population health remains an emphasis on accountability for value over volume. This unique feature separates population health from other health approaches. But what is the value? First, define the concept and then explain the value equation.
3. Given the enormous burden of health care costs, population health is helping the health industry transition from fee-for-service to value-based care. Describe the types of transitions that will need to be accomplished for the volume to value transformation to be completed.
4. To implement population health's value approach, health payments and reimbursements also needed to transition to an accountability arrangement that spreads the risk between payer, provider, and the patient/consumer. Figure 10.7 and Table 10.1 introduce the four types of payment options. Compare that continuum with the risks and benefits presented in Figure 10.8.
5. Financial considerations only form one-quarter of the accountability focus for population health. Attaining quality health care delivery services also includes safe and equitable care. List the six domains of quality and give an example of a positive health result for each.
6. Population health is an approach to delivering quality health care that is based on performance outcomes. Describe the four activities within the Plan-Do-Check-Act cycle that can be used to improve diverse types of health outcomes.

References

Agency for Healthcare Research and Quality. (2018). *The six domains of quality*. https://www.ahrq.gov/talkingquality/measures/six-domains.html

American Society for Quality. (2022). *What is the Plan-Do-Check-Act (PDCA) cycle?* https://asq.org/quality-resources/pdca-cycle

Bhargav, R. (2021, February 17). *History and evolution of Six Sigma*. https://www.simplilearn.com/history-and-evolution-of-six-sigma-article

Buehler, J., Snyder, R., Freeman, S., Carson, S., & Ortega, A. (2018). It is not just insurance: The Affordable Care Act and population health. *Public Health Reports, 133*(1), 34–38. https://www.ncbi.nlm.nih.gov/pmc/articles/PMC5805102/

Donabedian, A. (2003). *An introduction to quality assurance in health care*. Oxford University Press.

Fee for Service. (n.d.). *Fee for service. What is fee-for-service?* HealthInsurance.org. https://www.healthinsurance.org/glossary/fee-for-service/

Guinan, S. (2022, August 12). *Medicare vs. Medicaid: The important differences to know*. https://www.valuepenguin.com/medicare-vs-medicaid#:~:text=There%20are%2064%20million%20people,are%20also%20enrolled%20in%20Medicaid

Hayes, S., Collins, S., & Radley, D. (2019, May 23). *How much U.S. households with employer insurance spend on premiums and out-of-pocket costs: A state-by-state look*. Commonwealth Fund. https://www.commonwealthfund.org/publications/issue-briefs/2019/may/how-much-us-households-employer-insurance-spend-premiums-out-of-pocket

Health Research & Educational Trust. (2014, March). *The second curve of population health*. http://www.hpoe.org/Reports-HPOE/SecondCurvetoPopHealth2014.pdf

Higbea, R., Jashiewics, L., & Cline, G. (2022). Financing healthcare in the USA. In T. Clobe (Ed.), *Introduction to the United States healthcare system*. Affordable Learning Solutions & California Alliance for Open Education.

Institute for Healthcare Improvement. (2020). *Plan-Do-Study-Act (PDSA) worksheet*. http://www.ihi.org/resources/Pages/Tools/PlanDoStudyActWorksheet.aspx

Institute for Healthcare Improvement. (2005). *Innovation series 2005: Going lean in health care*. https://www.entnet.org/wp-content/uploads/files/GoingLeaninHealthCare-WhitePaper-3.pdf

Institute of Medicine. (2001). *Crossing the quality chasm: A new health system for the 21st century*. https://doi.org/10.17226/10027

Institute of Medicine. (2000). *To err is human: Building a safer health system*. National Academies Press.

Johns, M. (2017). Accountability practice. In *Leadership development for healthcare: A pathway process, and workbook* (p. 21). American Health Information Management Association Press.

Joshi, M. (2019). Part I: The foundation of healthcare quality. In D. Nash, M. Joshi, E. Ransom, & S. Ransom (Eds.), *The healthcare quality book: Vision, strategy, and tools* (4th ed.; p. 2). Health Administration Press/Association of University Programs in Health Administration.

LaPointe, J. (2018, July 11). *Key terms, components of payer contracts providers should know*. TechTarget. https://revcycleintelligence.com/news/key-terms-components-of-payer-contracts-providers-should-know

Lockner, A. (2018, September 26). *Insight: The healthcare industry's shift from fee-for-service to value-based reimbursement*. Bloomberg. https://news.bloomberglaw.com/

health-law-and-business/insight-the-healthcare-industrys-shift-from-fee-for-service-to-value-based-reimbursement

McIntyre, D., Rogers, L., & Heier, E. J. (2001). Overview, history, and objectives of performance measurement. *Health Care Financing Review, 22*(3), 7–21. https://www.ncbi.nlm.nih.gov/pmc/articles/PMC4194707/

Medicaid.gov. (n.d.). *Managed care.* https://www.medicaid.gov/medicaid/managed-care/index.html

MedlinePlus. (2019, August 30). *Managed care.* https://medlineplus.gov/managedcare.html

Miller, A., & Woodard, T. (2022). Alternative payment systems: Volume to value-based care. In A. Hewitt, J. Mascari, & S. Wagner (Eds.). *Population health management: Strategies, tools, applications, and outcomes* (pp. 14–41). Springer Publishing.

National Association of ACOs. (n.d.). *Learn all about ACOs.* https://www.naacos.com/#:~:text=As%20of%20January%202022%2C%20there,serving%20over%2011%20million%20beneficiaries

National Committee for Quality Assurance. (n.d.). *HEDIS and performance measurement.* https://www.ncqa.org/hedis/

Ndugga, N., & Artiga, S. (2021, May 11). *Disparities in health and health care: 5 key questions and answers.* https://www.kff.org/racial-equity-and-health-policy/issue-brief/disparities-in-health-and-health-care-5-key-question-and-answers/

Niles, N. (2021). *History of managed care: Basics of the U.S. health care system* (4th ed.). Jones & Bartlett Learning.

North Carolina Department of Health and Human Services. (2022, August 25). *Healthcare-associated infections (HAIs).* https://epi.dph.ncdhhs.gov/cd/hai/figures.html

Office of Inspector General. (2022, June 6). *Adverse events.* https://oig.hhs.gov/reports-and-publications/featured-topics/adverse-events/#:~:text=Adverse%20Event%20%2D%20An%20event%20in,intervention%2C%20or%20contributed%20to%20death

Olden, P. (2019). Controlling and improving performance. In *Management of healthcare organizations* (3rd ed.; p. 295). Health Administration Press/Association of University Programs in Health Administration.

SingleCare Administration. (2022, January 2022). *Medication errors statistics 2023.* https://www.singlecare.com/blog/news/medication-errors-statistics/

Struijs, J., de Vries, E. F., Baan, C., van Gils, P., & Rosenthal, M. (2020, April 6). *Issue briefs: bundled-payment models around the world: How they work and what their impact has been.* https://www.commonwealthfund.org/publications/2020/apr/bundled-payment-models-around-world-how-they-work-their-impact

Townsend, R. (2022, August 12). *Largest health insurance companies of 2022.* https://www.valuepenguin.com/largest-health-insurance-companies

UnitedHealthcare Community Plan. (2021, April 2). *Medicaid versus Medicare: You can have both.* https://www.uhccommunityplan.com/dual-eligible/eligibility/

medicaid-medicare-have-both#:~:text=The%20difference%20between%20Medic-aid%20and%20Medicare%20is%20that%20Medicaid%20is,younger%20people%20to%20get%20Medicare

U.S. Government Accountability Office. (1978, March 3). *Implementation of the Health Maintenance Organization Act of 1973, as amended*. https://www.gao.gov/products/105122

Vocabulary.com. (n.d.). *Value*. https://www.vocabulary.com/dictionary/value

Wagner, S. (2018). The future and medical practice innovation. In *Fundamentals of medical practice management* (pp. 155, 334). Health Administration Press/Association of University Programs in Health Administration.

Credits

Fig. 10.1: Generated with FreeWordCloudGenerator.com.

Fig. 10.2: Copyright © 2020 Depositphotos/AndreyPopov.

Fig. 10.4a: Copyright © 2021 Depositphotos/designer491.

Fig. 10.4b: Copyright © 2017 Depositphotos/designer491.

Fig. 10.6: Adapted from A) Stephen Wagner, *Fundamentals of Medical Practice Management*, p. 155, 334. Copyright © 2018 by Health Administration Press. Anne Hewitt, Julie Mascari, and Stephen Wagner, *Population Health Management: Strategies, Tools, Applications and Outcomes*. Copyright © 2022 by Springer Publishing Company.

Fig. 10.9: Copyright © 2020 Depositphotos/HayDmitriy.

Fig. 10.11: Source: https://www.ahrq.gov/talkingquality/measures/six-domains.html.

Fig. 10.14: Source: Adapted from https://asq.org/quality-resources/pdca-cycle.

CHAPTER ELEVEN

Delivering Population Health Care

Today's Models

Chapter Description

Chapter 11 showcases recent frameworks and strategies that are both innovative and patient centric. Just as new payment models enabled rewards for value-based outcomes, care delivery processes need to reflect better ways of delivering care to all Americans. Coordinated chronic care and transition-of-care models emerged along with patient-self management programs and became widely used options for treating the most vulnerable senior populations. To improve quality, access, and cost, health experts now focus on realigning payors, providers, and consumer's roles to ensure better-quality care and greater satisfaction. The expanded continuum of care provided the opportunity for the health care sector to offer new options for delivery of care,

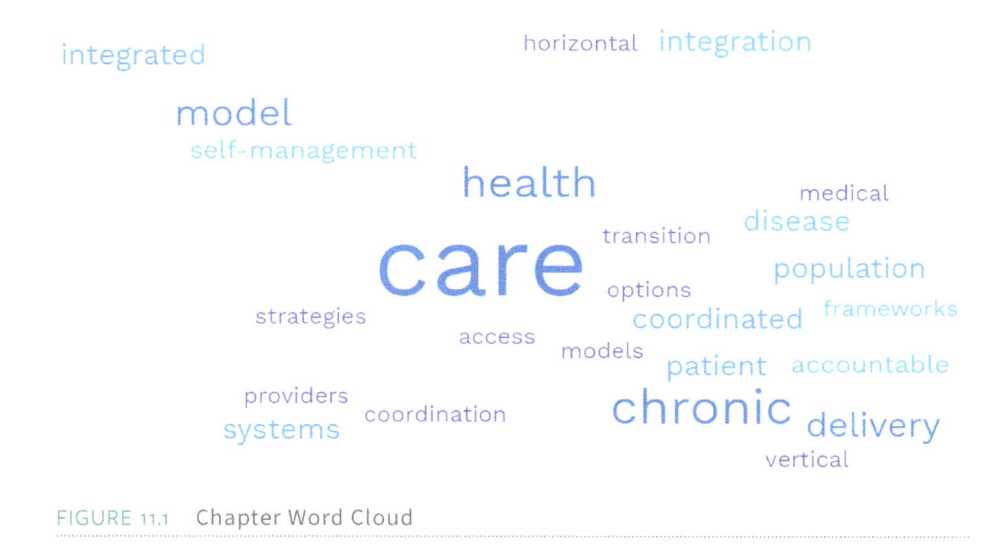

FIGURE 11.1 Chapter Word Cloud

199

created easier access to specialty health providers, and improved the transition to integrated care. Today, hospitals and other health care providers operate integrated health systems as flexible frameworks for coordinated care delivery. This chapter describes two major models of population health delivery processes: the patient-centered medical home (PCMH) and the newer accountable care organization (ACO). It also illustrates the impact PCMHs and ACOs have made on improving patient outcomes, especially for those populations with chronic conditions.

Chapter Objectives

After completing this chapter, students will be able to:

1. Describe the challenges of chronic care populations
2. Explain the importance and value of the transition-of-care model for population health
3. Share an application (example) of the transition-of-care model
4. Briefly discuss and diagram an integrated health system that includes examples of horizontal and vertical integration
5. Share an application (example) of the chronic care coordination model
6. Describe the characteristics of PCMHs
7. Summarize the role and benefits of ACOs

Key Words

Accountable care organization

ACO Realizing Equity, Access, and Community Health (ACO REACH)

Chronic care model

Chronic Disease Self-Management Program

Clinical decision support system (CDSS)

Continuum of care

Coordinated care

Decision support

Horizontal integration

Integrated care delivery networks and systems

Patient-centered medical homes

Transition-of-care model

Vertical integration

Population Health Strategies to Improve Chronic Care Coordination

Over the years, the American health care system received immense criticism for operating in silos (see Chapter 1) with fragmented delivery systems that failed to meet patients' needs and contributed to immense duplication of efforts, unnecessary treatments, and inflated the cost of care (World Economic

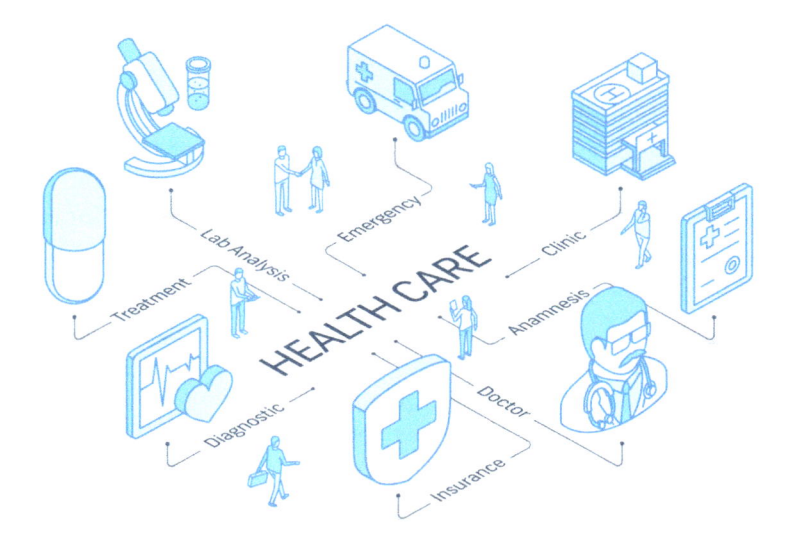

Chapter Eleven Delivering Population Health Care | 201

FIGURE 11.2   Integrated Health Care

Forum, 2020). Today's population health approach seeks to address those concerns with innovative health care processes and unique models that implement access, quality, and cost changes simultaneously. As discussed in Chapter 5, both the passage of the Patient Protection and Affordable Care Act (PPACA) and technological advances facilitated development of health information systems and enabled dramatic and positive changes to occur in patient care. The opportunity to transition from an acute care focus to an expanded preventive and chronic care delivery model finally occurred.

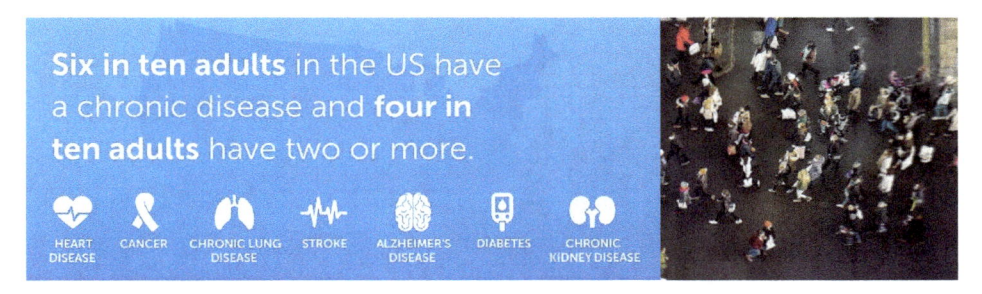

FIGURE 11.3   Chronic Disease in U.S. Adults

One of the primary groups to benefit from these new health care delivery systems were populations with chronic conditions who often lack **coordinated care** plans or experienced gaps in care due to the current fragmented health care system. A chronic condition or disease is one that lasts for 3 months or longer, cannot be prevented by vaccines or cured by medication, and does not disappear

(MedicineNet, 2016). Convincing evidence suggests that individuals with major diseases and conditions constitute the chronic care subgroup that requires systematic and continuous health care and medical interactions. Chronic conditions treated improperly, such as diabetes, heart disease, and cancer, result in unnecessary hospitalizations and poor health outcomes (National Center for Chronic Disease Prevention and Health Promotion, 2022). The Centers for Disease Control and Prevention (CDC) reports that 90% of the nation's $3.5 trillion in annual health care expenses are for people with chronic or mental health conditions (CDC, 2020). This undesirable situation occurs when individuals lack a primary care provider, need care management or coordination, and/or fail to follow through with their care plan. As the American population continues to age, managing chronic care outcomes becomes a meaningful priority for the entire health care sector.

So, what do we mean by a fragmented health care delivery system for those populations with chronic conditions that require care from multiple providers?

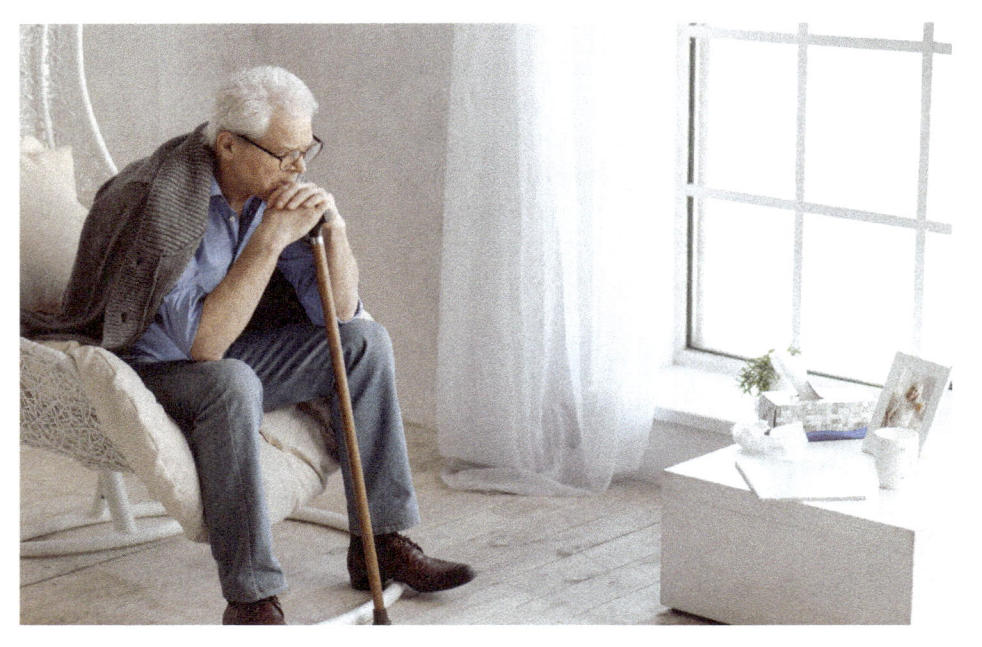

FIGURE 11.4   Example: Senior Patient With Chronic Condition

To illustrate the need for coordinated care, meet Walter. Walter is a 73-year-old man with arthritis, diabetes, and asthma. Due to his chronic diseases, he often complains of joint pain and shortness of breath. He relies heavily on his one adult child to schedule, transport, and accompany him to appointments.

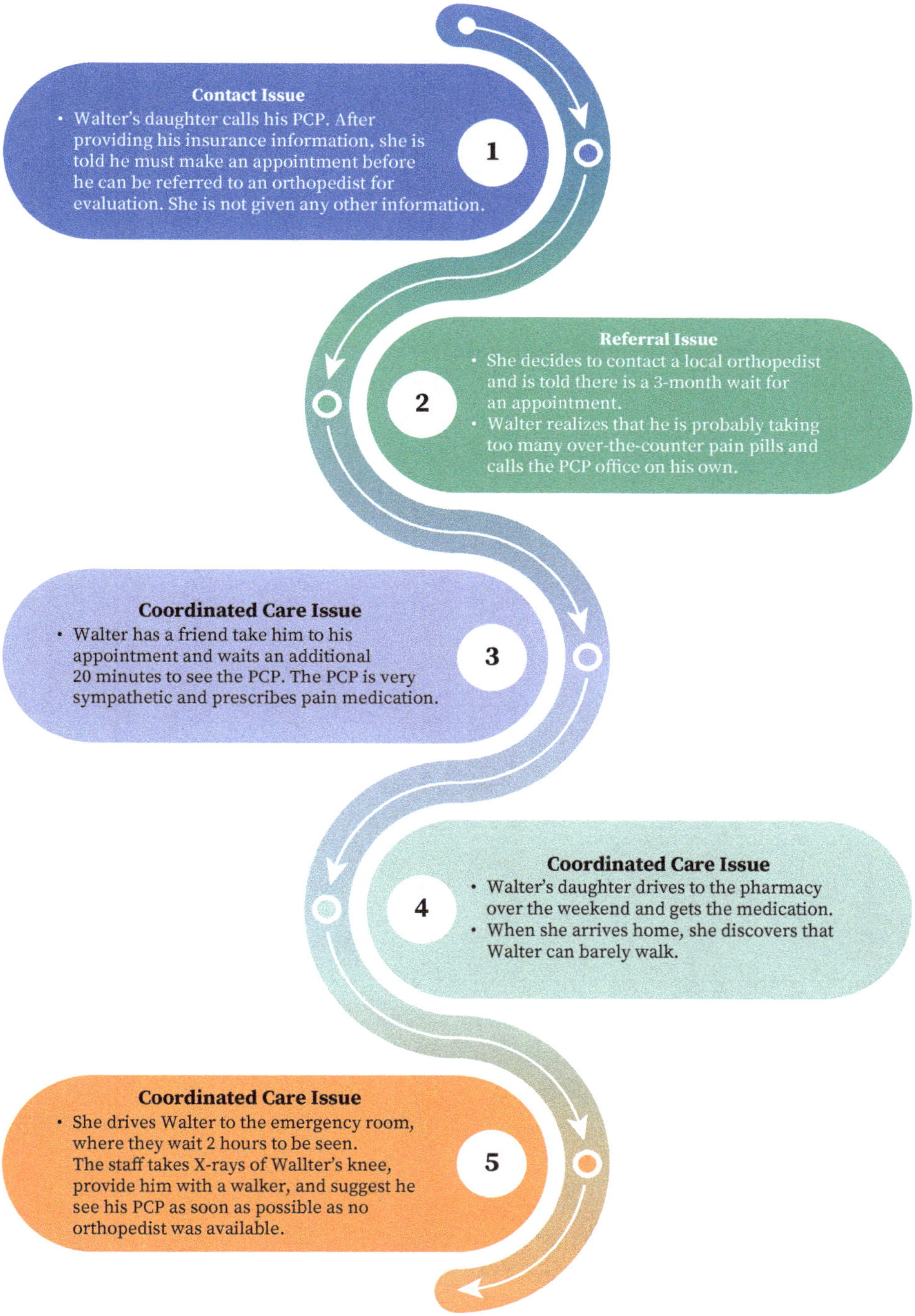

Chapter Eleven Delivering Population Health Care | 203

1. Contact Issue
- Walter's daughter calls his PCP. After providing his insurance information, she is told he must make an appointment before he can be referred to an orthopedist for evaluation. She is not given any other information.

2. Referral Issue
- She decides to contact a local orthopedist and is told there is a 3-month wait for an appointment.
- Walter realizes that he is probably taking too many over-the-counter pain pills and calls the PCP office on his own.

3. Coordinated Care Issue
- Walter has a friend take him to his appointment and waits an additional 20 minutes to see the PCP. The PCP is very sympathetic and prescribes pain medication.

4. Coordinated Care Issue
- Walter's daughter drives to the pharmacy over the weekend and gets the medication.
- When she arrives home, she discovers that Walter can barely walk.

5. Coordinated Care Issue
- She drives Walter to the emergency room, where they wait 2 hours to be seen. The staff takes X-rays of Wallter's knee, provide him with a walker, and suggest he see his PCP as soon as possible as no orthopedist was available.

FIGURE 11.5　Fragmented Care Patient Pathway

The above scenario shows a classic example of uncoordinated care with appointment difficulties, transportation concerns, missed self-management opportunities, unmanaged follow-up, and a lack of an overall care plan for a senior with multiple chronic conditions.

Chronic Care Model

At-risk populations, who suffer from chronic conditions, can experience rapid health status changes, especially if regular health care and/or self-management of a chronic disease is lacking. The Health Resources and Services Administration (n.d.) defines a **chronic care model** as one that includes "key elements of a health care system that encourage high-quality chronic disease care: the community, the health system, self-management support, delivery system design, decision support and clinical information systems." The Institute for Health Improvement (IHI) outlined six health delivery components essential for any chronic care coordination model (IHI, 2022; see Figure 11.6).

Self-Management Support	Delivery System Design	Decision Support
Clinical Information Systems	Organization of Health Care	Community

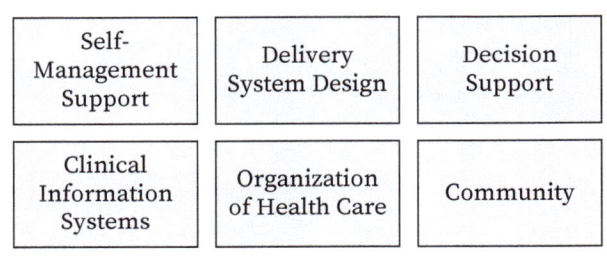

FIGURE 11.6 Recommended Changes for Chronic Care Improvement

You may think these six strategies appear unrelated, but dividing these recommendations into two main groups, internal health organizational changes and external sector changes, helps align their overall purposes. Internal strategies include decision support, clinical information systems, and delivery system design, and they all concentrate on improving decision-making. Health managers use the term *decision support* to describe computer programming and data analysis activities that produce tailored and valuable information to make an assessment. Both decision support and clinical information systems rely on interoperability capabilities and real time access to summarize relevant patient and consumer data. **Clinical decision support systems (CDSS)** combine computer-based programs (clinical information systems) that analyze data from electronic health records to provide reminders that assist health care providers at the point of care (Division for Heart Disease and Stroke Prevention, 2021). Delivery system design includes creating step-by-step processes and flow charts for providing care coordination to maximize improved chronic patient outcomes.

External sector strategies, essential for coordinating chronic care, emphasize broader stakeholder inputs such as payor involvement, community support, and patient/consumer participation. Payors may need to revise their reimbursement strategies to cover additional care transitions such as home visits. Community initiatives can include safety net programs that fill gaps in needed services such as transportation or free vaccine clinics. Other efforts include encouraging consumers to participate in community programs that focus on healthy lifestyle options such as safe walkways and more greenspaces. Patients, especially those living with multiple chronic conditions, should enroll in self-management programs to assist them in completing daily tasks for maintaining a healthy life. Consumers will also need to seek the appropriate care at the right time, at the right place, and with the right provider. Reengineering and reimagining the overall organization of health care involves the complex alignment of financial models, regulatory actions supporting new models of care, increased access, and availability of needed care services.

Self-Management of Chronic Disease

An important **chronic care model** component requires patients to engage in self-management of their symptoms and health condition. Patients with chronic diseases such as diabetes and arthritis need to participate daily in healthy supportive activities such as monitoring their insulin levels or changing lifestyle patterns by becoming more active. Self-management education (SME) programs serve as an additional transition strategy to address a patient's condition. SME programs educate patients in ways to help manage their chronic symptoms and diseases such as asthma, arthritis, diabetes, COPD, and chronic pain. Simple self-help education and techniques can easily improve the quality of life for those suffering from chronic disease. The CDC's **Chronic Disease Self-Management Program** features an interactive workshop for people with all types of chronic conditions (CDC, 2019). This evidence-based program helps people gain confidence so that they can oversee the day-to-day changes. Participants learn to manage their various symptoms with the goal of improving not only their physical condition, but also their psychological well-being to aid in preventing depression and despair. The positive impact is a reduction in demand for unnecessary primary care visits, decreased emergency department visits, and improved quality of life for chronic disease patients.

Practical Skill: The Chronic Disease Self-Management Program

Explore the CDC's website (CDC, 2018) at https://tinyurl.com/4sc62at2.

First, select one of the following chronic diseases: asthma, cancer, chronic obstructive pulmonary disease (COPD), depression, diabetes, or heart disease. Then complete the following questions:

1. Identify the various interactive learning techniques that are appropriate for your at-risk population.
2. Provide at least three examples of the types of symptoms management activities that are specific for your selected chronic disease.

Transition-of-Care Model

Transition of care refers to activities that provide linkages between primary, acute, and post-acute care and the selection of the appropriate health care delivery option for the at-risk population. The **transition-of-care model**, based on Coleman's four pillars of transition of care (see Figure 11.7), outlines four requirements that address the care process (Coleman, 2007).

Think of each of the following care change requirements as a question that the population health care coordinator would need to ask before selecting the best care option:

- Are the patients able to reliably manage all their medications without assistance?
- Do the primary care provider and patients have access to a personal health portal that contains a health record and opportunities for communication?
- Is there a care pathway that fully integrates and aligns both primary and specialty care for follow-up?
- Which monitoring systems exist that would assess in real time if a patient's health condition began to deteriorate quickly?

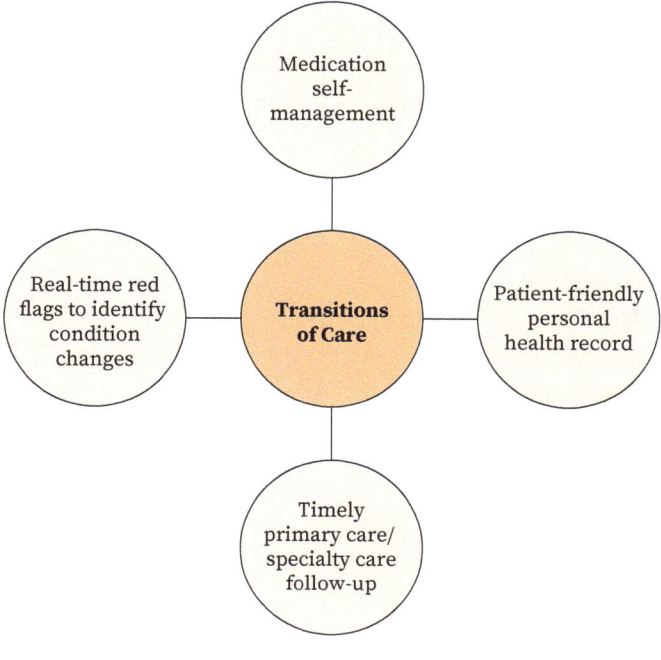

FIGURE 11.7   Transition-of-Care Model

Implementing Coordinated Care

In population health, diverse health professionals often function as teams to provide active organization and implementation of coordinated chronic care for vulnerable subgroups. Either care or case management, with care management focusing on ensuring patient's routine care and case managers often tailoring care for individuals with complex needs such as rehabilitation services, can serve this oversight function (Hewitt, 2022). Although these important population care delivery roles can overlap, significant differences do exist. Care management ensures direct patient care with support services and creates a smooth transition between different treatments and stages of care. Case management involves broader responsibilities such as planning, delivery, analysis, and assessment of the coordinated care plan. Together, all the care components merge to create a successful patient journey (*American Journal of Case Management*, 2018; Cuddeback & Fisher, 2016). Care and case management professional roles differ in education and certification requirements as well as who determines the scope of work. Payment methodologies also vary depending on the position location, whether in health care organizations (hospitals), health provider agencies, or health insurance companies (Aging Outreach Services, 2023). Care coordinator positions represent a hybrid type of model between these two current roles. In newer population health models, embedded care coordinators have become part of on-site office teams and are most often nurses (Hines & Mercury, 2013).

Post-Acute Care Strategies of Care

A particularly difficult hand-off facing care coordinators involves the patient's journey from acute to post-acute care as options for these types of care require complex coordination. Alternative sites for post-acute care have expanded beyond traditional nursing homes to include skilled nursing facilities, rehabilitation options, and enhanced home-health programs. Palliative and hospice care have also experienced greater interest from patients concerned with end-of-life care options. Improved electronic medical records with additional access for primary and acute care health providers and patient portal availability enhance the timely and useful flow of real-time data for patients' transitions of care. Two new coordination care strategies, companion-care, and hospital-at-home care delivery are useful options for smoothing this difficult transition stage for chronic care patients.

Back to Walter ...

Now, let us reimagine Walter's patient journey. What if a coordinated care pathway involving both the chronic care model and transition-of-care best practices occurred from the very beginning and the fragmented primary care provider (PCP) and emergency department visits did not need to happen?

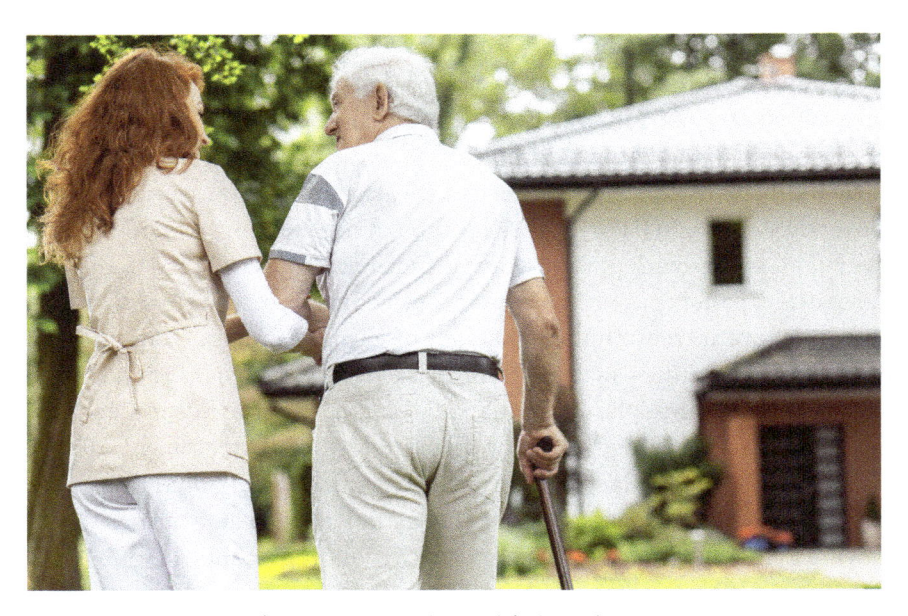

FIGURE 11.8 Senior Chronic Care Patient With Caregiver

Walter's care worker, Sylvia, arrives on a typical Monday morning at his home for her biweekly check-in visit. Instead of greeting her as usual, Walter shouts to just come in as the door is open. She notices dirty dishes in the sink with uneaten food and at least three bottles of different over-the-counter pain medication are on the kitchen table, along with Walter's unfilled weekly pill box organizer. She quickly texts his daughter for an update and learns she was out of town and did not get to check in with her dad over the weekend.

Sylvia performs her routine visit, checking his vital signs and reviewing his condition. She notices that Walter looks tired, appears out of breath, and is moving with extreme difficulty due to pain in his swollen knee. All this information Sylvia transfers to Walter's electronic health record and to Scott, his PCP's advanced practitioner, who Sylvia has alerted via text. Scott quickly reviews the information.

Sylvia sets up a virtual visit, and Scott joins both Walter and his daughter for a telehealth consultation. They discuss the current situation, and Walter shares that he has fallen and has a slight bump on his head. Scott checks Walter's medications and arranges for a refill medication delivery by Walter's pharmacy. He also arranges for a senior transport van to take him to his PCP, located in a PCMH location on the following day. The PCMH transport coordinator will call with the exact time of pickup. Walter's daughter will check in with him later that night and tomorrow morning. He assures both Walter and his daughter that a pain specialist or an orthopedist if needed will be available for him at the PCMH. He notes the need for an updated evaluation by his home health case manager.

Practical Skill: Coordinated Care Pathways

1. Can you identify the care coordination strategies in the second version of the Walter story?
2. Give one example of integrated care.
3. Why was a PCMH the right option for Walter?

Frameworks for Integrated Care

Improving coordinated care by enhancing delivery options and adopting chronic care models and transition of care best practices demonstrate effective care coordination changes. The largest challenge remains the continuing redesign and transformation at the organizational level. *Health care integration* refers to a system in which care providers have organized relationships for working and communicating across health conditions, services, and care settings (Institute of Medicine, 2001). Definitions of integrated care may depend on health professionals' different perspectives:

- The health system with a continuum-of-care system goal
- A population health manager's viewpoint of organizing all elements of service delivery
- A holistic social science approach to ensuring quality of life
- A patient or person-centered focus (Goodwin, 2016)

Today's integrated care is a combination of these viewpoints with the goal to develop an **integrated health system** that aligns all care and delivery components into a unified coordinated system (Goodwin, 2016). **Integrated care networks** operate as provider systems coupled with various sites of care able to deliver health care services. The term *integrated delivery networks* **(IDNs)** refer to multiple options for integrating care, whether within a system, an organization, or groups of organizations (Miller, 2022). Combining hospitals, physicians, other health care providers, transport services, and post-acute care and aligning them with community health providers and support services remains a major challenge. Two alignment strategies can aid the development of a population health integrated health delivery system.

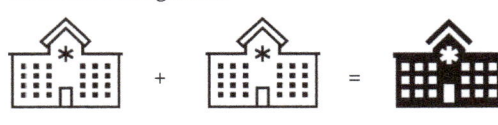

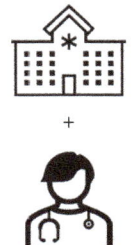

FIGURE 11.9   Examples of Horizontal and Vertical Integration

Horizontal and Vertical Integration

Horizontal and vertical integration strategies are two commonly used coordinated care alignment options. **Horizontal integration** occurs when similar organizations at the same level either consolidate, merge, create an alliance, or become acquired (Langabeer & Helton, 2021). This step produces a "system" that benefits from centralized services, governance, and management all working together. If one hospital purchases another or a primary care group aligns with another, the strategy is known as horizontal integration. **Vertical integration** occurs when health organizations or agencies

Chapter Eleven Delivering Population Health Care | 211

at distinct levels integrate to provide care (Miller, 2022). An example is when a hospital purchases physician practices or a nursing home. And, of course, complex integrated systems may have both horizontal and vertical integration. Health care planners decide to choose care delivery options using these strategies to improve patient care and create efficiency.

> **Practical Skill: Designing Integrated Delivery Systems**
>
> Take the time to create your own diagram of an integrated health system that exhibits both horizontal and vertical integration. Now you should be able to design a multi-hospital system, an independent practice association (IPA), which is a group of providers, and a multispecialty group practice, a term that refers to a group that includes primary and secondary physicians with common management. A physician-hospital organization is a partnership between a hospital and affiliated physicians (Shiver & Cantiello, 2016). These integration organization alignments may occur between multiple competitors or cooperative agencies and organizations with the shared goal of improving health care.

Two important integrated health care delivery models are ACOs and PCMHs. Both frameworks illustrate organizations that include provider reimbursement directly tied to positive health outcomes for priority at-risk populations.

Accountable Care Organizations

ACOs became a population health organizational model when the PPACA offered the infrastructure flexibility for a new care delivery option that combined an alternative payment system with a total emphasis on patient outcomes. ACOs are networks of providers who coordinate whole patient-centered care, with the PCP at the center of the network (LaPointe, 2019). ACOs can coordinate care of populations to reduce redundant emergency department visits and decrease unnecessary tests and treatments. Doctors who choose to form an ACO must meet stringent government requirements, including registering at least 5,000 assigned beneficiaries, creating a formal legal structure to receive and distribute shared savings, integrating processes that promote evidence-based medicine, and reporting and assessing necessary data for quality, cost metrics, and coordinated care outcomes (CMMS, 2021). ACO physician benefits are both managerial and financial and can lead to reduced patient costs and better outcomes. Practitioners must meet established clinical and performance (quality) benchmarks for their patients to receive monetary rewards, so a significant monetary risk is involved. The Medicare Shared Savings Program relies on 33 quality indicators to demonstrate improved population health outcomes (CMMS, 2022b).

Over time, federal regulations have revised requirements and initiated diverse alternative payment systems for ACOs (see Chapter 10). ACO Realizing Equity, Access, and Community Health (ACO-REACH) relies on the latest payment model from CMMS beginning in 2023. The acronym *REACH* underscores the need for ACOs to better coordinate and improve care offered for the Medicare population, especially those from underserved communities. ACO-REACH organizations must provide a specified action plan to improve equity of care (CMMS, 2022a). To address important social determinants of health (SDOH) that contribute to health inequities, ACOREACH organizations may choose to adopt companion care as a support strategy for at-risk populations with chronic conditions. Companion care addresses SDOH factors by assisting with daily living activities such as grocery shopping, providing transportation for medical care, organizing care, and even performing daily chores such as light cleaning (Brown et al., 2022). Companion care professionals are not health care providers, but the services they offer, especially companionship for senior patients, can extend the ACO's outreach to improve the lives of the chronic care patients and help providers lower costs. The newer ACO version will also require greater transparency of patient progress outcomes, mandate a level of physician and other health care provider' participation in organizational leadership, and direct governance such as board membership. One major benefit for participating ACOs will be a more predictable revenue stream.

Patient-Centered Medical Homes

PCMHs can easily be confused with ACOs, but their approach is for individual practices and not a network of providers. **PCHMs** include multiple providers under one organization banner that offers interdisciplinary, community-based primary care teams that provide culturally informed patient-centered care (Primary Care Innovations, 2020). PCMHs serve as a model for population health care coordination, and in 2020, the National Committee for Quality Assurance (NCQA) recognized 13,000 practices with 67,000 clinicians (NCQA, 2020).

The PCMH model successfully combines all the coordinated care elements outlined in Figure 11.10. The twin goals of PCMH accountability and patient support require not only diverse relationships and agreements among all partners, but also necessary communication connectivity. This means multiteam alignment among community agencies, hospitals, and medical specialists. Only these types of arrangements will eliminate the current fragmented system that so many chronic care individuals face daily. Each organization must deliver

FIGURE 11.10   PCMH Care Coordination Model

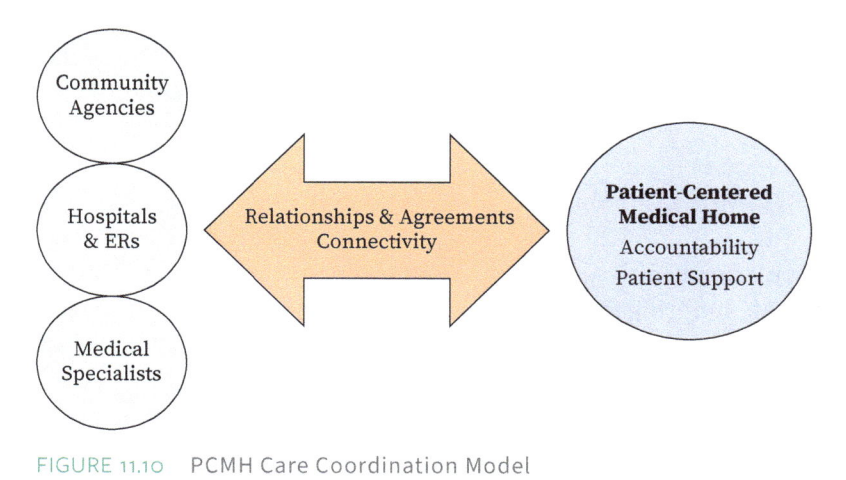

primary care that includes five core functions: patient-centered, comprehensive, coordinated, accessible, and with a quality and safety focus. The Agency for Healthcare Research and Quality (AHRQ) offers a certification option for PCMHs with three levels of recognition (1 to 3), which, if completed, successfully has the potential added benefit of increasing reimbursement rates (AHRQ, 2014). Unlike ACOs, which receive incentives or penalties from external sources based on performance, PCMH are primarily accountable to themselves, but they can also benefit from value-based reimbursement arrangements.

One significant point to remember concerning multi-provider joint ventures, whether they include physicians or hospitals, is that a financial risk agreement will be involved (Shiver & Cantiello, 2016). There are sophisticated models and care pathways, but they all encourage financially tying patient outcomes to providers' reimbursement to achieve significant savings (Kaufman et al., 2019).

Summary

The most vulnerable American population includes seniors with multiple chronic conditions, and they often face the most challenges navigating today's fragmented health care system. The population health response to this dilemma generated the development and implementation of coordinated care initiatives such as the chronic care model, the transition-of-care framework, chronic disease self-management programs, and the adoption of companion care. To implement care coordination goals, health organizations adopted an integrated system approach using both horizontal and vertical integration options to form fully integrated health networks that deliver care with better outcomes at a lower cost. ACOs and PCMH health organizations successfully demonstrate the alignment of care with communities and other diverse partners. They also demonstrate fiscal accountability while remaining patient-centered.

Discussion Questions

1. Population health seeks to help patients most in need, usually those individuals suffering from chronic conditions. Identify common barriers that hinder those with chronic conditions from participating in self-management or receiving care coordination.
2. Population health designs health care delivery and relies on chronic care coordination. Examine the case study of Walter in the text. For each of the coordinated care issues, describe the gap in coordinated care.
3. The original transition-of-care model identified medical self-management as the first action step when assisting chronic care patients. What recent initiatives and options are currently available to address this issue?
4. Coordinated care for chronic disease patients requires integrated health systems, care, and delivery networks. Explain the differences between horizontal and vertical integration. How would you describe a fully integrated health system?
5. List the distinctive characteristics of the latest ACO model: ACO-REACH. Which characteristics differ between this model and the traditional ACOs?

References

Accelerating Care Transition. (2010). *Moving research into action together.* https://www.act- center.org/application/files/8016/3111/1974/Model_Care_Coordination.pdf

Agency for Healthcare Research and Quality. (2014, June). *Chapter 3: Care Coordination Measurement Framework.* https://www.ahrq.gov/ncepcr/care/coordination/atlas/chapter3.html

Aging Outreach Services. (2023). *Care managers vs. case managers: understanding differences and duties* (June 6). https://agingoutreachservices.com/aging-outreach-services/care-vs-case-managers/

American Journal of Case Management. (2018). *Care management versus case management: Differences and similarities.* https://ajcasemanagement.com/care-case-management-differences-roles-need-rehabilitation/#:~:text=Care%20management%20is%20solely%20focused,to%20create%20one%20successful%20journey

Brown, C., Jefcoat, C., & Barlow, J. (2022, June 29). *Addressing social determinants of health with companion care.* https://www.ecgmc.com/thought-leadership/blog/

addressing-social-determinants-of-health-with-companion care?utm_source=newsletter&utm_medium=email&utm_content=tl-bg-addressing-social-determinants-of-health-with-companion-care&utm_campaign=hmi%20newsletter

Centers for Disease Control and Prevention. (2018, December 17). *Managing chronic conditions (any)*. https://www.cdc.gov/learnmorefeelbetter/programs/general.htm

Centers for Disease Control and Prevention. (2019, October 18). *Chronic Disease Self-Management Program*. National Center for Chronic Disease Prevention and Health Promotion, Division of Population Health. https://www.cdc.gov/arthritis/interventions/programs/cdsmp.htm#:~:text=About%20the%20program%3A%20The%20Chronic,%2Dsolving%2C%20and%20action%20planning

Centers for Disease Control and Prevention. (2020). *Health and economic costs of chronic diseases*. National Center for Chronic Disease Prevention and Health Promotion. https://www.cdc.gov/chronicdisease/about/costs/

Centers for Medicare & Medicaid Services. (2022b, June 1). *About the program*. https://www.cms.gov/Medicare/Medicare-Fee-for-Service-Payment/sharedsavingsprogram/about

Centers for Medicare & Medicaid Services. (2021, December 1). *For providers*. https://www.cms.gov/Medicare/Medicare-Fee-for-Service-Payment/sharedsavingsprogram/for-providers#:~:text=ACOs%20must%20have%20at%20least,in%20the%20Shared%20Savings%20Program.

Centers for Medicare & Medicaid Services. (2022a, February 24). *Accountable Care Organization (ACO) Realizing Equity, Access, and Community Health*. https://www.cms.gov/newsroom/fact-sheets/accountable-care-organization-aco-realizing-equity-access-and-community-health-reach-model

Coleman, E. (2007). *Care transitions model*. John A. Hartford Foundation. https://www.johnahartford.org/ar2007/pdf/Hart07_CARE_TRANSITIONS_MODEL.pdf

Cuddeback, J. & Fisher, D. (2016). Information technology. In D. B. Nash, R. J. Fabius, A. Skoufalos, & J. L. Clarke (Eds.), Population health: Creating a culture of wellness (2nd ed.; pp. 231–255). Jones & Bartlett Learning.

Division for Heart Disease and Stroke Prevention. (2021). Implementing clinical decision support systems. https://www.cdc.gov/dhdsp/pubs/guides/best-practices/clinical-decision-support.htm#:~:text=Clinical%20decision%20support%20systems%20(CDSS,at%20the%20point%20of%20care.

Goodwin, N. (2016). Understanding integrated care. *International Journal of Integrated Care, 16*(4). https://www.ncbi.nlm.nih.gov/pmc/articles/PMC5354214/

Health Resources and Services Administration. (n.d.). *Chronic care model*. https://www.hrsa.gov/behavioral-health/chronic-care-model

Hewitt, A. (2022). Population health models—Part II. In A. Hewitt, J. Mascari, & S. Wagner (Eds.), *Population health management: Strategies, tools, applications, and outcomes* (pp. 155–172). Jones & Bartlett Publishing.

Hines, P., & Mercury, M. (2013). Designing the role of the embedded care manager. *Professional Case Management, 18*(4), 182–187. https://alliedhealth.ceconnection.com/files/DesigningtheRoleoftheEmbeddedCareManager-1372337047139.pdf

Institute for Healthcare Improvement. (2022). *Changes to improve chronic care.* https://www.ihi.org/resources/Pages/Changes/ChangestoImproveChronicCare.aspx

Institute of Medicine. (2001). *Crossing the quality chasm: A new health system for the 21st century.* https://nap.nationalacademies.org/catalog/10027/crossing-the-quality-chasm-a-new-health-system-for-the

Kaufman, B. G., Spivack, B. S., Stearns, S. C., Song, P. H., & O'Brien, E. C. (2019). Impact of accountable care organizations on utilization, care, and outcomes: A systematic review. *Medical Care Research and Review, 76*(3), 255–290.

Langabeer, J. R., II, & Helton, J. (2021). *Health care operations management: A systems perspective* (3rd ed.). Jones & Bartlett Learning.

LaPointe, J. (2019, December 18). *Understanding the fundamentals of accountable care organizations.* Revcycle Intelligence. https://revcycleintelligence.com/features/understanding-the-fundamentals-of-accountable-care-organizations

MedicineNet. (2016). *Definition of chronic disease.* http://www.medicinenet.com/script/main/art.asp?articlekey=33490

Miller, A. (2022). Population health models—Part 1. In A. Hewitt, J. Mascari, & S. Wagner (Eds.), *Population Health Management: Strategies, Tools, Applications, and Outcomes* (pp. 122–123). Jones & Bartlett Publishing.

National Center for Chronic Disease Prevention and Health Promotion. (2022). *About chronic diseases.* Centers for Disease Control and Prevention. https://www.cdc.gov/chronicdisease/about/index.htm#:~:text=Chronic%20diseases%20such%20as%20heart,in%20annual%20health%20care%20costs

National Committee for Quality Assurance. (2020, August 12). *Patient-centered medical home (PCMH).* https://www.ncqa.org/programs/health-care-providers-practices/patient-centered-medical-home-pcmh/

Primary Care Innovations. (2020, August 20). *Primary care innovations and PCMH map by state.* https://www.pcpcc.org/initiatives/state

Shiver, J., & Cantiello, J. (2016). Integrated health care delivery models. In *Managing integrated health systems* (pp. 1–22). Jones & Bartlett Learning.

World Economic Forum. (2020, November). *Silos in healthcare are bad for us: Here's the cure.* https://www.weforum.org/agenda/2020/11/healthcare-silos-are-bad-for-us-heres-the-cure/

Credits

Fig. 11.1: Generated with FreeWordCloudGenerator.com.

Fig. 11.2: Copyright © 2020 Depositphotos/r.Hilch.

Fig. 11.3: Source: https://www.cdc.gov/chronicdisease/about/index.htm#:~:text=Chronic%20diseases%20such%20as%20heart,in%20annual%20health%20care%20costs.

Fig. 11.4: Copyright © 2017 Depositphotos/Dmyrto_Z.

Fig. 11.5a: Copyright © 2020 Depositphotos/biw3ds.

Fig. 11.8: Copyright © 2018 Depositphotos/photographee.eu.

Fig. 11.9a: Copyright © by Microsoft.

Fig. 11.9b: Copyright © by Microsoft.

Fig. 11.9c: Copyright © by Microsoft.

Fig. 11.10: Source: Adapted from https://www.act-center.org/application/files/8016/3111/1974/Model_Care_Coordination.pdf.

PART IV

Pivoting Toward New Directions

Part IV contains the final two chapters that address both challenges and needed transformations that will affect future population health strategies and outcomes. Chapter 12 concentrates on two health care delivery areas: patient engagement and virtual care. The chapter provides clarifications and examples of patient empowerment, engagement, experience, and satisfaction, which can help students appreciate the complexity of the ever-changing patient journey. Students will learn that net promoter scores, commonly used to measure customer satisfaction with the patient experience, can affect health practitioners' reimbursements and financial incentives. The chapter also supplies evidence supporting the tremendous explosion in virtual care as a popular health consumer alternative to face-to-face interactions. Digital health strategies such as wearables, remote patient monitoring, digital assistants, and the newest health delivery option—hospital at home—are featured. Chapter 13 introduces students to strategies needed to manage the grand challenges and wicked problems potentially facing population health. Students will learn the three-step innovation model and practice design thinking using an empathy map and ideation skills. Other concepts introduced will enable students to recognize potential disruptors in the health sector and find ways to seek multisectoral collaborations that lead to the co-production of health. Chapter 13 concludes with examples of management and models for reducing resistance to change. Agile leadership strategies appropriate for population health will provide beneficial skills to overcome future health challenges and ensure quality population health for all.

CHAPTER TWELVE

New Population Health Strategies

Patient Engagement and Virtual Care

Chapter Description

Chapter 12 explores and documents the rapid changes occurring in healthcare delivery approaches. Just as new payment models enabled rewards for value-based outcomes, health delivery processes need to reflect better ways of providing care to all Americans. **Patient empowerment** explains the concepts and skills necessary for delivering the "high-touch" patient–health professional interaction strategy. The chapter explains the basics of the patient–health care provider interaction continuum, including developing patient engagement, meeting expectations to reach patient satisfaction, and improving the overall patient experience. Learning examples include descriptions of the patient engagement capacity model and patient activation measure tool. *Virtual care*, a term that describes "high-tech" as new digital interaction pathways, integrates

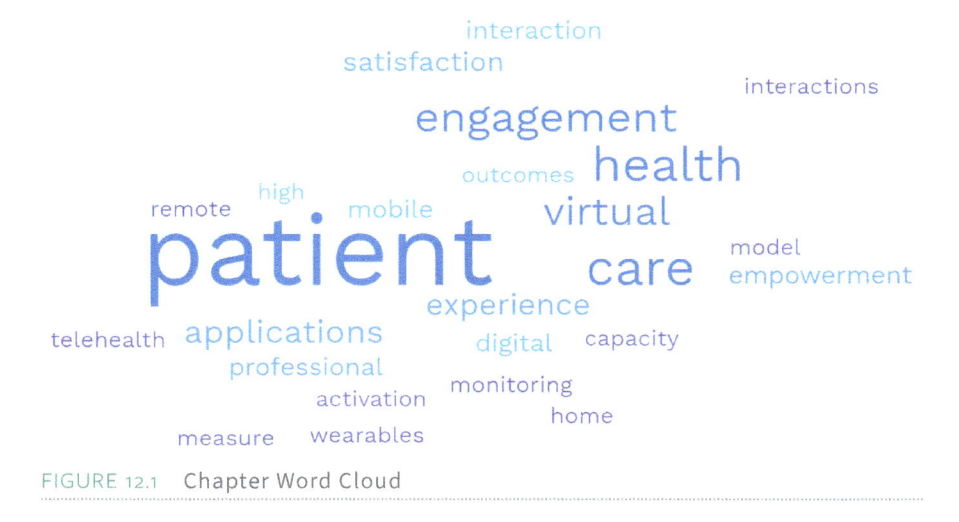

FIGURE 12.1 Chapter Word Cloud

221

not only telehealth and telemedicine concepts, but also the use of wearables, mobile applications, and remote monitoring care. Enhanced digital health applications also provide increased flexibility and cost savings for health care practitioners, freeing them from administrative tasks to spend more time on patient-provider interactions.

Chapter Objectives

After completing this chapter, students will be able to:

1. Explain the importance of patient–health professional interactions
2. Provide examples that illustrate patient experience, satisfaction, and engagement
3. Apply the patient activation and empowerment models to vulnerable populations
4. Briefly discuss the virtual care concept of health care delivery
5. Share examples for each of the seven levels of virtual care
6. Describe each of the five phases of digital patient engagement
7. List the benefits of technology innovations for health care workflows

Key Words

Adherence	Net promotor score	Patient experience	Patient satisfaction
Compliance	Patient Activation Measure	Patient–health professional interaction	Remote patient care monitoring
Digital assistant	Patient empowerment		Telehealth
Health education	Patient engagement	Patient journey	Virtual care
Hospital-at-home	Patient engagement capacity model	Patient-reported outcomes (PROs)	Wearable technology
Mobile health applications			

Patient–Health Care Professional Interactions

Health care remains a primary service industry, and although patients are also consumers, they engage in unique interactions with a variety of health care professionals. Positive patient-practitioner relationships serve as an essential component for the success of the entire health care industry. Over the years, this relationship was characterized by a medical model approach, as patients were considered not responsible for creating their problems or for solving them (Lewis et al., 1998). The health care provider assumed that the patient could not

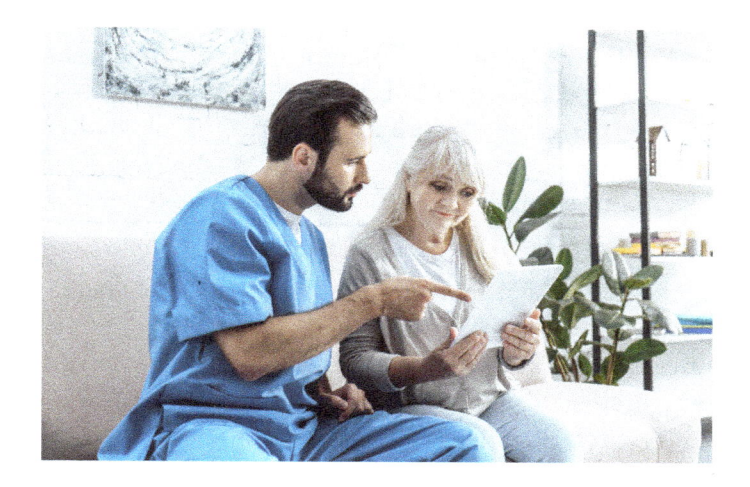

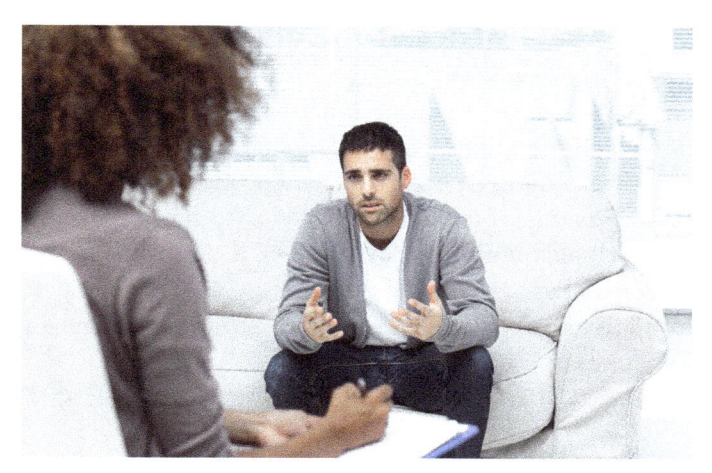

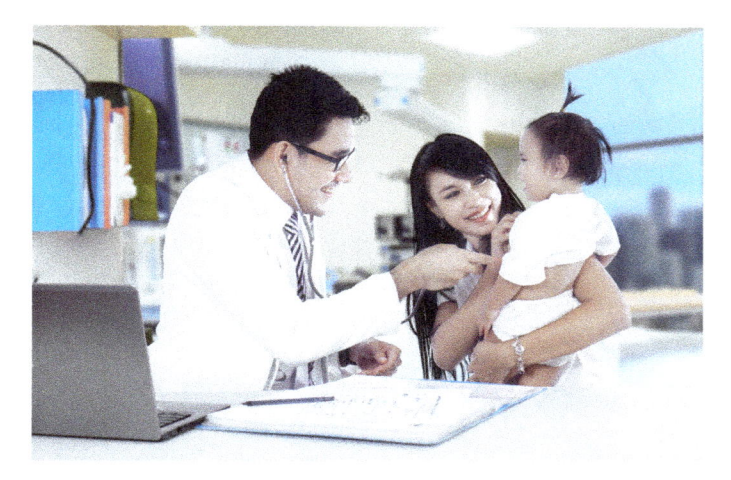

FIGURE 12.2   Understanding the Value of Patient-Provider Interactions

be treated or cured without their intervention and that patients needed only to follow their directions. Unfortunately, this type of treatment and counseling approach neglected to recognize patients' rights, their capability or self-efficacy, and their expectation to be an active partner in the healing relationship (Purtilo & Haddad, 1996). As a result, the health care sector today experiences the following types of unfortunate situations:

- Approximately 50% of patients with chronic illnesses that require long-term use of medications do not take them as prescribed (Brown & Bussell, 2011).
- An average of 42% of medical appointments result in a no-show, and estimates suggest that missed appointments cost the United States $150 billion annually (Pfeifer, 2022).
- Despite decades of health education to encourage smoking cessation, fewer than one in 10 adult cigarette smokers succeed in quitting each year (Centers for Disease Control and Prevention, 2022).

These examples illustrate the value and the need for positive patient–health care practitioner collaborations to ensure quality and cost-effective population health care. But what characteristics create a positive health interaction? The concept of **patient-health professional interactions** refers to interpersonal, face-to-face, and/or virtual communication between a health care practitioner and a patient (Parvanta et al., 2018). We know that two-party partnerships are the foundation for successful patient satisfaction, experiences, and engagement.

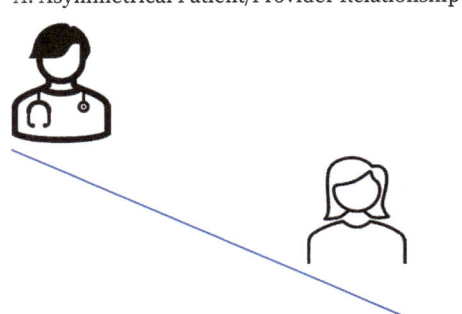

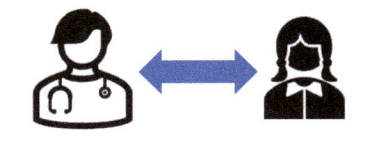

FIGURE 12.3 Asymmetrical to Symmetrical Provider-Patient Interactions

Population Health: Reframing the Talk

Why is one of the most difficult challenges in population health care the management of nonadherent patients? Evidence suggests that noncompliance costs the U.S. health care system more than $300 billion per year (Iuga & McGuire, 2014). Population health professionals now recognize that the term *patient compliance* is not appropriate for describing the care process (Culbertson, 2020). **Compliance** refers to an asymmetrical relationship between the health practitioner and the patient, in which the provider selects the course of treatment, and the patient is expected to follow their directions. Health care professionals also use the term *adherence* to infer a patient's obedience to their directives. Population health instead focuses on developing interactive relationships that are symmetrical between the patient and the health care provider. The population health challenge is to move away from the adherence approach and to engage patients and consumers in partnerships for collaborative and successful health care decision-making.

Patient interactions can occur between (a) a patient (consumer) and the health care practitioner and/or (b) the patient and any representative of the health care organization. These nonclinical essential interactions can significantly influence consumers' perspectives and expectations of health care treatment outcomes. Quality metrics assess patients' satisfaction levels, experiences, and level of engagement to identify gaps in patient perceptions, expectations, and outcome satisfaction.

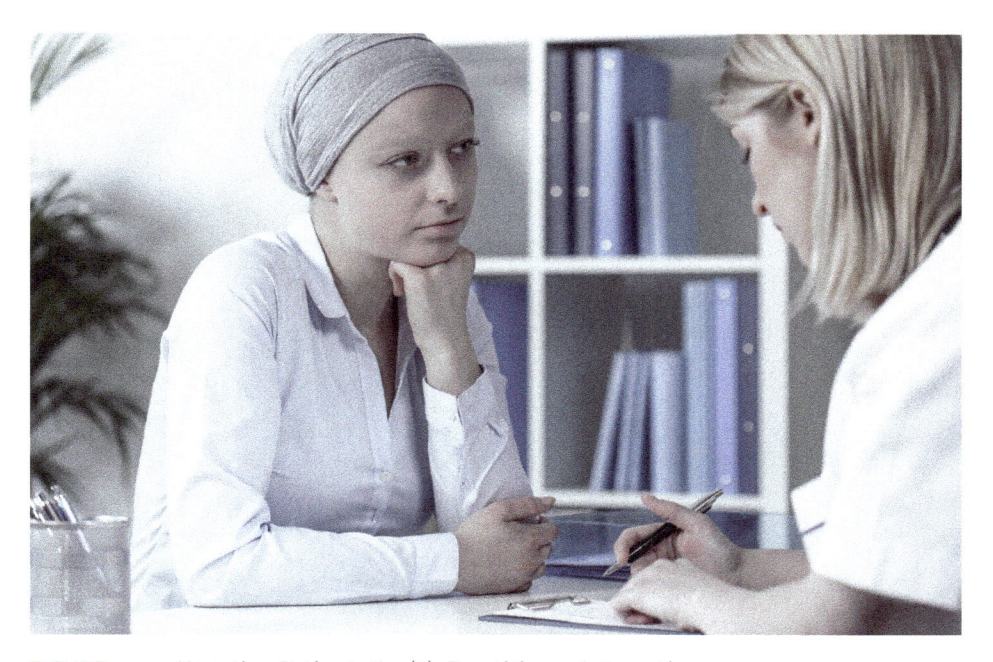

FIGURE 12.4 Negative Patient–Health Practitioner Interaction

Patient Engagement and Patient Empowerment

Patient engagement programs constitute an important part of population health's strategies to assist individuals attain optimum health status. In a recent *Patient Engagement Executive Handbook* survey, more than one-third of health care organizations indicated strong involvement in patient experience initiatives, especially in those focused on vulnerable populations and families not speaking English as a first language (Hagland, 2022). **Health education** is a complex set of activities that provide diverse opportunities to acquire knowledge and the skills to make quality health decisions (Joint Committee on Terminology, 2012). Health care practitioners consistently provide awareness, education, and skill-building activities to keep patients informed, increase self-management of conditions, and aid in overall health decision-making processes. The importance of health education cannot be underestimated, and patient experience managers now recognize that consumers prefer to receive their health communications in a variety of ways, including social media, texts, and videos.

Patient Engagement	Patient Satisfaction	Patient Experience
Patient participation and cooperation with health providers to ensure optimum health outcomes	Patient's feelings and attitude regarding their health expectations and outcomes	Patient's perception of the total health care interaction experience

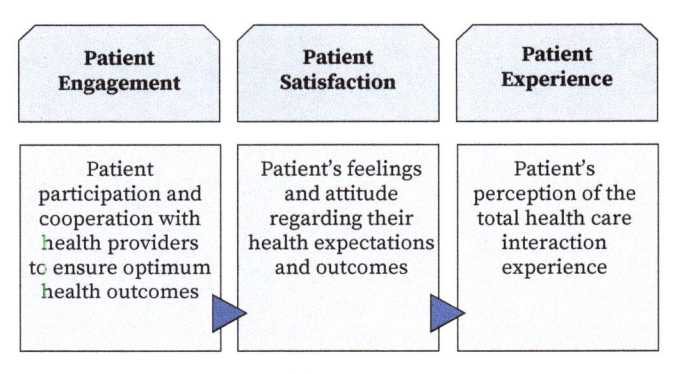

FIGURE 12.5   Definitions of Patient Engagement, Satisfaction, and Experience

Practical Skill: Why Isn't Health Education Enough?

Population health focuses on patient-centered and coordinated care, but the first step is helping the patient become aware of a health condition via health education. You ask almost any elementary student why they should eat fruits and vegetables and they will respond, "Because they are good for you." But transforming knowledge into action is often the reason health education does not succeed. How many fruits and vegetables do you eat in a day? Do you even count them? If health is a priority, why don't American's respond to health education? There are many reasons, and they are diverse depending on the individual, but until an individual is empowered to make a change and becomes engaged to make health a priority, their health behaviors will not change. What do you think?

Health care professionals have known for years that health education alone will not change patient behavior or health outcomes. Successful patient engagement requires health awareness, education, and *provider support* to encourage patient empowerment. **Patient empowerment** occurs when individuals are encouraged to exercise their authority and autonomy to build self-confidence (Purtillo & Haddad, 1996). Once patients acquire the skills and the confidence to participate in health discussions, they become active in their health care processes, and outcomes improve. One size does not fit all, as not all chronic care patients may want responsibility or accountability of their own care processes. Data indicates that for most populations, positive patient interactions lead to improved patient empowerment and greater health engagement as individuals become invested in their own health care.

Patient engagement is often described as activities or efforts to involve an individual in their own care (Graffigna & Barello, 2018) and is a broader term than patient empowerment as it includes all efforts for encouraging patients to participate in their personal care plans and work in partnership with health care providers. Patient engagement activities span the **continuum of care** from prevention to chronic disease palliative care. Simple health promotion and disease prevention behaviors such as getting an annual flu shot or completing monthly self-mammogram checks indicate positive patient engagement. More complex activities may require on-going or daily participation such as joining support sessions for smoking cessation or substance abuse prevention efforts. Actively engaged consumers have better outcomes and lower costs (Scott, 2019).

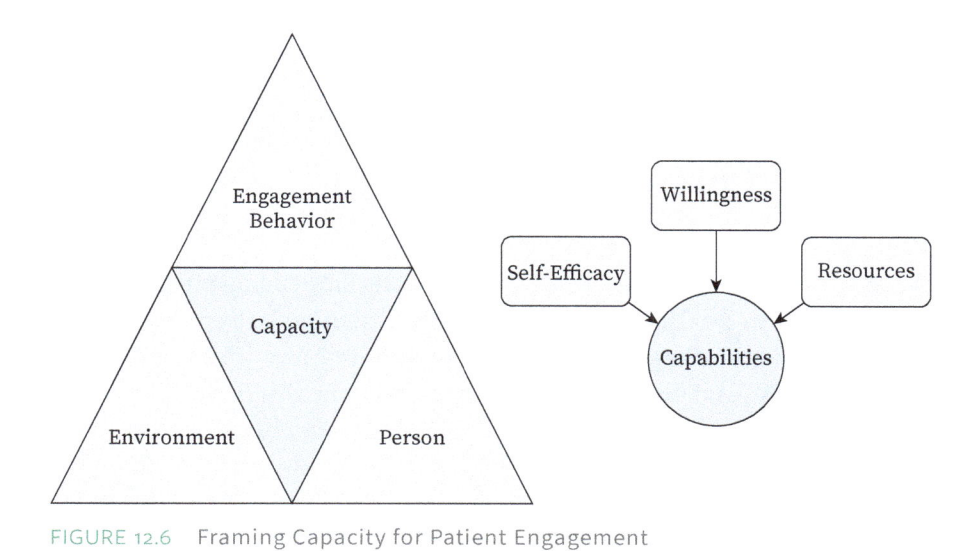

FIGURE 12.6   Framing Capacity for Patient Engagement

How do we know which patients will respond and become engaged in their own care? Which at-risk population group will need additional support? The

patient engagement capacity model helps population health practitioners assess two sets of overlapping factors: internal capabilities and external impacts on capacity (Sieck et al., 2019). The external impacts of the environment, personal characteristics, and engagement behavior interact to affect the individual's circumstances or capacity to change and engage. For example, if an individual has diabetes and strives to alter their diet, the family situation (i.e., environment) needs to be supportive and help the family member consume healthier foods either by planning a better diet or providing food choices that reduce the amount of sugar consumed. The second set of impact factors refers to internal or personal capabilities and includes three distinct components: willingness, resources (personal), and self-efficacy. If we use our individual with diabetes as an example, *willingness* refers to their desire to change dietary habits, and *self-efficacy* measures their confidence that they can consistently complete daily checkups of blood glucose levels. *Resources* refers again to the availability of necessary motivation required for change to occur. Together, these assessments form a patient engagement capacity framework that can inform the health care professional on the best activities to recommend.

> **Practical Skill: What Is Your Engagement Capacity?**
>
> Imagine that your health care practitioner has recommended a lifestyle change to improve your health status. Review the patient engagement capacity model. Which do you think would be the most important in helping you change your health behavior? Would it be difficult to change the environmental impact factors? Or would it be more difficult to change internal considerations, such as willingness to change or the belief that you could change? Describe your perceptions of the situation.

As you can imagine, if 40% to 50% of individuals lack engagement or empowerment, negative health situations develop. Effective patient engagement requires **patient activation**, and when a patient shows that they have the knowledge, skill, and confidence to manage their health care, they are said to be activated (Heath, 2019). Activation differs from compliance, in which individuals are told by health care providers on what to do. Hibbard and colleagues (2004) have developed a survey, called the **Patient Activation Measure® (PAM)**, to assess an individual's level of engagement (Phreesia, 2023). After completing the survey tool, an individual's score (100 points total) can identify areas for improvement and help tailor interactions and communications that will encourage participation and strengthen their engagement for better health outcomes (Heath, 2017). Patients may be asked to complete the PAM tool once they have a meeting with their health provider and health systems have begun integrating this information into the individual's electronic health record. Results suggest a 50% reduction in hospital visits when using an activation survey tool to categorize patients needing additional support (Phreesia, 2023).

Other patient engagement strategies focus on adopting best practices, such as (a) ensuring inclusion of patient/family/caregiver education on the specific disease/condition, (b) embedding care navigators in primary care or specialist offices, (c) enabling patient-centered interactions through patient portals or mobile technology, and (d) encouraging targeted analysis of patient-generated data that occurs in real time (Health Information Network [HIN], 2019). Adding SDOH assessments to electronic records aids in identifying potential barriers to patient engagement activities as well. The primary goal is for population heath managers to select and implement the best tailored strategies that will directly contribute to improvements in quality health care and lower costs.

Patient Satisfaction and Patient Experience

Patient satisfaction serves as a key indicator for determining which health care provider a consumer will choose. Individual patients or groups of consumers can be activated and engaged in their care, but if they are not satisfied with their health outcomes, they may delay or stop treatment, change health care practitioners, or simply decide to not participate in any health care activities. **Patient satisfaction** measures two patient perspectives: patients' health expectations and their health outcomes. Can you identify the key issue in patient satisfaction? It is simply that each patient has their own feelings and attitudes, and those may not match the reality of the actual encounter. A patient may feel the health care practitioner did not listen to their issues as they spent "too little" time with them, or they may stop taking a prescribed medication because they expected quicker results. Only effective patient engagement protocols can prevent these types of misunderstandings and perceptions.

How does patient satisfaction differ from patient experience? ***Patient experience*** refers to an individual's perceptions of the entire or total health care interaction, beginning with the initial contact with the health care organization or practitioner office, the scheduling of an appointment, the convenience of the appointment, the parking, and the friendliness of the office staff. These interaction points refer to a pathway known as the ***patient journey***. Patient experiences are more than just clinical interactions, and all these interactions help form the patient's perception of the health experience before they even interact with the health care provider.

Patient Experience

How do we assess patients' and consumers' satisfaction with their health care interactions? The following are three common assessment opportunities that most health organizations use regularly:

1. Standard post-interaction surveys and/or phone call follow-ups
2. Detailed third-party surveys administered post-discharge from a hospital stay
3. Mailed or virtual surveys that include a net promotor score question

Most consumers and patients are familiar with follow-up surveys, whether they are delivered digitally, on paper, or via a phone call. These surveys usually occur within a week after the patient-provider interaction. Health care consumers may also receive a detailed third-party survey that covers the entire health care interaction and experience. Results from these surveys are shared with health care practitioners as well as the health care organizations with the quality goal of improving care options and identifying barriers to optimum experiences. One of the largest performance improvement measurement firms collects outpatient satisfaction survey data and has the world's largest database of patient feedback (PressGaney, n.d.). Population health managers use these data to compare their outcomes with other peer organizations.

Net promoter scores (NPS) are based on a standard question that asks whether consumers would recommend a health care company, product, or service to a friend or colleague. The NPS is a customer experience and market research metric used to measure customer satisfaction and loyalty. Respondents are categorized as promoters (happy patients who rate the organization between 9 and 10), passive (neutral patients who are pleased but not enthusiastic and rate the organization between 7 and 8), and detractors (unhappy patients who rate the organization between 0 and 6) (Nice Systems, 2021). When aggregating the data, follow this simple equation: % promoters – % detractors = net promoter score.

TABLE 12.1   Net Promoter Scoring

Not Likely					Neutral				Extremely Likely	
1	2	3	4	5	6	7	8	9	10
Detractor						Passive		Promoter	

As population health seeks to improve health outcomes, patient experience strategies will aid in overcoming barriers to successful patient-provider interactions and transitioning to patient-centric care. Recent health technology innovations can also positively affect the patient's health care journey.

Chapter Twelve New Population Health Strategies | 231

Virtual Care for Successful "High-Tech" Population Health Outcomes

What does the term ***virtual care*** mean to you? Could you describe the difference between a digital front door and a virtual storefront to a classmate? What is the role of a digital navigator? How would you explain the concept of a **hospital-at-home** program? These new population health care delivery terms reflect the rapid adoption and impact of recent technological innovations that

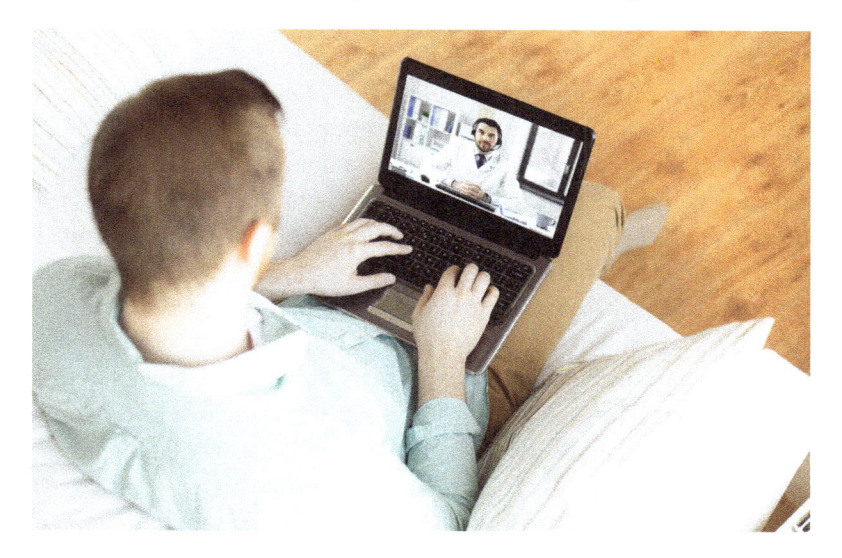

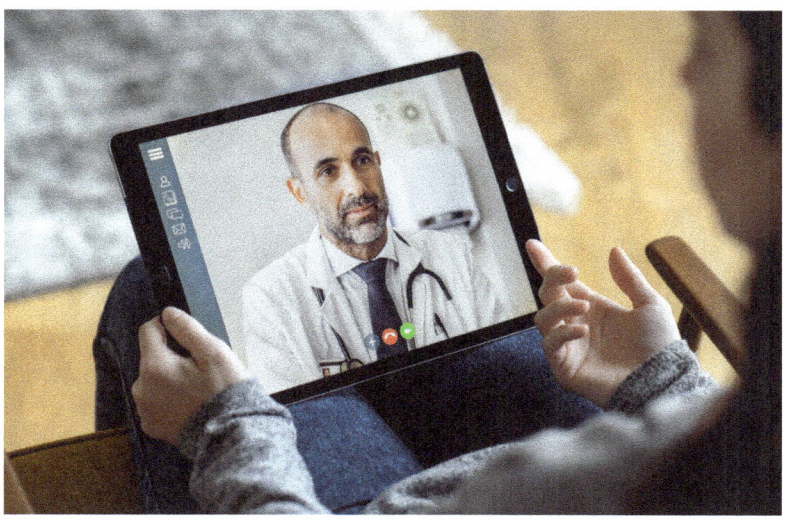

FIGURE 12.7   Virtual Care and Telehealth; Next-Day Appointments Are Too Far Out to Wait!

collectively illustrate virtual care. Understanding virtual care begins with recognizing opportunities for diverse types of digital interactions between a health provider and patient. Health professionals use the term **telehealth** to describe a digital platform with a variety and combination of options, such as audio-only, audio-video, chat-based, and store-and-forward options, the latter of which refers to transmission of health data through secure communications (Trilliant Health, 2022). Two other forms of telehealth include digital consultations among diverse health professionals and remote patient monitoring. The American Telemedicine Association (ATA) simply describes *telehealth* as the use of medical information exchanged from one site to another via secure communications to improve a patient's health status (ATA, 2020). Regardless of the term's description, the common foundation for these types of digital interactions is the ability for patients and consumers to interface with health care systems without physically being present at a health care location.

Virtual care denotes a broad health care approach that encompasses the entire continuum of care and a wide variety of digital health options (Teledoc Health, 2021). How important is virtual care? Experts suggest that digital health will reshape the entire health care sector, especially patient engagement activities, care delivery workflows, and payment models (Mohammed & Libby, 2020). Over time, the health care industry has been slowly adopting elements of telehealth and telemedicine technology on a limited scale. Telehealth and telemedicine options have proven valuable when health care specialists become unavailable at a particular site especially in rural health situations or during extremely high consumer demand situations for specialists, such as behavioral health

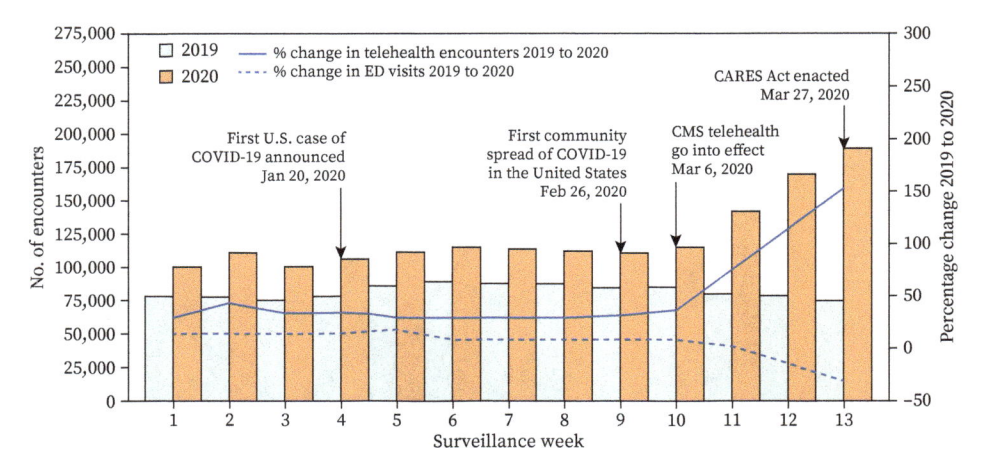

FIGURE 12.8 Number of Telehealth Patient Encounters Reported by Four Telehealth Providers That Offer Services in All States and Percentage Change in Telehealth Encounters and Emergency Department Visits—United States, January 1–March 30, 2019 (Comparison Period) and January 1–March 28, 2020 (Early Pandemic Period)

practitioners. Ask yourself, what type of global event or situation occurred that reconfigured health care delivery to move beyond limited telehealth and triggered such an important and rapid technological transformation of health care in only four weeks?

The primary catalyst for virtual care integration into the health care sector was the COVID-19 pandemic, when face-to-face health care almost halted and health systems overnight transformed to include digital care delivery options. In 2020, virtual visits increased significantly and almost doubled during the initial pandemic phase (O'Shea, 2020). Figure 12.8 shows the 150% increase in telehealth visits in four short weeks to address the COVID-19 impact on care delivery (Koonin et al., 2020). Not surprisingly, the two service areas with the largest increases were behavioral health to manage increased substance misuse and abuse (Raths, 2020) and chronic care for patients with multiple comorbidities. Due to virtual care's ability to provide continuous access and support for mental health, at least 80% of behavioral health care providers now deliver care virtually at least 60% of the time (Qualifacts & National Council of Behavioral Health, 2020). The convenience factor, a primary consumer requirement and major driver of change, also encouraged health systems to enhance and expand virtual interactions across the patient's journey. Virtual care visits are no longer alternative care delivery options but have emerged as integrated components of coordinated care management.

Aligning Virtual Care With Population Health: Mobile Applications

A widely adopted virtual care strategy for patient engagement is the use of **mobile health applications** to provide tailored and consistent support messages for at-risk groups of vulnerable populations. Another term often mentioned is *connected health,* which also seeks to encourage positive health behaviors by integrating smartphone applications that provide supportive recorded messages, patient monitoring options, and text messages (Trilliant Health, 2022). In fact, recent research shows today's university students use mobile health applications primarily for wellness, such as tracking physical activities and counting caloric intake (Jabour et al., 2021). How popular are mobile health applications? Google currently estimates during the third quarter of 2022, the number of health care and medical apps available on the Google Play store was above 50,000 (Ceci, 2022)!

Today, consumers and patients can access mobile applications that cover a range of health topics, from general wellness questions and disease prevention advice to self-management of chronic disease symptoms. The most popular mobile health applications include those that provide information on specific health conditions and symptoms, medication and pill reminders, and exercise and dietary trackers (Knerl, 2021). One reminder for all consumers is that mobile applications are not designed to replace interactions with health care providers and practitioners when necessary.

Mobile Applications and Patient Engagement

The National eHealth Collaborative (Perna, 2013) recognized the potential for aligning mobile health applications and developed a patient engagement framework that combined provider support with mobile health applications.

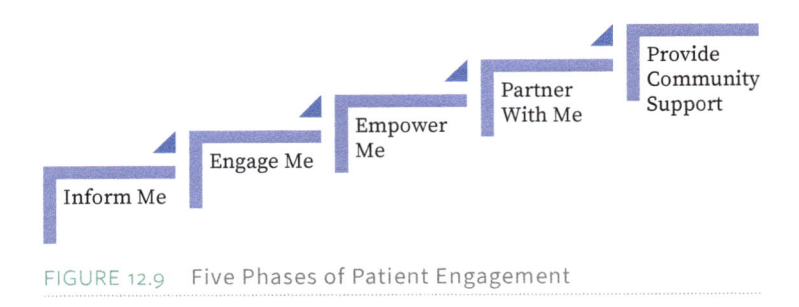

FIGURE 12.9   Five Phases of Patient Engagement

As you see, these five phases also represent the high-touch components discussed earlier in the chapter. Each sequenced step focuses on engaging the patient through the health care delivery journey and suggests digital tools and strategies that are tailored for each stage.

- Phase 1 involves introducing the patient and consumer to useful health information or educational materials delivered electronically.
- This step is quickly followed in Phase 2 with mobile communications sharing of related ideas and activities tailored to the individual's specific interest of health concern to not only attract but also retain their interest.
- A crucial opportunity occurs in Phase 3, where the shift of power transfers from the health care professional, aided by digital interaction platforms where the priority population can see, download, and even transmit personal directly with the health care provider. Mobile health-patient interactions may include the use of special apps and/or daily text reminders.
- As the patient/consumer progresses along the continuum to Phase 4, the interoperability and cooperation of a symmetrical relationship between the patient and any number of health care professionals leads to an increased number of successful engagement outcomes. In the final phase, the empowered patient is capable and confident of identifying and sharing their support community with the providers.

> **Practical Skill: Health Care Mobile Apps**
>
> Review the five phases of patient engagement in Figure 12.9. Can you see the relationship between awareness, health education, and patient empowerment in the first three phases? Which population activities would be useful to complete the "partner with me" and "provide community support"?

Population Health Virtual Care Decision-Making Strategies

Population health leaders can expect continued and rapid transformations of health technology to regularly impact health care service delivery, patient expectations and experiences, and health outcomes (Chernikoff, 2022). The evolving day-to-day clinical and nonclinical health care delivery processes and accompanying explosion of mobile applications and wearable devices place constant pressure on population health decision-makers. In addition to increasing technology costs and the loss of health care workers during COVID-19, the health care industry also faces a need for digital health workforce training and health information technology (HIT) employees. A 2020 report suggests that digital training should be a top workforce priority (Lytle, 2020). Fortunately, industry experts recently introduced a virtual care framework to aid health systems in planning their virtual care strategies. When reviewing the virtual care framework, remember that for every level, all Health Insurance Portability and Accountability Act of 1996 (HIPAA) regulations must be met, and that includes mandatory secure messaging and communication.

Level 1, based on a strong HIT foundation, requires electronic medical record (EMR) access and integration with basic business workflow processes such as scheduling, payments, and alignment with other core services. At the beginning of the chapter, the terms *digital front doors* and *virtual storefronts* were introduced. Now, you can define *digital front doors* as patient portals where consumers can access their personalized health information including lab results and communications from health professionals. *Virtual storefronts* refer to the main webpages of a health care system or hospital where all the diverse options for patient/consumer interactions appear in an extensive choice menu (AllBusiness.com, n.d.).

Level 2 provides convenient options to digitally connect (via computer or mobile phone) with a variety of health care providers, including both primary care and specialists. These virtual interactions, scheduled via sophisticated workflow platforms, allow both patients and health care practitioners to move beyond patient portal information and connect for general health conversations,

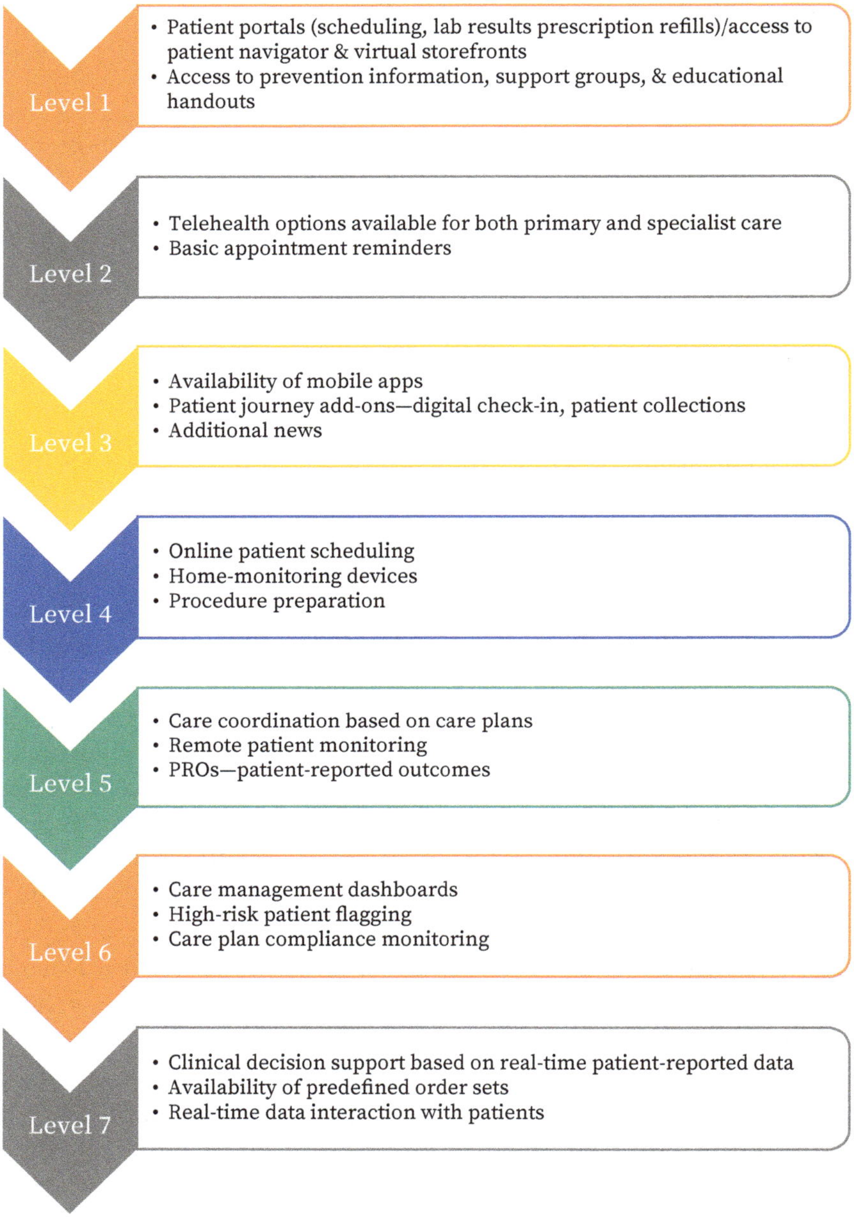

Level 1
- Patient portals (scheduling, lab results prescription refills)/access to patient navigator & virtual storefronts
- Access to prevention information, support groups, & educational handouts

Level 2
- Telehealth options available for both primary and specialist care
- Basic appointment reminders

Level 3
- Availability of mobile apps
- Patient journey add-ons—digital check-in, patient collections
- Additional news

Level 4
- Online patient scheduling
- Home-monitoring devices
- Procedure preparation

Level 5
- Care coordination based on care plans
- Remote patient monitoring
- PROs—patient-reported outcomes

Level 6
- Care management dashboards
- High-risk patient flagging
- Care plan compliance monitoring

Level 7
- Clinical decision support based on real-time patient-reported data
- Availability of predefined order sets
- Real-time data interaction with patients

FIGURE 12.10   Seven Levels of Virtual Care Framework

discussions of treatment options, care plan concerns, and review of treatment outcomes. Mobile applications allow consumers to conveniently interact with health care providers to schedule appointments and receive assistance in managing personal health records (Treichler, 2022).

Levels 3 and 4 elevate the types and number of virtual care interaction options by adopting sophisticated data analytic applications. These enhancements allow health systems to rapidly and accurately identify at-risk and vulnerable population subgroups who can benefit from the use of integrated data applications. Instead of being handed multiple papers on a clipboard at a face-to-face appointment, patients now have the convenience of checking in virtually, even if a personal interaction or treatment is needed. Level 3 options also support the sharing of an individual's care plan with all health care providers needed to ensure a thorough and successfully coordinated plan.

Level 4 enables the consumer to schedule appointments online, which eliminates the multiple phone calls and lengthy process of reaching the appropriate individual to arrange an appointment. Level 4 also provides technology to support wearables as a virtual care option for collecting health status data such as blood pressure, temperature changes, and/or other diverse health status indicators.

One of the major benefits of advanced HIT is the ability to not only affect the patient's health care but also improve the ease and quality of the provider's work processes. In **Level 5**, we begin to see the benefits of virtual care technology to decision-making as multiple providers and patients can collaborate on care plans simultaneously for better care coordination. The addition of home monitoring offers a sense of security and can be of extreme importance to a chronically ill individual. Imagine knowing that your personal heart monitor is assessing and sending data directly to the specialist for monitoring. Integrated remote home health monitoring (RHM) can aid in reducing emergency department visits, admissions for chronic care populations, and was proven to be instrumental for follow-up of COVID-19 patients (HIN, 2018; Minemyer, 2020). RHM involves complex management decisions such as deciding which patients need a service, when to integrate patient engagement options, which groups would benefit from either in-house and external health practitioner training, and how to improve overall scheduling and workflow plan (HIN, 2015).

Level 6 features virtual care techniques to advance and improve management strategies. For example, in Level 5 the patient who has the wearable device also is sharing data known as **patient-reported outcomes (PROs)**. In Level 6, that PRO information can be analyzed to create a care management dashboard that not only monitors adherence to the care plan but also can identify those patients at elevated risk. A population health care plan dashboard is a visual representation of five to seven indicators of health status. Health care providers select indicators that measure the success of a population health program. A sample dashboard might include data on the number of times an individual monitored their blood pressure, the number of days they took their medication, the number of days they exercised, and even the number of steps that were tracked. The dashboard enables the care or case manager to determine whether changing the individual's care plan is the best decision and helps flag those individuals that are becoming at elevated risk. Think how valuable this is for population health group managers who have thousands of individuals to develop and supervise care plan monitoring.

The most advanced virtual care options and population health interventions occur at **Level 7**. Given the cost of the supporting technology, personnel requirements, and potential expense of highly sophisticated sensors and wearable electronics, not all health systems will be able to maintain a presence at this level. For the patient, Level 7 provides the highest level of real-time patient-reported data available for health care provider clinical decision-making. For the health care provider, the capability to develop a predefined order set for treatment or medication and have it followed if the patient's information indicates change shows the impact of sophisticated technology on workflow ease and speed. Currently, the interoperability of health systems, monitoring devices, and decision-making and implementation tools requires Level 7 technological expertise.

Virtual Care: Population Health Technology Applications

Before you begin this section, take the time to complete a quick scan of your class and count the number of individuals who either own a smartwatch or are using a mobile application to monitor their health. A Google search for the top 10 health wearables produced 100 million results in 53 seconds (Google, 2022). Newer technologies, such as wearables, mobile health applications, and biometric remote care monitoring devices, stand out as currently available options that meet the needs of patients, health care providers, and the health care sector. Population health managers need to weigh the benefits and challenges of each type of care option.

Wearable Technology: Wellness, Monitoring, and PROs

Wearable technology refers to any type of electronic devices designed to be worn on the user's body, such as jewelry, accessories, medical devices, and clothing or elements of clothing (Yasar & Wigmore, n.d.). Health consumers have responded positively to wearables or devices that are physically worn and allow the individual to track and analyze their personal data (Daley, n.d.). Even the most basic of the wearable devices available can assist the individual in monitoring a health condition, a symptom, or even a positive health lifestyle such as the number of steps taken in a day. In fact, it is estimated that one-quarter of adult Americans now use a wearable health-related device.

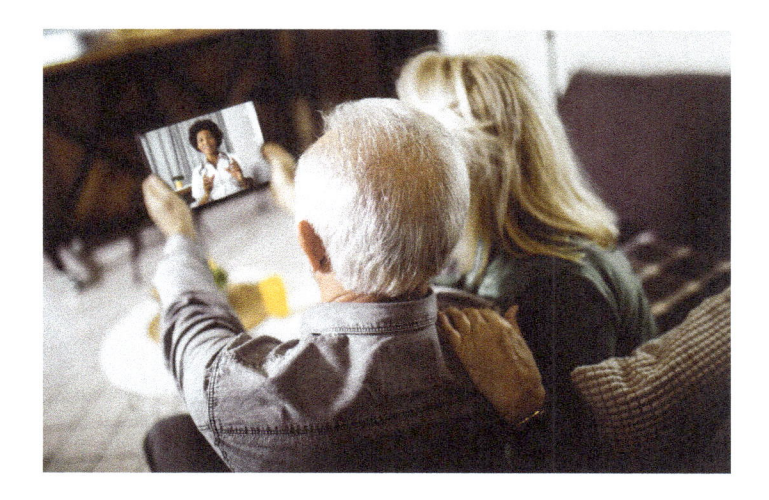

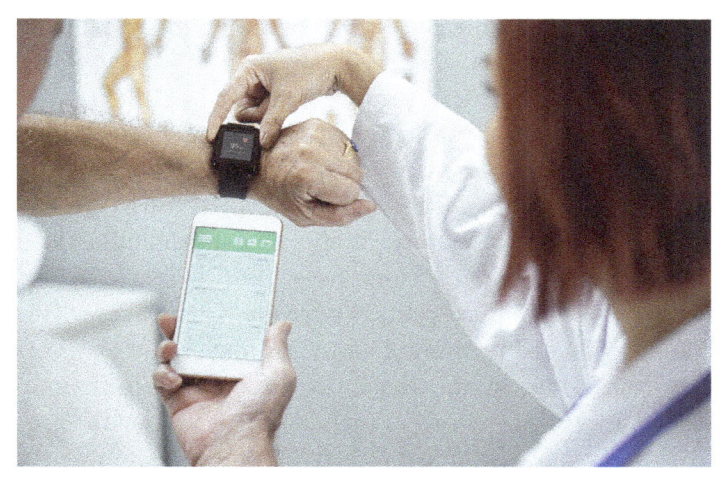

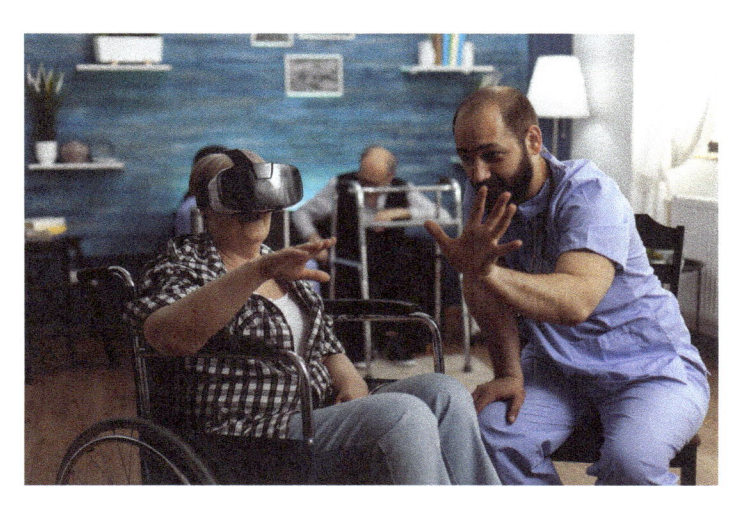

Chapter Twelve New Population Health Strategies | 239

FIGURE 12.11   Wearable and Mobile Applications

Lifestyle behavior monitors such as smartwatches and activity trackers are not the only digital options available, as now consumers can wear rings that track sleep patterns and body temperature. Although rings lack immediate feedback features, their convenience continues to increase their popularity (Kelly, 2022). The term *wearable computing* implies processing data or data communication capabilities, but the level of the computing sophistication among wearables can vary. Virtual reality, augmented reality technology, smart jackets, and a wide variety of other sophisticated tech gadgets and devices are leading us toward a better-connected and healthy lifestyle. One of the most talked-about potential technology applications, the Metaverse, is a collective virtual shared space, created by the convergence of enhanced physical and digital reality (Wile, 2022). Experts suggest multiple health opportunities within this platform that could further expand options for patient–health practitioner interactions (McKinsey, 2022). Will the Metaverse be the next space for patient-provider health interactions? We will have to wait and see.

Today, the use of biometric wearables benefits health care providers by enabling access to both quicker and more reliable data that facilitate accurate diagnostic decisions and treatment for an at-risk patient in real time. Now consumers can easily adopt self-management skills for monitoring chronic diseases with devices such as glucose monitors that transmit data via a digital device that helps health care providers assess the impacts of eating, exercise, and blood sugar levels. **Remote patient care monitoring** refers to the use of connected tools to record personal health and medical data in one location for review by a provider in another location at a different time (Trilliant Health, 2022). Research provides evidence of the successful prevention of heart failure and hospital admissions attributed to the home use of remote care monitoring devices such as blood pressure cuffs, scales, and pulse oximeters (O'Shea, 2020).

Practical Skill: Population Health: Hospital at Home

A recent population health innovation, the hospital-at-home concept, incorporates both remote health monitoring and wearables strategies that enable a select group of patients to remain in the comfort of their home. Not all health systems have the technological infrastructure or trained personnel to undertake this type of virtual care. The home hospital concept, using remote care monitoring as a post-acute care approach, attempts to reduce the costs of acute care episodes and reduce 30-day readmissions by providing the necessary treatment and follow-up in the patient's home (Vaidya, 2020). Early studies report significant progress in providing quality care at a lower cost which also supports a value-based management strategy.

Chapter Twelve New Population Health Strategies | 241

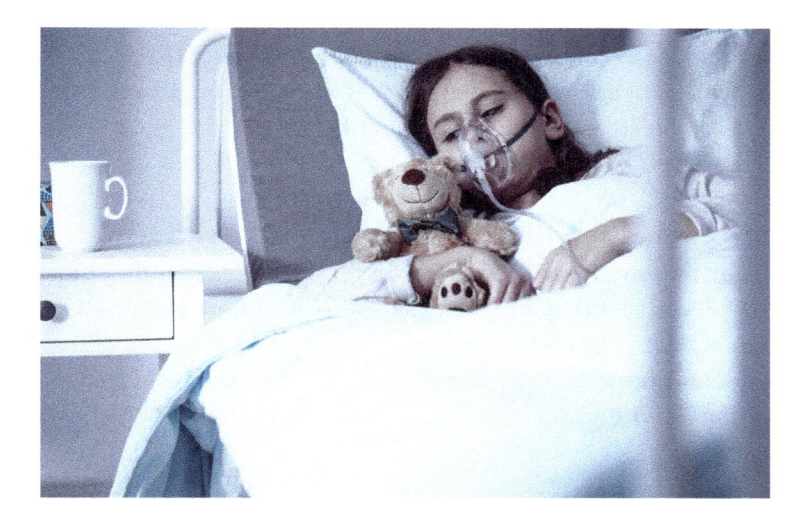

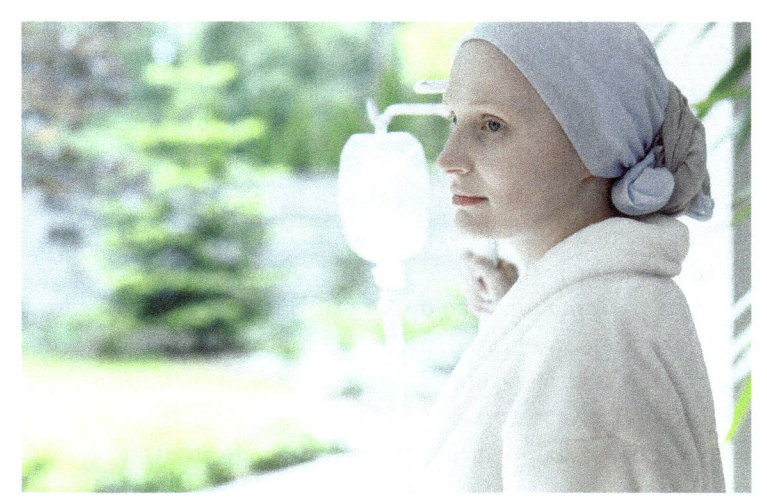

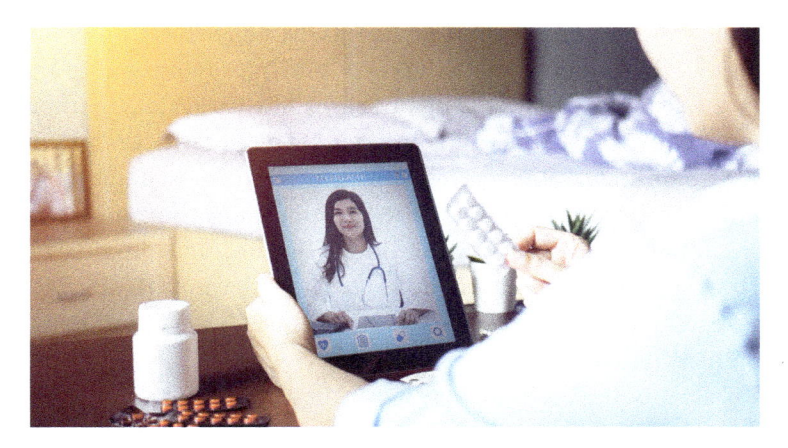

FIGURE 12.12   Hospital at Home

Medical devices and wearables represent only one of three health impact technology categories. Experts suggest that information and communication technologies can also positively affect health care providers and other professionals (Excel Medical, 2022).

Impacting Population Health Management Workflows

Current information and communication technologies together can increase the sophistication, speed, quality, and safety of workflow processes. The initial benefits begin when population health managers can leverage and align EMR real-time data for both the healthcare provider and patients' decision-making. More sophisticated technologies can provide additional workflow benefits such as:

- Improved response time for both clinical and nonclinical decision-making
- Providing flexibility and increasing efficiency of health care personnel by standardizing basic tasks such as scheduling and billing
- Aiding decision-making with real-time reporting that enhances the speed and accuracy of the risk segmentation process
- Satisfying patient's consumer needs and desires for preferred type of communication to encourage greater patient engagement
- Reducing waste as patients can be directed to the right provider at the right time and the right place
- Improving patient safety as opportunities for greater interaction and feedback become integrated into patient journeys
- Standardizing health and staff training to ensure virtual and digital coaching skills are uniform across a system
- Increasing medication safety protocols and automated checklists for improved safety and quality

Today, we know that the right technology can assist with increasing efficiency, empowering patients, reducing costs, and improving quality and patient safety. Why? Because it allows the health care delivery system to improve care transitions, keep care at the home and not at the health care practitioner's office, and streamline inappropriate care away from emergency departments. As nonhealth care industries enter the health sector, the concept of virtual clinics for common ailments and conditions has become a reality taking the next step beyond individual interactions and consultations (Landi, 2022). Each one of these achievements aids care delivery quality and results in lowered population health care costs.

Digital assistants and their impact on workflow represent another example of new technological innovations applied to improve population health workflows. Efficiencies occur when resources are put to their best use. Digital assistants'

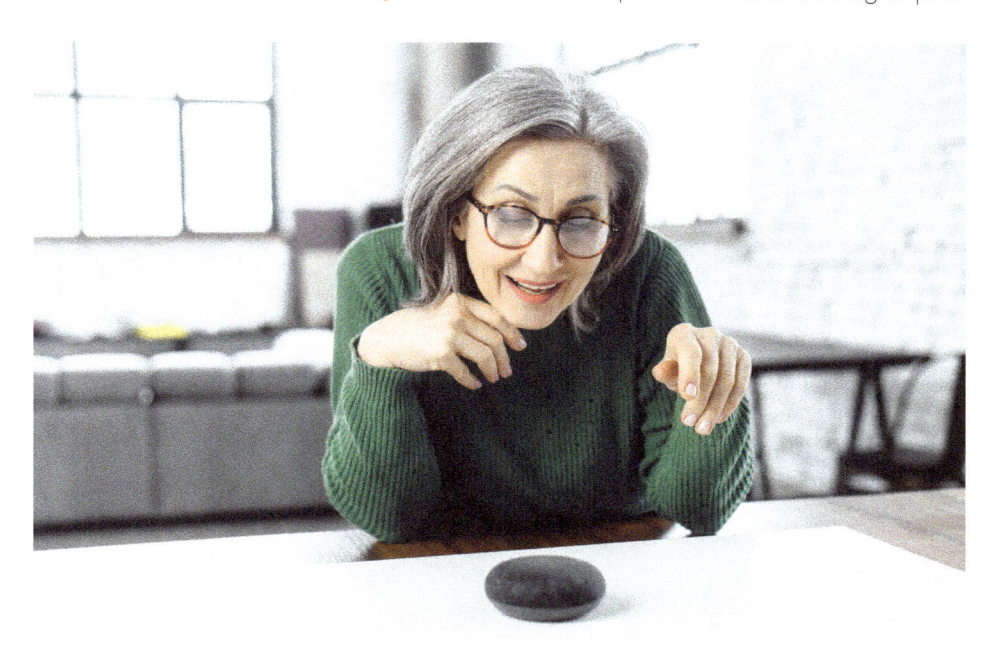

Chapter Twelve New Population Health Strategies | 243

FIGURE 12.13   Virtual Care and Digital Assistant Applications

Practical Skill: Digital Assistants

Digital care journeys can mimic face-to-face pathway versions as patients move through the continuum of care. A **digital assistant**, or virtual assistant, provides technology designed to aid users by answering questions and processing simple tasks (Workgrid, n.d.). You might think of them as like Siri or Alexa as they respond and complete easy connections. In health care, digital assistants help users navigate routine virtual care functions that do not require human interaction. For example, they can assist in scheduling an appointment, or arranging transportation if needed, or ensure that medications will be delivered (Dua, 2022). At-risk populations often include seniors with chronic diseases, digital assistants can be extremely valuable in ensuring continuity of care and care coordination. Digital assistants also free up health providers to spend less time away from patient care.

free up health providers to spend more time with their patients and practice medicine instead of administrative duties to increase efficiency. As described by the Institute for Healthcare Improvement, the workflow benefit is matching the work with the worker (Institute for Healthcare Improvement, n.d.). As virtual care becomes more embedded in the population health approach, additional and unexpected health benefits have appeared.

> **Practical Skill: Population Health: Will Digital Health Close Gaps in Health Equity? An Unexpected Benefit?**
>
> Health experts are noticing an important benefit of digital health as evidence appears that virtual care can contribute to closing gaps in health equity. A recent industry study, showed positive outcomes in reducing health inequities for new digital care models (Virta Health, 2022) that included the following major population health components in the intervention:
>
> - Enabled access to health care providers
> - Continuous oversight and engagement of care plans
> - Food-as-medicine approaches to reverse, not manage, diabetes
> - Behavioral support and community involvement
>
> Instructions:
>
> 1. Review the following article:
>
> Virta Health. (2022). *Is digital health closing gaps in health equity?* Fierce Healthcare, December 5, 2022. https://tinyurl.com/yuhpzumc
>
> 2. Answer the following questions:
>   a. Identify the health metrics and the statistics used as the assessment tools to prove an impact on health equity.
>   b. Discuss which factors of the Virta Health intervention led to success.

Digital health and virtual care options increase daily, and hold promises for improving population health outcomes for all Americans.

Virtual Care Challenges

Adoption of new health technological innovations can raise concern for either patient safety or privacy. However, strong regulating legislation such as HIPAA, evidence-based requirements for appropriate clinical use, and adoption protocols have led to high consumer participation. Growing patient and health care practitioner trust seems to suggest that current efforts not only are widely accepted but also produce positive health outcomes. Consumer surveys report up to 75% of patients who had never tried telehealth visits expressed an interest in participating (Wike, 2015), and other survey results showspecific digital applications provide improved access and patient/provider flexibility (HIN, 2018). Seniors especially will benefit as insurance companies begin the addition of home health services as supplemental benefits (King, 2022).

However, health care practitioners express concern over the uncertainty of current payment reimbursement as based on the use of COVID-19 waivers. Physicians particularly are focused on establishing a standard for payment for virtual care time (Adams et al., 2022). These concerns over payment may be alleviated soon as major health systems begin to charge patients for clinical time and expertise needed when reviewing patient portal messages (Dyrda, 2022). These payment strategies envision charging patients for telehealth that covers patient-provider messaging if the message takes longer than 5 minutes or requires medical expertise (Muoio, 2022). Depending on the type of review necessary by the health care provider, specific types of messaging may trigger additional costs to the patients' insurance (Raths, 2022). Virtual care will continue to be an additional care coordination model available for health care providers.

Summary

Innovative population health care delivery models require convenient, patient-centered interactions facilitated by high-tech and high-touch options. Wearables, mobile applications, and remote patient monitoring options provide opportunities to increase patient engagement and empowerment that result in improved health care outcomes, better utilization of care, and lowered costs. Today's patients expect consumer amenities to accompany their health care journeys and telehealth options such as patient portals, online scheduling, and digital consultations offer a complementary strategy that increases patient satisfaction and enhances the entire health care experience. Virtual care is not the future; it is now and already on a trajectory to become the health care delivery norm as it provides greater convenience and flexibility for not only the patient, but the health professional and partnering organization as well. This chapter explained four types of digital health application strategies, including:

1. Aligning the HIT infrastructures to improve data access and workflow via the adoption of EMRs
2. Applying advanced analytics for population health tasks such as risk segmentation
3. Adopting digital decision-making applications available for all stakeholders
4. Integrating e-health applications such as wearables, mobile applications, and personalized health care (Olla & Tan, 2023)

Digital health applications have increased health care practitioner flexibility to interact with patients by revising traditional workflow processes such as appointment scheduling, patient billing and payments, and medication ordering. Today, we know that the right technology can assist with increasing efficiency, empowering patients, reducing costs, and improving quality and patient safety. Engaging patients beyond hospital walls with consumer convenient technology will improve patient-provider interactions and health care practitioner workflow processes.

Discussion Questions

1. Compare the differences between patient engagement, satisfaction, and experience.
2. Describe the role of patient empowerment. Does focusing on adherence and compliance influence patient empowerment?
3. Self-efficacy is a concept presented as part of the patient engagement capacity model and is also included in the health belief model. Why is the component so critical to patient engagement?
4. When would it be appropriate to use the net promoter score question? What valuable information can you learn? Why are there three categories?
5. Explain the virtual care perspective in comparison to the use of telehealth.
6. Do you use mobile health applications on your smartphone? Share a summary of the capabilities of the app and your experiences.
7. Review the seven levels of virtual care framework. Which components of the first four levels would you consider to be essential for any health care practitioner or organization?

References

Adams, K., Gonzalez, G., & Diaz, N. (2022). *Three reasons physicians resist telehealth*. Becker's Hospital Review, April 1, 2022. https://www.beckershospitalreview.com/telehealth/3-reasons-physicians-resist-telehealth.html?origin=CIOE&utm_source=CIO-E&utm_medium=email&utm_content=newsletter&oly_enc_id=1450I5993723C6U

AllBusiness.com. (n.d.). *Definition of a virtual storefront*. https://www.allbusiness.com/barrons_dictionary/dictionary-virtual-storefront-4960671-1.html

American Telemedicine Association. (2020, September 21). *ATA's standard telehealth terminology and policy language for states on medical practice*. https://www.americantelemed.org/wp-content/uploads/2020/10/ATA-_Medical-Practice-10-5-20.pdf

Bolbjerg, M. (2022, October 17). *The seven levels of virtual care. Getting leaner and boosting revenue.* Qure4u. Blog. https://www.qure4u.com/the-7-levels-of-digital-care-getting-leaner-and-boosting-revenue/

Brown, M. & Bussell, J. (2011). Medication adherence: WHO cares? *Mayo Clin Proc.* Apr. 86(4): 304–314. Doi: 10.4065/mcp.2010.0575 https://www.ncbi.nlm.nih.gov/pmc/articles/PMC3068890/#:~:text=Although%20these%20medications%20are%20effective,take%20their%20medications%20as%20prescribed

Ceci, L. (2022, November 8). *Google Play: Number of available medical apps as of Q3 2022.* Statista. https://www.statista.com/statistics/779919/health-apps-available-google-play-worldwide/#:~:text=Google%20Play%3A%20number%20of%20available%20medical%20apps%20as%20of%20Q3%202022&text=During%20the%20last%20measured%20period,compared%20to%20the%20previous%20quarter

Centers for Disease Control and Prevention. (2022). *Smoking cessation: Fast facts.* https://www.cdc.gov/tobacco/data_statistics/fact_sheets/cessation/smoking-cessation-fast-facts/index.html

Chernikoff, D. (2022). *The rapid transformation of healthcare.* enterprise.nxt, February 16, 2022 https://www.hpe.com/us/en/insights/articles/the-rapid-transformation-of-healthcare-2104.html

Culbertson, G. (2020, January/February). Ethical community engagement: Lessons learned. *Healthcare Executive,* 40–44.

Daley, S. (n.d.). *What is wearable technology? Examples of wearables.* Builtin. https://builtin.com/wearables

Dua, D. (2022, June 27). *How a digital health assistant improves outcomes and reduces member churn.* Fierce Healthcare, June 27, 2022. https://www.fiercehealthcare.com/payers/optum-launches-new-solution-aimed-driving-down-unnecessary-testing

Dyrda, L. (2022). *What physicians, patients think of charging for MyChart messages.* Becker's Hospital Review, November 18, 2022. https://www.beckershospitalreview.com/ehrs/what-clinicians-patients-think-of-charging-for-mychart-messages.html

Excel Medical. (2022, September 23). *The impact of patient care technologies on the quality and cost of healthcare.* https://www.excel-medical.com/the-impact-of-patient-care-technologies-on-the-quality-and-cost-of-healthcare/

Google. (2022, December 11). *The top ten health wearables in 2022.* https://www.google.com/search?q=the+top+10+health+wearables+2022&rlz=1C1GCEA_enUS1018US1018&sxsrf=ALiCzsZRNu24gHr4Cv49Dy7OvYL6kJMwXw:1670767446838&ei=VuOVY7_PMvbV-5NoP6ISg4A4&start=0&sa=N&ved=2ahUKEwi_0q7h3fH7AhX2KlkFHWgCCOw4ChDy-0wN6BAgHEAQ&biw=1280&bih=649&dpr=1.5

Graffigna, G., & Barello, S. (2018). Spotlight on the Patient Health Engagement model (PHE model): A psychosocial theory to understand people's meaningful engagement in their own health care. *Patient Prefer Adherence, 12,* 1261–1271. https://www.ncbi.nlm.nih.gov/pmc/articles/PMC6056150

Hagland, M. (2022). *Leaders are advancing the patient experience—across diverse environments*. Healthcare Innovation Group, November 9, 2022. https://www.hcinnovationgroup.com/population-health-management/patient-engagement/blog/21286600/leaders-are-advancing-the-patient-experienceacross-diverse-environments?utm_source=HI+Daily+NL&utm_medium=email&utm_campaign=CPS221111063&o_eid=6978A6266356F5Z&rdx.ident[pull]=omeda|6978A626635 6F5Z&oly_enc_id=6978A6266356F5Z

Health Information Network. (2015). *Remote patient monitoring for chronic condition management*. https://hin.3dcartstores.com/Remote-Patient-Monitoring-for-Chronic-Condition-Management-a-45-minute-webinar-on-February-24-2015-now-available-for-replay_p_5012.html

Health Information Network. (2018). *Telehealth and remote patient monitoring in 2018*. http://www.hin.com/library/registerTelehealthRemoteMonitoring2018.html

Health Information Network. (2019). *Patient engagement in 2019: Positive payoffs from patients activated in their healthcare*. http://www.hin.com/library/registerPatientEngagement2019.html

Heath, S. (2017). *What is the patient activation measure in patient-centered care?* Patient Engagement HIT, September 12, 2017. https://patientengagementhit.com/news/what-is-the-patient-activation-measure-in-patient-centered-care

Heath, S. (2019). *Patient engagement strategies for improving patient activation*. Patient Engagement HIT, March 1, 2019. https://patientengagementhit.com/features/patient-engagement-strategies-for-improving-patient-activation

Hibbard, J. H., Stockard, J., Mahoney, E. R., & Tusler, M. (2004). Development of the Patient Activation Measure (PAM): Conceptualizing and measuring activation in patients and consumers. *Health Services Research*, *39*(4 Pt 1), 1005–1026. DOI: 10.1111/j.1475-6773.2004.00269

Institute of Health Improvement. (n.d.). *Across the chasm aim 5: Health care must be efficient*. https://www.ihi.org/resources/Pages/ImprovementStories/HealthCareMustBeEfficientAim5.aspx

Iuga, A. O., & McGuire, M. J. (2014). Adherence and health care costs. *Risk Management and Healthcare Policy*, *7*, 35–44. https://doi.org/10.2147/RMHP.S19801

Jabour, A., Rehman, W. Idrees, S., Thanganadar, H., Hira, K., & Alarifi, M. (2021, May 31). The adoption of mobile health applications among university students in health colleges. *Journal of Multidisciplinary Healthcare*, *14*, 1267–1273. https://www.ncbi.nlm.nih.gov/pmc/articles/PMC8178693/

Joint Committee on Terminology. (2012). Report of the 2011 Joint Committee on Health Education and Promotion Terminology. *American Journal of Health Education*, 43(2).

Kelly, S. (2022). *Forget smartwatches, consumers are snapping up these quirky alternatives*. CNN Business, December 3, 2022. https://www.cnn.com/2022/12/03/tech/alternative-wearable-devices/index.html

King, N. (2022). *Milliman: Home benefits surge in popularity among Medicare Advantage plans.* Fierce Healthcare, November 17, 2022. https://www.fiercehealthcare.com/payers/milliman-home-benefits-surge-popularity-among-medicare-advantage-plans

Knerl, L. (2021, June 15). *Twelve best healthcare apps for patients*. HP. https://www.hp.com/us-en/shop/tech-takes/best-healthcare-apps-for-patients

Koonin, L. M., Hoots, B., Tsang, C. A., Leroy, Z., Farris, K., Tilman, Jolly, B. T., Antall, P., McCabe, B., Zelis, C. B. R., Tong, I., & Harris, A. M. (2020). Trends in the use of telehealth during the emergence of the COVID-19 pandemic—United States, January–March 2020. *Morbidity and Mortality Weekly Report, 69*, 1595–1599. http://dx.doi.org/10.15585/mmwr.mm6943a3external icon

Landi, H. (2022, November 15). *Amazon's latest push into digital health: A virtual clinic for common conditions like allergies and hair loss.* Fierce Healthcare., https://www.fiercehealthcare.com/health-tech/amazon-care-amazon-clinic-online-retail-giant-rolls-out-virtual-care-common-conditions

Lewis, J., Lewis, M. D., Daniels, J. A., & D'Andrea, M. J. (1998). Community counseling and the counseling process. In *Community counseling: Empowerment strategies for a diverse society* (2nd ed.; pp. 122–170). Brooks/Cole Publishing Co.

Lytle, T. (2020, February 24). *The healthcare industry's top HR challenges*. ShRM.H https://www.shrm.org/hr-today/news/hr-magazine/spring2020/pages/health-care-industry-top-hr-challenges.aspx

McKinsey Digital. (2022, March 29). *What is the Metaverse—and what does it mean for business?* https://www.mckinsey.com/capabilities/mckinsey-digital/our-insights/what-is-the-metaverse-and-what-does-it-mean-for-business

Minemyer, P. (2020). *A look inside Geisinger's new remote monitoring program for COVID-19 patients.* Fierce Healthcare, June 11, 2020. https://www.fiercehealthcare.com/hospitals/a-look-inside-geisinger-s-new-remote-monitoring-program-for-covid-19-patients?utm_medium=nl&utm_source=internal&mrkid=931686&mkt_tok=eyJpIjoiT-0dZM01UY3labVkwWVdGaSIsInQiOiJkQXJFZGs0N0lYUWhHUlN0c1NuOWFcL1FX-Z2tHOFJxYkg1Zk4xbnkxOElqVGF3Rzd5YXpLMTU1TlNNbHNcL0FlUnFGT25pTXAx-WElBbUpVZWJzMjJqZUVUR0ttN2JONmhkejZJTXUwdlwvbXhsaFQ0Zk9VWjFQb-WU5cTRcL2NHV1BGcmwifQ%3D%3D

Mohammed, A. S., & Libby, D. (2020, November 18). *Digital health will reshape patient engagement, care delivery and payment models.* ECG Management Consultants. https://www.ecgmc.com/thought-leadership/whitepapers/we-believe-series-digital-health-will-reshape-patient-engagement-care-delivery-and-payment-models

Muoio, D. (2022). *As major hospitals now bill for some patient-provider messaging, the move could usher wider adoption.* Fierce Healthcare, December 2, 2022. https://www.fiercehealthcare.com/providers/major-providers-decision-bill-time-consuming-electronic-patient-messages-could-usher

Nice Systems. (2021). *What is a net promotor?* https://www.netpromoter.com/know/

Olla, P., & Tan, J. (2023). *Digital health care: Perspectives, applications, and cases*. Jones & Bartlett Publishing.

O'Shea, D. (2020). *How health care providers can use technology to help improve patient care and their practices*. Modern Healthcare, December 18, 2020. https://www.modernhealthcare.com/technology/how-health-care-providers-can-use-technology-help-improve-patient-care-and-their

Parvanta, C., Nelson, D., & Harner, R. (2018). *Public health communication: Critical tools and strategies*. Jones & Bartlett Publishing.

Perna, G. (2013). *5 steps to patient engagement, a NEHC framework is created*. Healthcare Innovation, April 10, 2013. https://www.hcinnovationgroup.com/clinical-it/clinical-documentation/article/13020460/5-steps-to-patient-engagement-a-nehc-framework-is-created

Pfeifer, E. (2022). *Ah no! A no-show! Why patients do not show up for appointments, and how to reduce patient no-shows*. Equiscript. https://www.equiscript.com/blog/patient-no-shows

Phreesia. (2023). *Patient Activation Measure®*. https://www.phreesia.com/patient-activation-measure/

PressGaney. (n.d.). Putting human experience at the heart of healthcare. https://www.pressganey.com/company/

Purtilo, R., & Haddad, A. (1996). *Health professional and patient interaction*. W. B. Saunders Publishing.

Qualifacts & National Council of Behavioral Health. (2020). *The new role of virtual care in behavioral healthcare*. https://naccme.s3.amazonaws.com/Qualifacts+August+2020+WP/The_New_Role_Of_Virtual_Care_In_Behavioral_Healthcare__Qualifacts.pdf?__hstc=233546881.9eaa5e568f758a79e21a1a75923e4184.1603991852815.1603991852815.1603991852815.1&__hssc=233546881.1.1603991852816&__hsfp=3055432663

Raths, D. (2020). *Highmark adds tele-addiction, peer support services to SUD recovery approach*. Healthcare Innovation, December 28, 2020. https://www.hcinnovationgroup.com/population-health-management/behavioral-health/article/21204045/highmark-adds-teleaddiction-peer-support-services-to-sud-recovery-approach?utm_source=HI+Daily+NL&utm_medium=email&utm_campaign=CPS201231003&o_eid=6978A6266356F5Z&rdx.ident%5Bpull%5D=omeda%7C6978A6266356F5Z&oly_enc_id=6978A6266356F5Z

Raths, D. (2022). *Health systems begin charging for some portal message responses*. Healthcare Innovation, November 16, 2022. https://www.hcinnovationgroup.com/clinical-it/patient-portals/article/21287423/health-systems-begin-charging-for-some-portal-message-responses?utm_source=HI+Daily+NL&utm_medium=email&utm_campaign=CPS221117084&o_eid=6978A6266356F5Z&rdx.ident[pull]=omeda|6978A6266356F5Z&oly_enc_id=6978A6266356F5Z

Scott, D. (2019). *Patient engagement in 2019: Will it impact patient outcomes?* Spok, July 11, 2019. 2 https://www.spok.com/blog/patient-engagement-in-2019-can-it-impact-patient-outcomes/

Sieck, C., Walker, D., Sheldon, R., & McAlearney, A. (2019). The patient engagement capacity model: What factors determine a patient's ability to engage? *NEJM Catalyst*, March 13, 2019. https://nam05.safelinks.protection.outlook.com/?url=https%3A%2F%2Fcatalyst.nejm.org%2Fpatient-engagement-capacity model%2F&data=01%7C01%7Canne.hewitt%40shu.edu%7C9ae44a0dba4c46706a1208d6b513b4c5%7C51f07c2253b744dfb97ca13261d71075%7C1&sdata=OSbrk3NbO1dierYT%2BcONz6RZmTXpk6%2BsOzxEAtI%2BOZc%3D&reserved=0

Teledoc Health. (2021). *Telemedicine vs. virtual care: defining the difference.* https://intouch-health.com/finding-the-right-term-for-modern-digital-healthcare/

Treichler, C. (2022, June 30). *Fourteen best online apps that make personal health easier.* https://www.onlinedoctor.com/15-best-online-medical-apps-that-make-personal-health-easier/

Trilliant Health. (2022, February). *Trends shaping the health economy*: *Telehealth.* https://www.trillianthealth.com/insights/reports/telehealth-trends-shaping-the-health-economy

Vaidya, A. (2020, December 1). *Biofourmis launches hospital-at-home solution nationwide.* MedCityNews. https://medcitynews.com/2020/12/brigham-and-womens-biofourmis-launch-hospital-at-home-solution-nationwide/

Virta Health. (2022, December 5). *Is digital health closing gaps in health equity?* Fierce Healthcare. https://www.fiercehealthcare.com/sponsored/digital-health-closing-gaps-health-equity

Wike, K. (2015). *Seventy-five percent of patients 'express interest' in using telemedicine.* Health IT Outcomes. https://www.healthitoutcomes.com/doc/of-patients-express-interest-in-using-telemedicine-0001

Wile, J. (2022, October 21). *What is the metaverse and should you be buying in*https://www.gartner.com/en/articles/what-is-a-metaverse

Workgrid. (n.d.). *What is a digital assistant?* https://www.workgrid.com/article/what-is-a-digital-assistant

Yasar, K., & Wigmore, I. (n.d.). *Wearable technology.* TechTarget. https://www.techtarget.com/searchmobilecomputing/definition/wearable-technology

Credits

Fig. 12.1: Generated with FreeWordCloudGenerator.com.

Fig. 12.2a: Copyright © 2018 Depositphotos/VitalikRadko.

Fig. 12.2b: Copyright © 2013 Depositphotos/Wavebreakmedia.

Fig. 12.2c: Copyright © 2014 Depositphotos/realinemedia.

Fig. 12.3a: Copyright © by Microsoft.

Fig. 12.3b: Copyright © by Microsoft.

Fig. 12.3c: Copyright © by Microsoft.

Fig. 12.4: Copyright © 2015 Depositphotos/photographee.eu.

Fig. 12.6: Adapted from Cynthia Siek, et al., "The Patient Engagement Capacity Model: What Factors Determine a Patient's Ability to Engage?," *NEJM Catalyst*. Copyright © 2019 by Massachusetts Medical Society.

Fig. 12.7a: Copyright © 2020 Depositphotos/Syda_Productions.

Fig. 12.7b: Copyright © 2020 Depositphotos/ridofranz.

Fig. 12.8: Source: https://www.cdc.gov/mmwr/volumes/69/wr/mm6943a3.htm.

Fig. 12.10: Source: Adapted from https://www.qure4u.com/the-7-levels-of-digital-care-getting-leaner-and-boosting-revenue/.

Fig. 12.11a: Copyright © 2020 Depositphotos/adriaticphoto.

Fig. 12.11b: Copyright © 2019 Depositphotos/DragonImages.

Fig. 12.11c: Copyright © 2023 Depositphotos/DragosCondreaW.

Fig. 12.12a: Copyright © 2019 Depositphotos/photographee.eu.

Fig. 12.12b: Copyright © 2017 Depositphotos/photographee.eu.

Fig. 12.12c: Copyright © 2020 Depositphotos/asiandelight.

Fig. 12.13: Copyright © 2021 Depositphotos/VadymPastukh.

CHAPTER THIRTEEN

Today's Challenges and Tomorrow's Opportunities

Chapter Description

This chapter captures the impact of a turbulent healthscape, beginning with the COVID-19 pandemic in early 2020, continuing with the amazing technological achievements, and advancing to the unprecedented service delivery transformations that dominate the health care sector today. As the industry struggles to overcome extreme workforce shortages and burnout, high inflation, and increased competition from nonhealth care sector disruptors, the primary population health goals remain improving quality and outcomes and lowering costs. This chapter provides potential solutions to these major challenges by identifying future trends that will directly affect population health

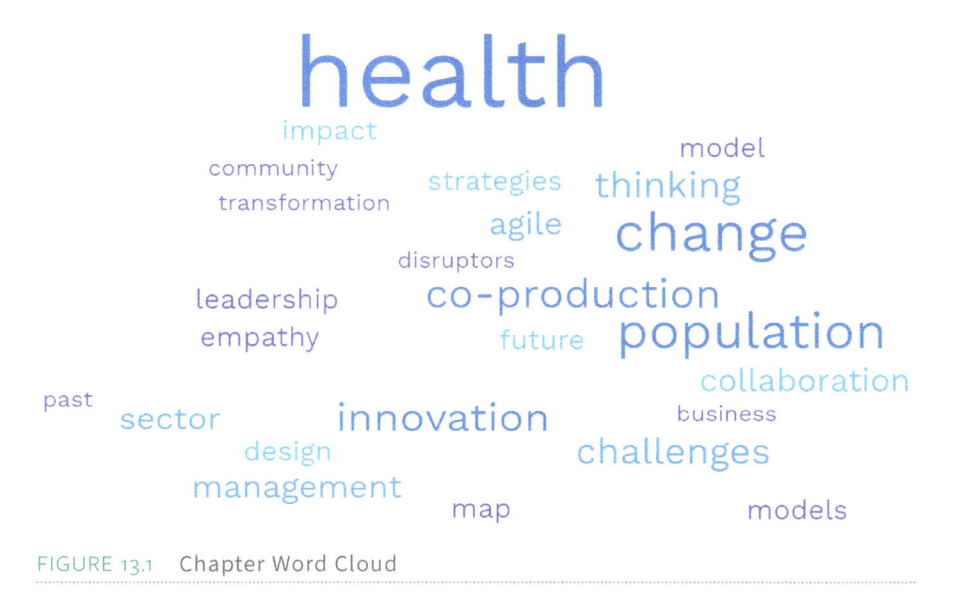

FIGURE 13.1   Chapter Word Cloud

253

care. Four population health strategies, which include design thinking for innovation, change management techniques, co-production of health options, and agile management, provide useful real-world skill sets to prepare for these unparalleled challenges.

Chapter Objectives

After completing this chapter, students will be able to:

1. Discus the major drivers of health sector transformation
2. Identify at least three future challenges for population health
3. Explain the five-step process of innovation
4. Complete an empathy map
5. Compare the levels of community cooperation with the business version
6. Provide recent examples of the co-production of health model
7. Share an application of the PAST model of change
8. Describe the characteristics of agile management

Key Words

Agile leadership	Design thinking	Grand challenge	Radical collaboration
Change management	Disruption	Ideation	Reengineering
Collaboration	Divergent thinking	Innovation	Reorganizing
Co-production of health	Empathy map	PAST change model	Wicked problem

Population Health: The Challenges Ahead

As recent national headlines illustrate, the barriers to quality health care continue as major obstacles for population health. In a recent Centers for Medicare & Medicaid Services (CMMS) report, U.S. health care spending increased by 2.7% to $4.3 trillion in 2021 (Robertson, 2022) an amount that represents 18.3% of the nation's economy (Martin et al., 2022). And yet, American's life expectancy, a prominent indicator of a nation's health status, dropped significantly from the 1996 level of 78.8 years to 76.4 years and effectively wiped out the gains of more than 20 years (Wernau & Kamp, 2022). The individual cost of health care over a lifetime, if paying for health insurance on your own, rose to $700,000, which is more than double what a person with employer-sponsored insurance is forecasted to pay (Grieve, 2022; Synchrony, 2022). The impact of COVID-19,

Chapter Thirteen Today's Challenges and Tomorrow's Opportunities | 255

U.S. Life Expectancy Fell to Lowest Level Since 1996

Covid-19 and opioid overdoses contributed to a 5% rise in death rate last year

Wernau, J. & Kamp, J. (2022, December 22). U.S. Life expectancy fell to lowest level since 1996. The Wall Street Journal. A3.

https://www.wsj.com/articles/u-s-life-expectancy-fell-to-lowest-level-since-1996-11671667059

How the Covid-19 Pandemic Changed Americans' Health for the Worse

Heart disease and drug overdoses are among afflictions exacting a higher toll than before

Abbot, B. (2022, August 4). How the Covid-19 Pandemic Changed American's Health for the Worse. Wall Street Journal, p. A6.

https://www.wsj.com/articles/how-the-covid-19-pandemic-changed-americans-health-for-the-worse-11659260165

National Health Care Spending in 2021: Decline in Federal Spending Outweighs Greater Use of Health Care

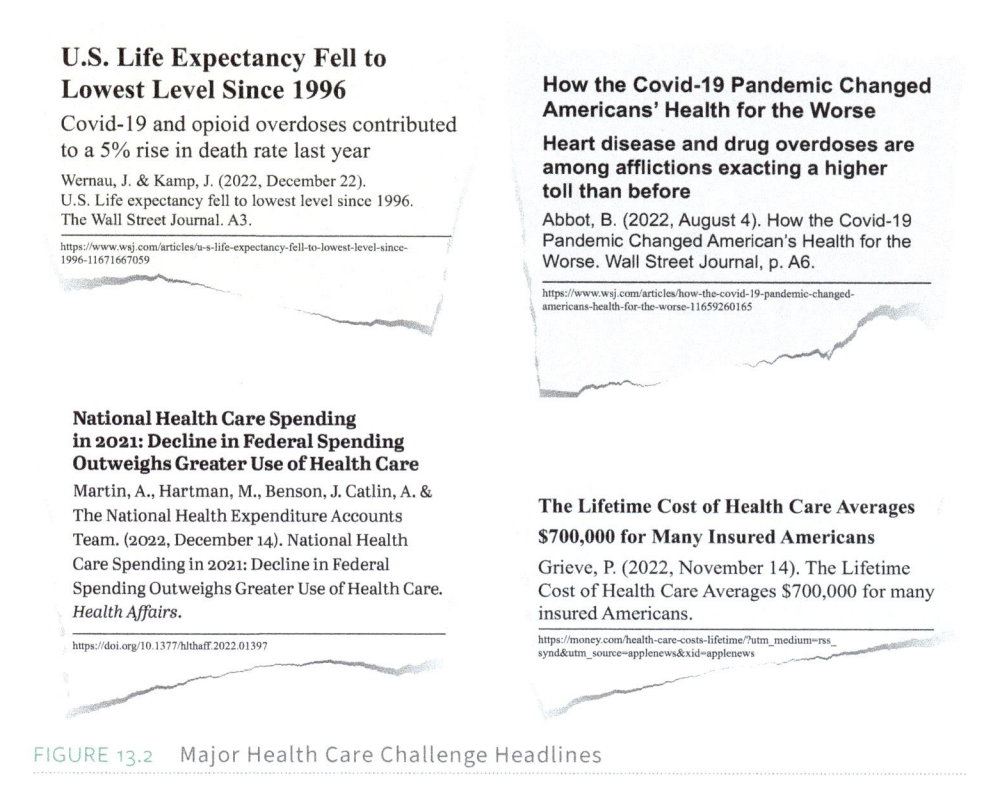

Martin, A., Hartman, M., Benson, J. Catlin, A. & The National Health Expenditure Accounts Team. (2022, December 14). National Health Care Spending in 2021: Decline in Federal Spending Outweighs Greater Use of Health Care. *Health Affairs*.

https://doi.org/10.1377/hlthaff.2022.01397

The Lifetime Cost of Health Care Averages $700,000 for Many Insured Americans

Grieve, P. (2022, November 14). The Lifetime Cost of Health Care Averages $700,000 for many insured Americans.

https://money.com/health-care-costs-lifetime/?utm_medium=rss_synd&utm_source=applenews&xid=applenews

FIGURE 13.2   Major Health Care Challenge Headlines

the worst global pandemic since 1918, caused a serious decline in U.S. kindergarten vaccination rates as well as a significant increase in the age-adjusted rate of U.S. drug overdoses from 22 to 28 per 100,000 population (Abbott, 2022), and the disease remains the third leading cause of death overall.

Experts refer to this type of environmental scenario as a *wicked problem* or a *grand challenge* because of the tremendous impact on entire populations and the resulting revolution for delivering health care. Challenges that have no easy solutions are known as **wicked problems** "because they involve many interdependent, changing, and difficult to define [sic] factors" (Nembhard et al., 2020). Over the years, health disparities have emerged as a wicked health problem despite continued national initiatives such as the Healthy People 10-year goals. **Grand challenges** also focus on large, unresolved problems (Colquitt & George, 2011; George, 2014), particularly those with complex interactions and substantial uncertainty (Ferraro et al., 2015). Wouldn't the recent COVID-19 pandemic fit this definition? An especially wicked problem is the extraordinary issue of global sustainability. Should population health also be concerned with environmental, social, and governance (ESG) issues (Perez et al., 2022)? Global sustainability fits the definition of a wicked problem to solve.

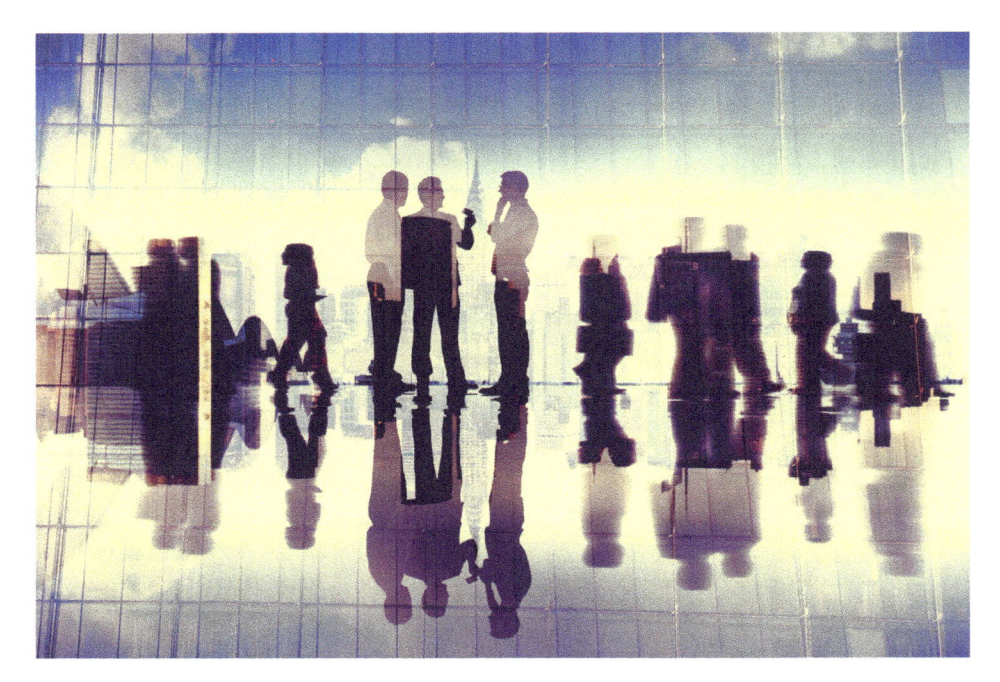

FIGURE 13.3   Solving Future Population Health Challenges

How will population health experts face these formidable obstacles? Where are the pathways of service delivery that have the most potential for the future? Which innovative solutions will result in improved quality of care? Each year, professional health care organizations, health care sector publications, consultants, and other health invested companies and stakeholders identify major trends to help guide the health sector. The summary table (Table 13.1) presents a collation of future health care trends identified by various expert sources.

Can you identify trends that would be appropriate for population health? Do you see any commonalities across all the recommendations? Review these three broad themes for health care change:

- Digital technology that affects clinical decisions, care delivery, and workflow:
    o Prioritize technological upgrades that provide value to all stakeholders
    o Address workforce overload and shortage to improve provider and staff satisfaction
    o Improve patient engagement and experience by emphasizing digital health equity and tracking social determinants of health indicators
    o Recognize role of consumerism

Chapter Thirteen Today's Challenges and Tomorrow's Opportunities | 257

TABLE 13.1   Predicted Future Trends for Health Care

Virtual Nurses, Bots, Artificial Intelligence (AI): Digital Health Predictions for 2023	American Hospital Association (AHA) Environmental Scan 2023	The Future of U.S. Health Care: What's Next for the Industry Post-COVID-19	A Look Ahead: Top Six Business Trends for Hospitals and Health Systems in 2023
Expanded usage of AI, robotic process, automation wearables	Financial stability	Financial sustainability	Technological upgrades
Patient pathway convenience—pre-service to follow-up	Workforce	Care delivery site options away from the hospital	Reimbursements under pressure
Hybrid care models	Behavioral health	Chronic disease burdens increase	Digital-first patient experiences in competitive health care marketplace
Financial cost and return on investment	Health equity	Profit impacts changes for payers, providers, pharmaceuticals, and technology services	Creative ways to address workforce shortages
Patient engagement	Affordability and access	Evolving models—new business building requiring innovation	Personalized health care
Technology-based virtual home-health and patient-sitting programs, digital front doors/AI chatbots	Quality and safety		Private equity investment fuels health care landscape consolidation
New diagnosis and predictive clinical models for inpatient/outpatient care settings	Value-based delivery models		
Consumerism	Rural health		
Continued trend of mergers/ megamergers with new entrants	Consumerism		
	Social and demographic trends (older and culturally affected populations)		

Sources: Bruce, G. (2022). Virtual nurses, bots, AI: Digital health predictions for '23. *Becker's Hospital Review*, December 21, 2022. https://www.beckershospitalreview.com/digital-health/virtual-nurses-bots-ai-digital-health-predictions-for23.html?origin=CIOE&utm_source=CIOE&utm_medium=email&utm_content=newsletter&oly_enc_id=1450I5993723C6U; American Hospital Association. (2022). Environmental scan 2023. https://www.aha.org/environmentalscan; Singhal, S., & Patel, N. (2022, July 19). The future of U.S. healthcare: What's next for the industry post-COVID-19. *McKinsey Digital*. https://www.mckinsey.com/industries/healthcare-systems-and-services/our-insights/the-future-of-us-healthcare-whats-next-for-the-industry-post-covid-19; Clearwave. (2022). A look ahead: Top six business trends for hospitals and health systems in 2023. https://s3.lightboxcdn.com/vendors/7a2140ce-78bb-4521-81e3-ce42907b9cd0/uploads/b5c13db9-c627-4952-b3b9-000d4688ed65/TrendsHospitalsHS2023.pdf

- Emerging population-centered health care delivery systems:
  - Integrate hybrid delivery models such as home-health, patient sitting
  - Continue focus on the increasing size and/or need of special vulnerable populations—seniors, behavioral health, rural health, culturally affected groups
  - Prioritize personalized health care

- Innovative operating models that ensure financial stability and sustainability:
  - Align with nontraditional partners or private equity to improve sustainability
  - Use return on investment thinking for new business models, with sensitivity to health policy legislation
  - Seek models that include both ESG targets, address the potential impact on climate change
  - Require proactive models that produce value-based care options

Figure 13.4 shows the major health drivers for population health innovation.

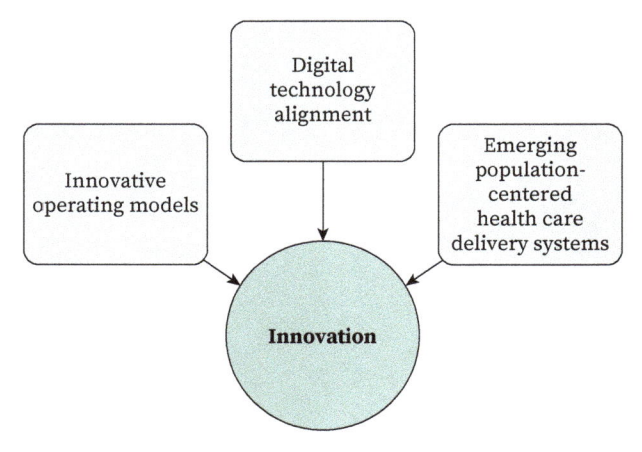

FIGURE 13.4 Health Drivers of Population Health Innovation

Practical Skill: Population Health Innovation

Review the outlined future trends in Table 13.1, the summary discussion, and Figure 13.3. Do you agree that these represent the future direction for population health? Are there any factors missing? What about new government laws and regulations? Are you concerned with consumer and patient concerns for their future care? Develop at least three additional potential future trends for population health.

Chapter Thirteen Today's Challenges and Tomorrow's Opportunities | 259

Introduction to Innovation

Implementing unique strategies and initiatives requires a new set of skills to create innovations, turn everyday reorganizing into reengineering, transition to transformation strategies, and maintain quality of care during relentless change. Future population health professionals, whether clinical or management, will benefit from learning these leadership skills to attain improved health outcomes for all.

Innovation → Reengineering → Transformation → Continual Change

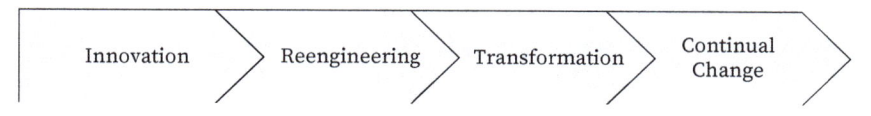

FIGURE 13.5 Strategies for Developing New Population Health Models

Population health often becomes the catalyst for change and a pioneer for new health care delivery and financial reimbursement models. Finding successful solutions necessitates thinking outside the box as either current status quo health care models need to be refined or recent technologies have provided opportunities for enhancement. How would you describe an innovation? **Innovation** can be either an individual or an organizational activity, the goal of which is executing (i.e., completing) an idea that addresses a specific challenge and achieves value for both company and the customer (Skillicorn, 2016). Given the wicked problems and grand challenges facing population health, the time is

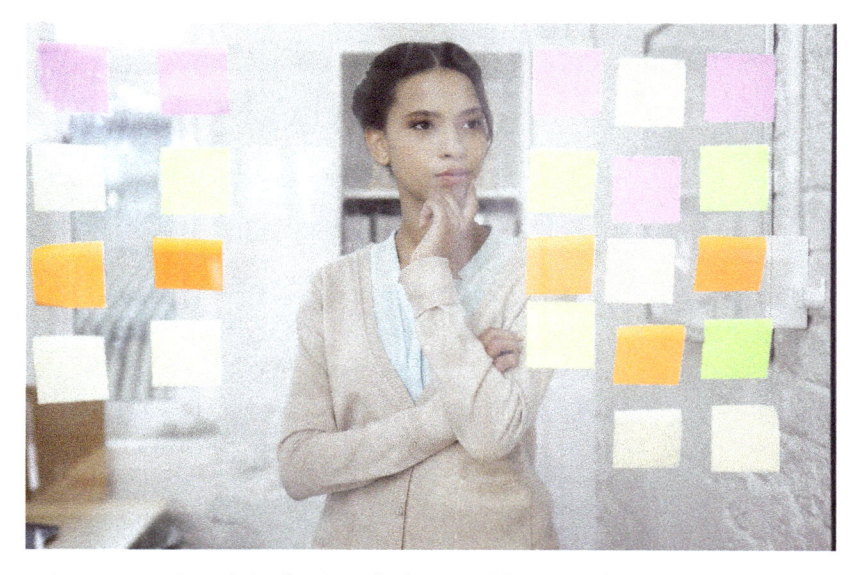

FIGURE 13.6 Creativity for Population Health Strategies

overdue to embrace innovation across the entire health care system. One caveat to remember is that innovation is not adopting the latest and the newest or the trendiest. Innovation is a new idea, a new way of thinking, or a new application of an approach or practice and not a passing fad, but rather a contribution that brings value by ensuring positive population health outcomes for all.

Why hasn't innovation been used as an active population health strategy? Was it because of the fragmented nature of health silos or the mindset of applying old solutions to new problems? Today's health sector, in general, remains behind other industries in using innovation as an established management strategy (Herzlinger, 2006). The lack of innovative health care solutions is often attributed to a chronic lack of creativity (Roberts, 2017).

Practical Skill: Population Health and Creativity

Are you a creative person? Creativity requires being present in the moment and the use of imagination. To be creative means not being judgmental of ideas and looking at problems in diverse ways (Johns, 2017). With all the various stimuli in our daily environment, finding time for undivided attention to finding solutions and allowing oneself to have open space to free up one's brain is not a common activity. The concept of innovation can easily be confused with creativity. Creativity is typically centered around original thought, knowledge, and imagination for generating innovative ideas (Johns, 2017). Innovation, on the other hand, is used to turn a creative idea into a viable solution (Stanford Online, n.d.).

Instructions: Complete the simple creativity assessments at the following links. What did you discover?

https://tinyurl.com/3ccw35r5

https://tinyurl.com/2yw4wmv2

Remember, there are many elements that are necessary for creativity, not just imagination and focus time. Barriers also exist at the organizational and system levels. For example, innovation will not occur if individuals are not rewarded or valued for their contributions, or the health organizations are resistant to change. Other external barriers may be that clinical standards or regulations prohibit certain processes or that a resource, such as technology, adds too much expense to the innovation (Wagner et al., 2022). Despite these obstacles, a recent report found more than 110 innovation centers have been established in health care delivery systems in the past 10 years (Bhattacharyya et al., 2022).

A Framework for Innovation: Design Thinking

A clear health care delivery lesson learned from population health initiatives over time is that patient-centered approaches and processes are the most effective and successful because they add value for the consumer and the health care professional. The human-centered approach to problem-solving parallels health care's patient-centered approach in its applications. **Design thinking** is a framework for problem-solving that emphasizes empathy, innovation, **collaboration**, and continual experimentation (Murtell, 2021). The original framework of design thinking dates to the mid-20th century, but the concept is relatively new to the health care industry (Linke, 2017) and is becoming adopted by health care professionals and in education (Abookire et al., 2020).

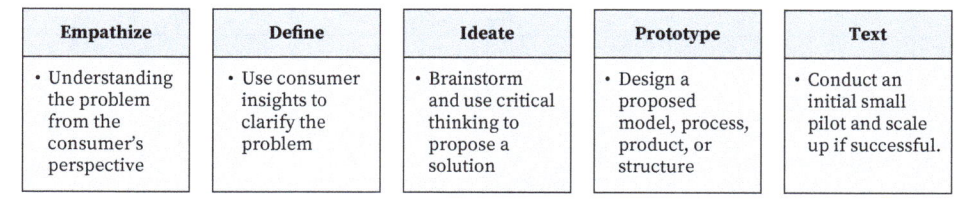

Empathize	Define	Ideate	Prototype	Text
• Understanding the problem from the consumer's perspective	• Use consumer insights to clarify the problem	• Brainstorm and use critical thinking to propose a solution	• Design a proposed model, process, product, or structure	• Conduct an initial small pilot and scale up if successful.

FIGURE 13.7   Design Thinking Framework

Design thinking provides a five step-by-step framework for problem-solvers: empathy, define, ideate, prototype, and test. Step 1 requires individuals to deeply learn about the problems by first gaining empathy for those who experience the pain point of a particular issue. Using the in-depth information from the empathy stage, Step 2 involves identifying and defining the true problem and not just the symptoms. In Step 3 of the design thinking frame, problem-solvers engage in developing ideas and, if successful, can move into the next phase of developing a prototype. Step 4, testing the prototype, is the last step to assess the effectiveness and viability of the innovation. The design thinking process is often repetitive until a satisfactory innovation emerges. Design thinking can be useful for workflow processes, products, and visualization of new organizational structures. To fully engage with the process, review the detailed discussions for each of the framework steps.

Step 1: Empathy

Management experts often share the saying "Asking the right question can be more important than finding the answer." We can apply this lesson to the first step of the framework as developing empathy requires us to see the problem from the perspective of the patient, consumer, and health care provider. ***Pain points*** are problems that occur during an experience and, in the case of health care, may pop up along the patient or consumer pathway. ***Empathy*** means having the capacity to understand another person's thoughts and feelings in a situation from their point of view and not your own. Empathy is unlike sympathy, in which you experience thoughts and feelings of another but maintain an emotional distance. Empathizing with others is a way to explore their feelings and immerse yourself in their experience. Creating an **empathy map** allows the problem-solver to document the consumer's perceptions by observing, listening, and feeling (Gray et al., 2010; Osterwalder et al., 2014). The goal is to answer probing questions such as "What makes the patient upset? What do they think is the solution? "When does the problem occur, and why?

For example, hundreds of health care articles have been published over the years seeking to improve emergency department (ED) experiences. To truly

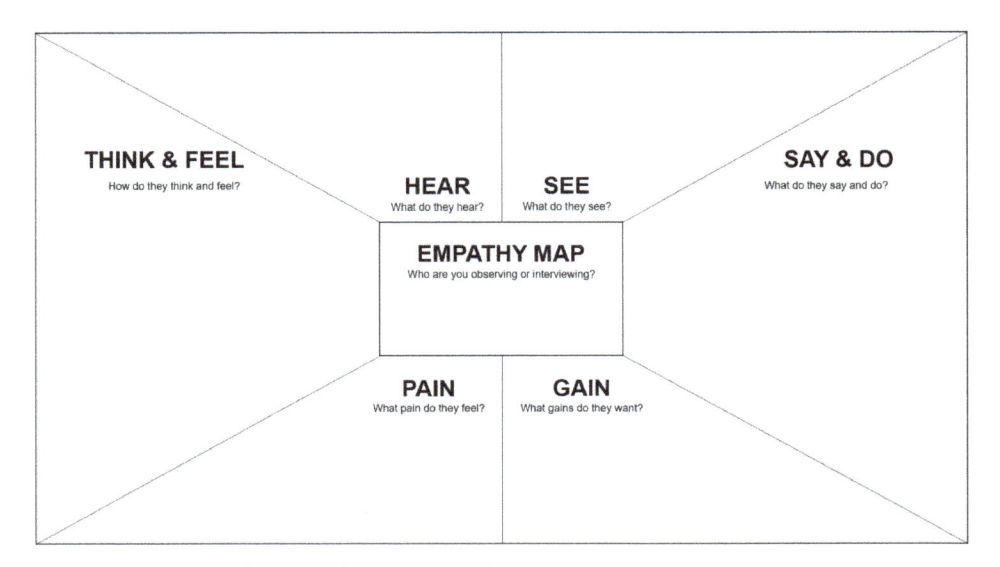

FIGURE 13.8   Sample Empathy Map Template

understand the problem, an innovation team collects information from patients, health care providers, staff, family members and caregivers, and diverse support personnel in radiology, the pharmacy, and other support areas.

Step 2: Define the Problem

Understanding consumer needs, barriers, attitudes, and aspirations is the only way to unlock innovative solutions (Murtell, 2021), and based on the data and experiences from developing the empathy map, the problem-solver identifies and defines the problem. This analytical step involves sifting through the information and prioritizing the findings. Like a research project, specific themes or patterns will emerge and detect the underlying problem. Using our ED example, a specific theme appropriate for the problem definition might be the size of the facility as it affects all end users, including patients, family, staff, and health care providers. Now that we know the challenge, we must move on to find the solution.

Step 3: Ideate

Moving from the problem to a solution idea is known as ***ideation***, which refers to dropping any boundaries for our thoughts and asking questions such as "Suppose that …," "What if …," and "Could we use. …" Being curious is a positive characteristic for this innovation step. By stretching the thinking process outside of the traditional way, it is possible to discover novel and breakthrough ideas. One technique often mentioned to encourage ideation is ***divergent thinking***, to produce as many ideas as possible (Institute for Healthcare Improvement, n.d.). In fact, we can remember this step as the post-it note activity, in which the ideas are shared for everyone to review. Referring to our ED scenario, ideas from the innovation team may include moving the ED to a larger area, reconfiguring or adding additional space, moving to a separate location from the hospital, using telehealth as an ED substitute, or investing in a mobile ED unit.

Innovation teams often complete this process multiple times to test their potential ideas and solutions.

Step 4: Design a Prototype

Once the problem-solver or innovation team selects a particular solution, a sample, or prototype, is created, and developed. Rapid sketching or quick designing is a simple technique to use in this stage and allows other problem solvers to piggy-back on an idea (Murtell, 2021). Just as you would alter your course in going through a maze, experimentation is a major component of constructing a prototype, whether it be a product, a process, or an idea. The innovation team has decided to construct a mobile ED vehicle and have created a mock-up prototype.

Step 5: Test the Prototype

The last step in the design-thinking cycle is to assess the effectiveness and success of the prototype. For example, a health system retrofitted an exceptionally large motor home (i.e., recreational vehicle) to resemble a mini-ED and deployed it within the community. The test proved successful—too successful, in fact—and the mobile unit was overwhelmed. This is also an experimentation phase as any failure is treated as a valuable learning experience and an opportunity to adjust and refine before testing again. One of the keys to successful innovation is known as *failing fast*, in which an innovation team works quickly to analyze areas for improvement and then experiment unto a proposed solution is successful. The question to ask is "What can be improved?"

Not every innovation will become a tremendous success, but the design thinking process is a crucial strategy and skill to improve population health care delivery processes and meet unprecedented future challenges.

Reorganizing to Reengineering: New Models for Population Health

Innovation provides opportunities for major transformations, but not all population health organizations require dramatic overhauls. Another future-oriented strategy to meet emerging challenges involves transitioning from reorganizing to reengineering.

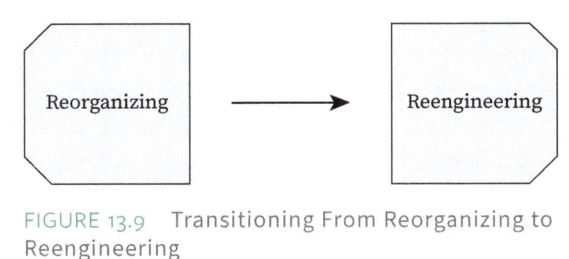

FIGURE 13.9   Transitioning From Reorganizing to Reengineering

Reorganizing, also referred to as *redesigning*, is a common organizational practice that focuses on an organization's configurations or structure. A reorganization may involve the creation of a new department for population health or hiring new personnel such as an epidemiologist. **Reengineering** is an activity that takes reorganizing to the next level and is a complete top-to-bottom reimagination of the entire organization (Moseley, 2018). Population health reengineering often focuses on improving operations which align with quality, cost, access, and consumer satisfaction. An excellent example is a health care organization that completely transitions away from fee-for-service payment to alternative payment strategies that represent value-based care. Both organizational strategies are useful to improve internal operations, but they may not consider external competitors and their future actions.

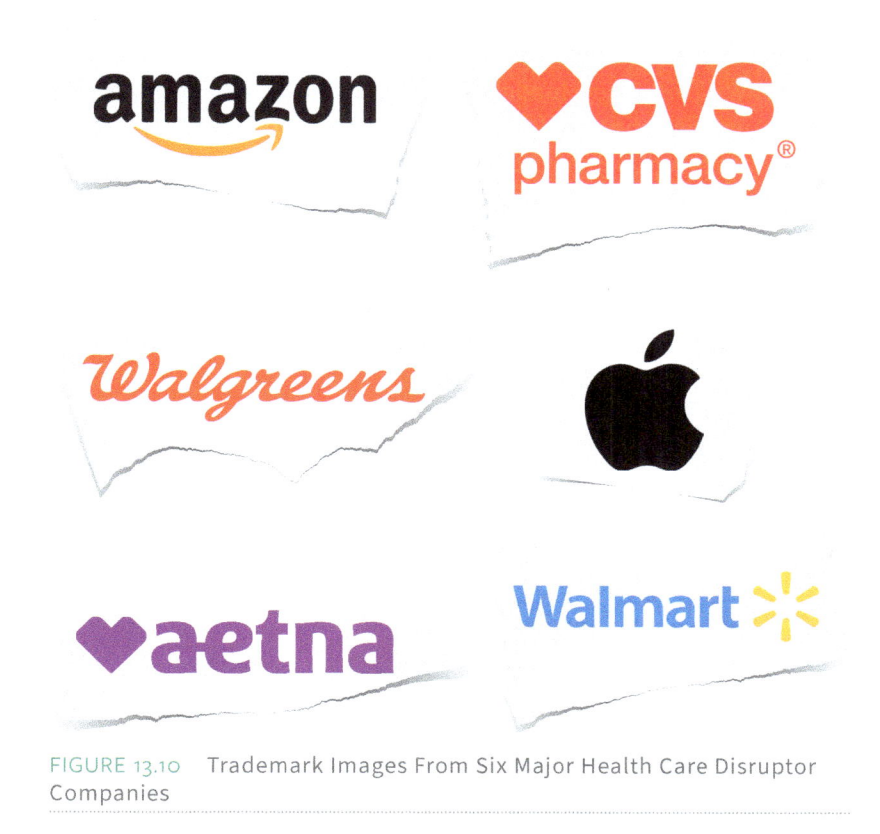

FIGURE 13.10   Trademark Images From Six Major Health Care Disruptor Companies

While the health care sector continues to innovate and reengineer, other nonhealth industries have begun to target the health care delivery marketplace. **Disruption** refers to an event that interferes with the everyday, whether that be a process, an activity, or a way of doing business. The AHA suggests that six major firms (Amazon, Apple, CVS/Aetna, Google/Alphabet, Walgreens, and Walmart) intend to disrupt the current health care market (AHA, 2020). In the current healthscape, *disruptors*, or nonhealth care sector companies that have entered the health care marketplace, include major retailers such as Amazon and Walmart (Landi, 2022; Schwartz, 2022). However, within-sector major health care organizations such as CVS, with its MinuteClinic® locations (CVS, n.d.), and Walgreens, with its CareCentrix® branding (Walgreens Health, 2022), have already begun to provide health services at their local retail sites.

A disruption becomes more significant when these companies begin to acquire already functioning and viable health care providers, practitioners, or facilities and convert them to their unique business model. For example, Amazon has already purchased a major primary care company, One Medical, for billions of dollars (Schwartz, 2022), and CVS has offered to purchase Signify, a major home-health provider (Signify Health News, 2022). Other disruptors also are targeting the two major health care service areas of home health and primary care. Will these new models lead to a return to physician home-health calls? Is it a surprise that health care seems to have come full circle from where it was years ago, when the local family doctor made home visits that constituted 40% of the overall doctor-patient interactions (Heilweil, 2022)? By leveraging their unique strengths in sophisticated technologies, size, scope, and consumer expertise, these disrupting companies are positioning themselves to provide quality health care at a lower cost. Is the question for the future whether health care will be able to compete with these disruptors (Bruce & Twenter, 2022)?

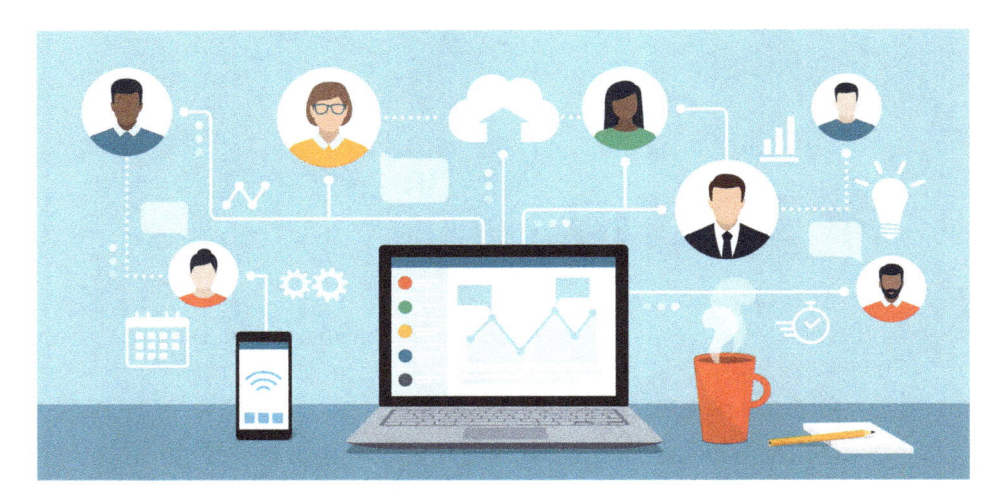

FIGURE 13.11   Opportunities for Health Care Sector Disruptors

Practical Skill: Disruptors for the Future

Can you imagine meeting a health care provider at Walmart? What about getting a flu shot at Best Buy? Would you order your prescriptions from Amazon? Disruption in the health care sector has the potential to significantly alter how and where we seek health care in the future. Did you plan to work in a hospital or clinic? What if you manage a series of health clinics for Google? What if your physical therapy facility were located inside Kroger's? These are only some of the potential scenarios that might occur in the future.

Transition to Transformation: Collaboration Shifts to the Co-Production of Health

The health care sector has recognized that the status quo was unsustainable and, like the disruptors, is also seeking new alignments. Why? The interdependence of the global marketplace and interoperability of today's health care systems were tested significantly and found lacking during the COVID-19 pandemic. The resulting impact served as both the catalyst and motivation to develop new health care models and implement diverse organizational strategies. A consensus reached by all health-related organizations was the necessity for improved and expanded relationships among stakeholders. Using a multisectoral perspective, the industry stakeholders would increase diversity and equity, improve connections to better coordinate care, and have greater outreach for vulnerable populations.

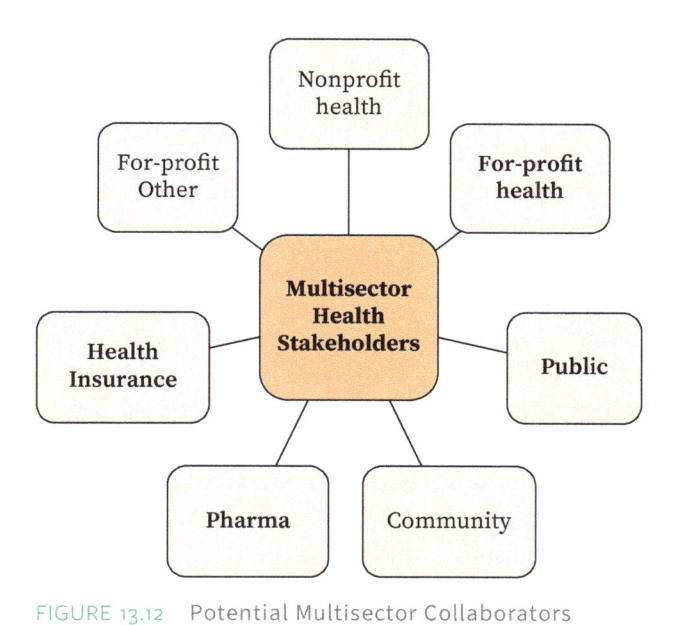

FIGURE 13.12   Potential Multisector Collaborators

The new model includes collaborators with vastly different business arrangements, including nonprofit, profit, public, community, and private organizations. Because of the diverse business missions, structures, and governance frameworks, transitioning informal to formal relationships that are needed to transform health care will be a challenge, especially for collaborations between for-profit and nonprofit organizations.

Relationship Continuum
Using a Business Perspective

← Loose Linkages   Formal Agreements →
Alliances → Joint Venture → Merger

Relationship Continuum Using a Community
Collaborative Perspective

← Loose Linkages   Formal Agreements →

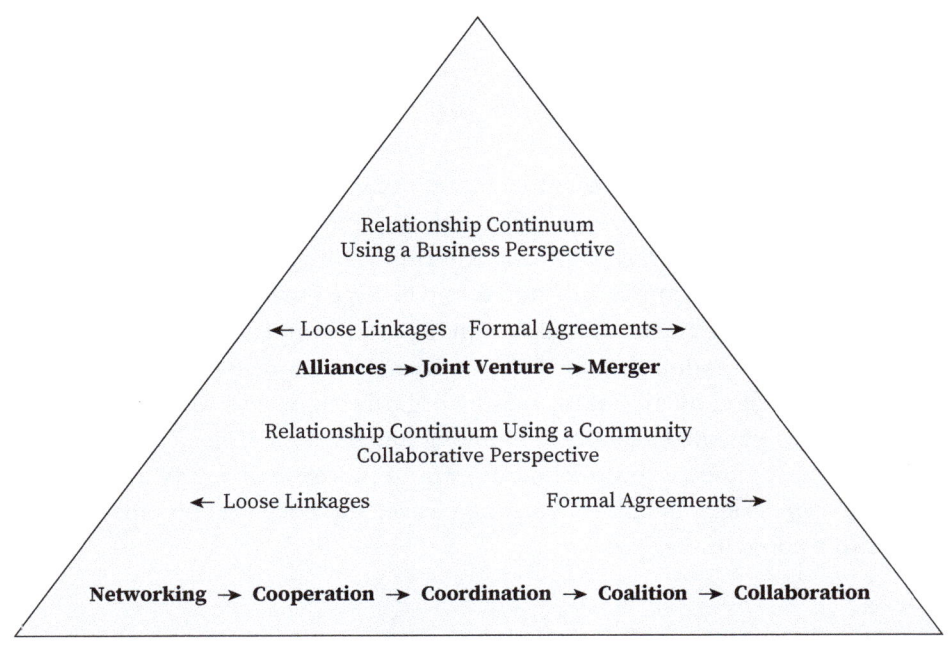

Networking → Cooperation → Coordination → Coalition → Collaboration

FIGURE 13.13   Relationship Levels: Community and Business Perspectives

As illustrated in Figure 13.13, when organizations form collaborations to achieve a common goal, the arrangements can vary from informal to formal relationships, and the more formal the arrangement, the stronger level of commitment and resources. The community relationship model has been established over the years, based on partnerships between hospitals, public health agencies, and community health organizations. However, the highest level of this perspective is *collaboration*, which can be described as working with others. In contrast, the business perspective ranges from loose linkages to formal agreements with only three options: alliances, joint ventures, and mergers. Each of these commitment levels indicates additional obligations, sharing of resources, and, of course, accountability. Notice that neither continuum uses the term *partnership* to denote an organizational relationship, although frameworks exist that equate cooperation with an alliance and coordination with a partnership (Association of State Public Health Nutritionists, n.d.).

Advancing Collaborations to the Co-Production of Health

Collaborative relationships with traditional health care organizations, while beneficial, may lack scope, strong consumer input, and function as outsourcing units for specific tasks. For example, a public health agency may receive a federal grant and contract with a local nonprofit to provide outreach services and with the local hospital to provide clinical screenings or treatment. Unlike population health, not all entities are held accountable for positive health outcomes. Another issue has been the reliance on local health sector stakeholders, which has limited the scope of outreach. With the current health care sector transforming to meet incredible and unprecedented challenges, new and unique partnerships will need to be formed with disruptors, competitors, venture capitalists, national nonsector organizations such as large retail companies, and other nonprofit agencies to meet population health needs for all. Together, these organizations will begin to transition from collaboration to co-production of health for the future.

The **co-production of health** involves the collaboration of patients, caregivers, health care providers, and payers to develop, implement, and evaluate relationships and actions that contribute to the improvement of health for individuals and populations (Radl-Karimi et al., 2018). Given the scope and size of grand challenges and using a population health-based perspective, the co-production of health requires more than just collaboration; it mandates an emphasis on co-design, delivery of health care services, and cost accountability for all. A new term, **radical collaboration**, adopted from design thinking for health care, describes an organizational strategy that involves working with nontraditional or unexpected organizations and includes shared decision-making and responsibility (Wagner & Hewitt, 2022; Collective Change Lab, 2020). For example, a radical collaboration might include aligning with new disruptors in the health care market, such as Amazon or Walmart, or even multiple hospital systems sharing the co-production of health's system of alignment versus a typical outsourcing arrangement, by which each party separately contributes skills, expertise, or other resources.

Let's review our previous example of a public health agency receiving a federal grant and contracting with a local nonprofit for outreach services and the local hospital to provide clinical screenings or treatment. Now, we add a for-profit digital therapeutic company that provides tailored text messages, offers televisits 24/7, and collects follow-up surveys based on a capitation fee. This time the payment is influenced by the number of clients and patients with improved outcomes and not solely a report listing the number of participants who were reached or screened. Population health integrates both accountability and cost reduction into the co-production of health model. In this case, benefits include a larger scope for the project and the ability to integrate local community services, along with patients, in the co-design and delivery of health care services.

Population Health and the Co-Production of Health Initiatives

Co-production of health initiatives, as described in the previous example, may encounter collaboration challenges such as when organizations lack capital or expertise or follow different governance structures. When partnering with smaller nonprofit agencies, obstacles such as a lack of technology expertise or interoperability between delivery systems and differing organizational communication and culture patterns occur frequently. Public health agencies also encounter these problems given that their funding mandates and their organizational structure are linked to the federal, state, and local governments. But barriers can exist when co-producing health with well-known and funded organizations. In 2018, three extremely successful nonhealth care organizations, Amazon, Berkshire Hathaway, and J. P. Morgan, agreed to form a health care company (Haven) with a prominent physician scholar as chief executive officer. Expectations for the co-production of health care were high. However, despite the company's strengths—as it covered 1.25 million lives and each partner had capital to invest and incredible consumer, business, and financial expertise (Gawande, 2019; Tozzi, 2019)—Haven eventually closed. The explanation was that much had been attained in developing health care solutions (LaMonica, 2021). Despite this outcome, the Haven example served as a catalyst for other companies to expand into the health care sector. Suddenly, co-production of health became an option not only within the health care sector, but also in other industry sectors and for diverse potential disruptors.

The co-production of health represents a true transformation of an industry as health care organizations can no longer cooperate only with other health-focused companies. To succeed, they need to make multisectoral collaborations.

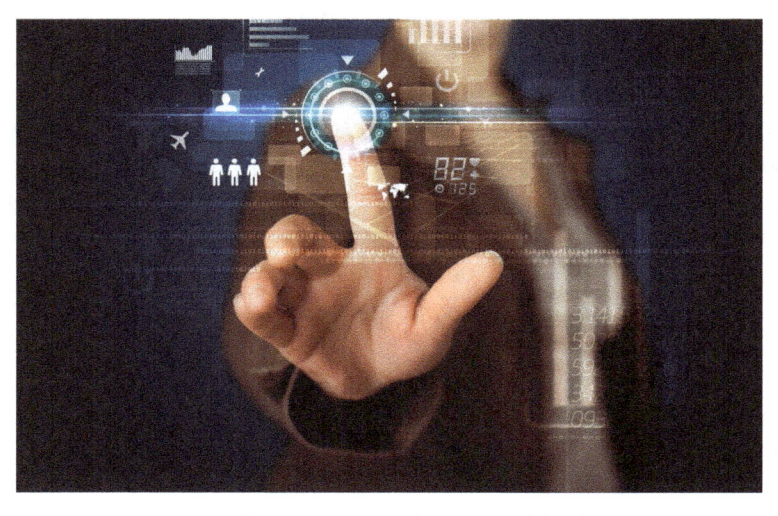

FIGURE 13.14   Managing Future Population Health Change

Hospitals will need to move past their longstanding relationships with local public health agencies and local nonprofits such as the United Way and branch out to align with other for-profit, nonhealth-sector companies, such as pharmaceutical organizations, national retail chains, drug stores, and other retail outlets. The AHA aligns the co-production of health with population health and recently stated, "The management of a population's health is promoted via a co-production of health model that emphasizes care coordination and patient engagement and is supported by appropriate fiscal models and evidence-based practice" (AHA, 2022).

Managing Change for Future Population Health Initiatives

Whether you plan to work or are already employed within the health care sector as a practitioner, staff member, or manager, the constant in your workspace will be change. The necessity for change can come from either external pressure, such as a recent national health policy (Inflation Reduction Act of 2022), payer reimbursement changes (ACO Realizing Equity, Access, and Community Health), or an internal company's strategic changes, such as altering workflow processes (telehealth) to improve quality. Change can be categorized as either a transition—the process of incremental shifts, or transformation—inspired and motivated change. Regardless of the type of change, the success of the population health organization will depend on its capacity to adapt and adopt new and revised processes.

Practical Skill: Understanding Change

Do you like change? Does change make you anxious? Is there a specific type of change that you dislike the most? Not everyone likes to change, and some individuals can be very resistant to it. Often it is because they think the change will reduce their satisfaction in some way or they do not understand the benefit of the change (Olden, 2019). Before beginning a partnership with a patient, family physicians often ask them to answer only the following two questions to assess their readiness to change:

1. "How important is it to you to make this change on a scale of 0 to 10, with 10 being extremely important?"
2. "How confident are you that you can make this change on a scale of 0 to 10, with 10 being extremely confident?"

The first question helps to identify the patient's action priorities and the second question directly aligns with their self-efficacy to complete any actions (*FPM* Journal Blog, 2018).

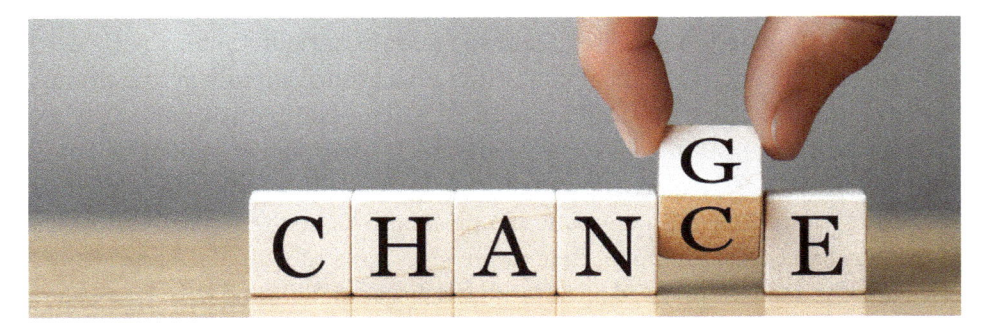

FIGURE 13.15   Population Health Future Changes

Managing Resistance to Change

Population health is concerned with vulnerable populations and identifying individuals who are resistant to change is primary. Equally important is the recognition that patients/consumers will not respond to change if health care managers and practitioners do not model the appropriate behaviors). Remember that change requires people to understand, accept, move forward, appreciate the change, and, finally, act (Wagner et al., 2022). A recognized change model that was originally developed to discuss grief for losing a loved one (Malik, 2022) includes five phases: shock/denial, anger, bargaining, depression, and acceptance. Over time, this model has been applied to the workplace, especially when major transformative changes are required.

To assist population health practitioners and other professionals overcome resistance to change in their worksite, health experts have developed multiple models. All these models have one commonality in that they view accepting

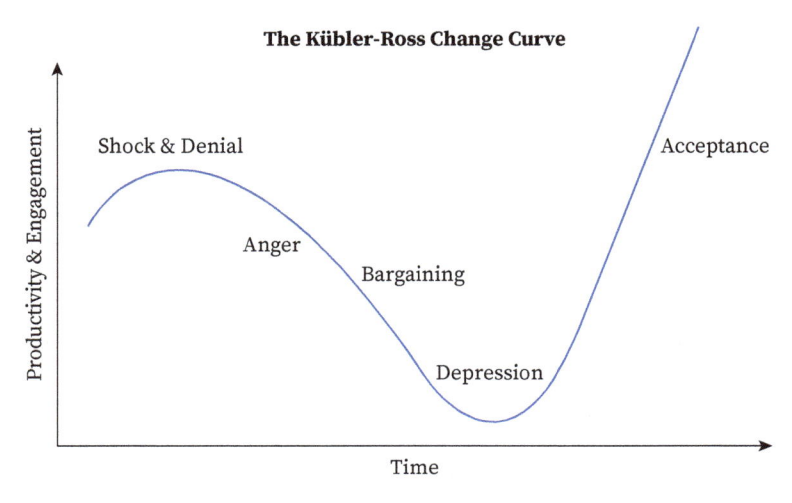

FIGURE 13.16   The Kübler-Ross Change Curve

change as a process and people progress along a continuum from doubt and overt resistance to acceptance and integration into their workflow. The **PAST change model** is an effective and easy change framework to implement.

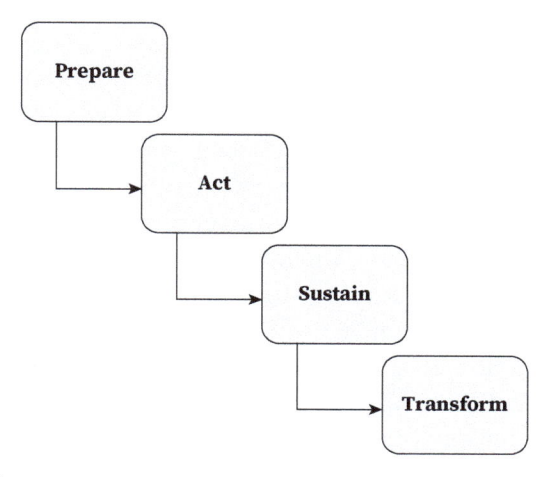

Prepare:
- Clearly define the necessary change
- Assess readiness to change
- Address emotions and gaps in readiness
- Rely on both informal and formal assessments of attitudes

Act:
- Access current situation
- Begin change implementation
- Measure to assess change and program status

Sustain:
- Use continuous reinforcement to prevent relapse
- Monitor all aspects of the program

Transform
- Setting expectations and standards for the entire program
- Developing rules, feedback, and accountability

FIGURE 13.17   The PAST Change Model

Agile Leadership for Population Health's Future

If population health innovations include new models and expanded strategies for health care delivery, then the need for better and more responsive leadership skills will certainly follow. New and original leadership theories often emerge in response to challenging situations. A management theory may have existed previously and not have been truly tested or an extreme situation, such as the COVID-19 pandemic, requires an immediate and demanding need for a change in leadership style emerges. **Agile leadership** began in the technology industry but recently emerged as a winning leadership strategy for the health care sector. Why? Because agile managers do not follow the more traditional leadership styles, such as bureaucratic (top-down), coaching, or adaptive (incremental change) options (Hewitt, 2022). Instead, the goal of agile leaders is to remove consumer barriers or obstacles as quickly as possible, solicit feedback, and continue innovating. In health care, these managers not only seek to eliminate patient and consumer pain points, but they also enable their teams by emphasizing adaptability, openness, and empowerment of others. A simple way to describe the difference is that agile leadership encourages shared decision-making, increases flexibility to meet unexpected challenges, and adds resilience for sustainability (Forbes, 2020; Van Dyke, 2022).

The grand challenges and wicked problems facing population health will not respond to top-down, single health organization decision-making based on authority or traditional **change management** strategies that usually focus on implementing one change at a time. Agility is not just about being faster as strategies for patient-centric inclusion, and quality execution of processes are primary components (Ratanjee, 2021). How do we implement agile leadership?

* Transformation of healthcare delivery
* Rapid adoption of co-production models
* Increasing number of non-traditional collaborations

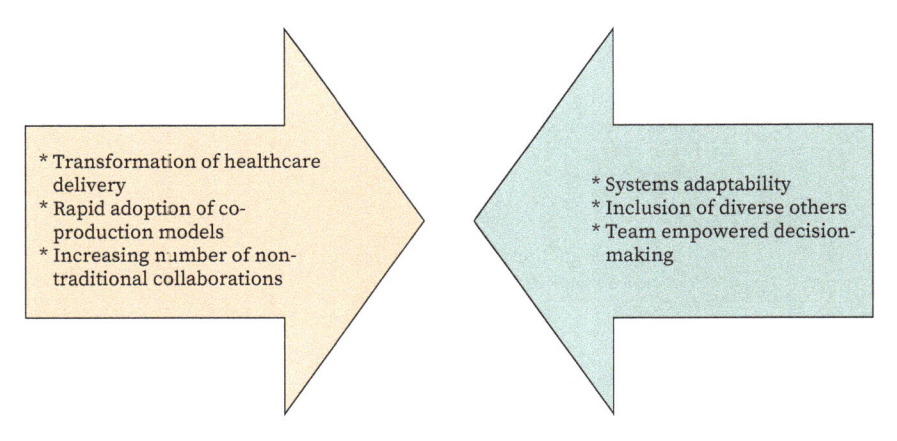

* Systems adaptability
* Inclusion of diverse others
* Team empowered decision-making

FIGURE 13.18   Leadership Drivers of Change and Agile Style Strategies

For example, if our team is playing football, the team members are diverse and make shared decisions on the plays. They can react rapidly to any changes made by their competitors or the environment, such as referee calls. But even more importantly, the revolving quarterbacks respond appropriately, while the coach remains on the sidelines. Now imagine that the opposing team is really made up of disruptors in the healthscape! For population health, whether a large or small company, the value added is meeting the patient's/consumer's and the organization's needs. Agile leadership is for all health professionals—you will get your turn being the agile quarterback!

Summary

The future for population health will bring continuing wicked problems and new grand challenges. Health experts suggest a diverse set of priorities that can be summarized into three categories: (a) digital technology that affects clinical decisions, care delivery, and workflow; (b) emerging population-centered health care delivery systems; and (c) innovative operating models that ensure financial stability and sustainability. Future activities will require adopting unique strategies such as increasing innovation, moving from reorganizing to reengineering, ramping up transitions to create actual transformations, and managing constant change. Skills described in this chapter include the five steps of innovation, design thinking, the PAST model of change management, a new model of co-production of health, and an introduction to agile management as an option for today's turbulent environment.

Discussion Questions

1. Review the concepts of grand challenges and wicked problems. Then examine the future trends table (Table 13.1). Which of the future trends do you think are most likely to solve any of the many grand challenges facing population health today?
2. Briefly explain three-part innovation model and identify an example.
3. Why are change management skills important to all future health care professionals?
4. Select one of the change management models and apply it to a current situation in your experiences.
5. Distinguish between reengineering and reorganizing. Which one would be most appropriate for organizational transformation? Why?
6. List at least three characteristics of an agile leadership style. Why does this leadership approach a match for change management?

References

Abbott, B. (2022, August 4). How the COVID-19 pandemic changed American's health for the worse. *Wall Street Journal*, A6. https://www.wsj.com/articles/how-the-covid-19-pandemic-changed-americans-health-for-the-worse-11659260165

Abookire, S., Plover, C., & Frasso, R. (2020, August). Health design thinking: Innovative approach in public health to defining problems and finding solutions. *Frontiers in Public Health*, 1–6. https://www.frontiersin.org/articles/10.3389/fpubh.2020.00459/full

American Hospital Association. (2022). *Environmental scan 2023*. https://www.aha.org/environmentalscan

American Hospital Association. (2022). *Population health management*. https://www.aha.org/center/population-health-management

Association of State Public Health Nutritionists. (n.d.). *ASPHN collaboration primer*. https://asphn.org/wp-content/uploads/2017/10/collaboration-primer.pdf

Bhattacharyya, O., Shapiro, J., & Schneider, E. (2022). Innovation centers in health care delivery systems: Structures for success. *Journal of Medical Internet Research, 24*(2), e33961. https://www.ncbi.nlm.nih.gov/pmc/articles/PMC8874810/#:~:text=Within%20the%20last%2010%20years,States%20%5B6%2C7%5D

Bruce, G., & Twenter, P. (2022). *Can health systems compete with disruption from CVS, Walgreens?* Becker's Hospital Review, December 19, 2022. https://www.beckershospitalreview.com/disruptors/can-health-systems-compete-with-disruption-from-cvs-walgreens.html?origin=BHRE&utm_source=BHRE&utm_medium=email&utm_content=newsletter&oly_enc_id=1450I5993723C6U

Clearwave. (2022). *A look ahead: Top six business trends for hospitals and health systems in 2023*. https://s3.lightboxcdn.com/vendors/7a2140ce-78bb-4521-81e3-ce42907b9cd0/uploads/b5c13db9-c627-4952-b3b9-000d4688ed65/TrendsHospitalsHS2023.pdf

Collective Change Lab. (2020). *What does radical collaboration really mean?* https://www.collectivechangelab.org/blog/radcollab

Colquitt, J., & George, G. (2011). Publishing in *AMJ*—Part 1: Topic choice. *Academy of Management Journal, 54*, 432–435. https://www.researchgate.net/publication/279401019_Publishing_in_AMJ--Part_1_Topic_ChoiceCVS. (n.d.). *Welcome to MinuteClinic*®. https://www.cvs.com/minuteclinic

CVS. (n.d.). Welcome to MinuteClinic®: In-person and virtual care 7 days a week. https://www.cvs.com/minuteclinic

Ferraro, F., Etzion, D., & Gehman, J. (2015). Tackling grand challenges pragmatically: Robust action revisited. *Organization Studies, 36*(3), 363–390. https://www.emerald.com/insight/content/doi/10.1108/S1474-823120210000020011/full/pdf?title=prelims

Forbes. (2020, June 17). *15 key qualities that define an "agile" leader*. www.forbes.com/sites/forbescoachescouncil/2020/06/17/15-key-qualities-that-define-an-agile-leader/?sh=3514c1de7f31

FPM Journal Blog. (2018). *Two quick questions to assess patients' readiness for change*. American Academy of Family Physicians, October 5, 2018. https://www.aafp.org/pubs/fpm/blogs/inpractice/entry/readiness_for_change.html

Gawande, A. (2019). *Haven*. Haven Healthcare. https://havenhealthcare.com/

George, J. M. (2014). Compassion and capitalism: Implications for organizational studies. *Journal of Management, 40*(1), 5–15.

Gray, D., Brown, S., & Macanufo, J. (2010). *Gamestorming: A playbook for innovators, rulebreakers, and changemakers*. O'Reilly Media.

Grieve, P. (2022). *The lifetime cost of healthcare averages $700,000 for many insured Americans*. Money.com, November 14, 2022. https://money.com/health-care-costs-lifetime/?utm_medium=rss_synd&utm_source=applenews&xid=applenews

Heilweil, R. (2022, September 8). *Why CVS is spending $8 billion to bring back physician house calls: The return of the doctor house call isn't a comeback. It's a harbinger.* Vox.com, September 8, 2022.https://www.vox.com/recode/2022/9/8/23342682/why-cvs-is-spending-8-billion-to-bring-back-physician-house-calls

Herzlinger, R. E. (2006). Why innovation in health care is so hard. *Harvard Business Review, 84*(5), 58–66.

Hewitt, A. (2022, Fall). Agile leadership: Leadership skills in future health professionals. *In the Lead*. p. 14-19. Seton Hall Publishing. tps://issuu.com/setonhallmagazine/docs/in_the_lead_magazine_fall2022

Hewitt, A., Wagner, S., Twal, R., & Gourley,h D. (2015). *Community hospitals with local public health departments: Collaborative emergency management*. In S. B. Hamner, S. Stovall, & D. Taha (Eds.), *Emergency Management and disaster response utilizing public-private partnerships*. IGI Global.

Institute for Healthcare Improvement Open School. (n.d.). *Divergent and convergent thinking. Part I*. https://www.ihi.org/education/IHIOpenSchool/resources/Pages/AudioandVideo/Whiteboard17.aspx

Johns, M. (2017). *Leadership development for healthcare: A pathway, process, and workbook*. AHIMA Press.

LaMonica, P. (2021). *Haven—the joint health care venture by Amazon, Berkshire and JPMorgan—is shutting down*. CNN Business. https://www.cnn.com/2021/01/04/investing/haven-shutting-down-amazon-jpmorgan-berkshire/index.html

Landi, H. (2022, September 15). *Healthcare plays by CVS, Walgreens and Amazon will drive more partnerships, tech investments, experts say*. Fierce Healthcare, September 15, 2022.https://www.fiercehealthcare.com/health-tech/healthcare-plays-cvs-walgreens-and-amazon-will-drive-more-partnerships-tech-investment?utm_source=email&utm_medium=email&utm_campaign=HC-NL-FierceHealthcare&oly_enc_id=5901H8477778D6Z

Linke, R. (2017, September 14). *Design thinking, explained*. https://mitsloan.mit.edu/ideas-made-to-matter/design-thinking-explained

Malik, P. (2022). *The Kübler-Ross change curve in the workplace*. Whatfix, February 24, 2022. https://whatfix.com/blog/kubler-ross-change-curve/

Martin, A., Hartman, M., Benson, J. Catlin, A., & the National Health Expenditure Accounts Team. (2022). National health care spending in 2021: Decline in federal spending outweighs greater use of health care. *Health Affairs*, December 14, 2022. https://doi.org/10.1377/hlthaff.2022.01397

Moseley, G., III. (2018). *Managing health care business strategy* (2nd ed.). Jones & Bartlett Learning.

Murtell, J. (2021). *The 5 phases of design thinking*. American Marketing Association, August 14, 2021. https://www.ama.org/marketing-news/the-5-phases-of-design-thinking/

Nembhard, I. M., Burns, L. R., & Shortell, S. M. (2020, April 17). Responding to COVID-19: Lessons from management research. https://catalyst.nejm.org/doi/full/10.1056/CAT.20.0111

Olden, P. (2019). *Management of healthcare organizations: An introduction* (3rd ed.). HAP Press.

Osterwalder, A., Pigneur, Y., Bernarda, G., & Smith, A. (2014). *Value proposition design*. John Wiley & Sons.

Perez, L. Hunt, V., Samandari, H., Nuttal, R., & Biniek, K. (2022, August 10). *Does ESG really matter—and why?* McKinsey Digital, August 10, 2022. https://www.mckinsey.com/business-functions/sustainability/our-insights/does-esg-really-matter-and-why?cid=other-eml-dre-mip-mck&hlkid=60bb86a2a106425080408c4d121e8316&hctky=12039362&hdpid=d27a6996-6caa-403a-a102-35b5530a5a7a

Radl-Karimi, C., Nicolaisen, A., Sodemann, M., Batalden, P., & von Plessen, C. (2018). Coproduction of healthcare service with immigrant patients: Protocol of a scoping review. *BMJ Open*, 8, e019519. https://bmjopen.bmj.com/content/8/2/e019519

Ratanjee, V. (2021, June 22). Contributor: Seven shifts to an agile culture in health care. *American Journal of Managed Care*. https://www.ajmc.com/view/contributor-seven-shifts-to-an-agile-culture-in-health-care

Roberts, J. (2017). Design thinking gains converts in health care after finding success in other fields. *H&HN Magazine*. http://www.hhnmag.com/articles/7812-how-design-thinking-could-transform-a-health-care-organization

Robertson, M. (2022). *Healthcare spending hit $4.3 trillion in 2021: 7 things to know.* Becker's Hospital Review, December 14, 2022. https://www.beckershospitalreview.com/finance/healthcare-spending-hit-4-3-trillion-in-2021-7-things-to-know.html?origin=BHRE&utm_source=BHRE&utm_medium=email&utm_content=newsletter&oly_enc_id=1450I5993723C6U

Schwartz, N. (2020). *How CVS, Amazon and Walgreens are pushing into primary care and home health*. Becker's Hospital Review, November 8, 2020. https://www.beckershospitalreview.com/disruptors/how-cvs-amazon-and-walgreens-are-pushing-into-primary-care-home-health.html

Schwartz, N. (2022). *Walmart's 5 biggest moves in healthcare*. Becker's Hospital Review, December 30, 2022. https://www.beckershospitalreview.com/disruptors/walmarts-5-biggest-moves-in-healthcare-in-2022.html?origin=CIOE&utm_source=CIO-E&utm_medium=email&utm_content=newsletter&oly_enc_id=1450I5993723C6U

Signify Health News. (2022, September 5). *CVS to acquire Signify Health*. https://www.signifyhealth.com/news/cvs-health-to-acquire-signify-health

Singhal, S., & Patel, N. (2022). *The future of US healthcare: What's next for the industry post-COVID19*. McKinsey Digital, July 19, 2022. https://www.mckinsey.com/industries/healthcare-systems-and-services/our-insights/the-future-of-us-healthcare-whats-next-for-the-industry-post-covid-19

Skillicorn, N. (2016). *Infograph: What is innovation? 15 experts share their innovation definition.* INC. March 18 2016. https://www.inc.com/nick-skillicorn/9-defining-characteristics-of-successful-innovation.html

Stanford Online. (n.d.). *Creativity and innovation management: How to inspire original ideas.* https://online.stanford.edu/creativity-and-innovation-management#:~:text=Creativity%20is%20typically%20centered%20around,with%20into%20a%20viable%20solution

Synchrony. (2022). *Insured American's lifetime healthcare expenses may top $700k, according to new Synchrony research.* Cision, PR Newswire, November 14, 2022. https://www.prnewswire.com/news-releases/insured-americans-lifetime-healthcare-expenses-may-top-700k-according-to-new-synchrony-research-301674859.html

Tozzi, J. (2019). *Amazon-JPMorgan-Berkshire health-care venture to be called Haven.* Bloomberg, March 6, 2019. https://www.bloomberg.com/news/articles/2019-03-06/amazon-jpmorgan-berkshire-health-care-venture-to-be-called-haven

Turakhia, P., and Combs, B. (2017). Using principles of co-production to improve patient care and enhance value. *AMA Journal of* Ethics, *19*(11), 1125–1131.

Van Dyke, M. (2022, November/December). Leadership for intense times: Why agility and responsiveness are more important than ever. *Healthcare Executive,* 8–14.

Vlismas, T. (2020, June 24). *What is empathy? Learn about 3 types of empathy.* https://take-altus.com/2020/06/empathy-1/

Wagner, S. (2017). *Fundamentals of medical practice management.* Health Administration Press.

Wagner, S., & Hewitt, A. (2022). Collaborations and coproduction of health. In A. M. Hewitt, J. L. Mascari, & S. Wagner (Eds.), *Population health management: Strategies, tools, applications, and outcomes.* Springer Publishing.

Wagner, S., Shay, P., & Schumacher, E. (2022). Leadership for the future sector: Transformation, innovation, and change for population health managers. In A. M. Hewitt, J. L. Mascari, & S. Wagner (Eds.), *Population health management: Strategies, tools, applications, and outcomes.* Springer Publishing.

Walgreens Health. (2022). *Healthcare solutions: Champions for patient health.* https://www.walgreens.com/healthcare-solutions/home

Wernau, J., & Kamp, J. (2022, December 22). U.S. life expectancy fell to lowest level since 1996. *Wall Street Journal,* A3. https://www.wsj.com/articles/u-s-life-expectancy-fell-to-lowest-level-since-1996-11671667059

Credits

Fig. 13.1: Generated with FreeWordCloudGenerator.com.
Fig. 13.2a: Copyright © 2015 Depositphotos/opicobello.
Fig. 13.3: Copyright © 2015 Depositphotos/Rawpixel.
Fig. 13.6: Copyright © 2015 Depositphotos/Wavebreakmedia.

Fig. 13.7: Source: Adapted from https://www.interaction-design.org/literature/article/5-stages-in-the-design-thinking-process.

Fig. 13.8: Anne Hewitt, Julie Mascari, and Stephen Wagner, "Leadership for the Future Health Sector: Transformation, Innovation, and Change for Population Health Managers," *Population Health Management: Strategies, Tools, Applications and Outcomes*, p. 238. Copyright © 2022 by Springer Publishing Company.

Fig. 13.10a: Copyright © by Amazon.com, Inc.

Fig. 13.10b: Copyright © by Walmart.

Fig. 13.10c: Copyright © by Walgreen, Co..

Fig. 13.10d: Copyright © by CVS.com.

Fig. 13.10e: Copyright © by Aetna Inc.

Fig. 13.10f: Copyright © by Apple, Inc.

Fig. 13.10g: Copyright © 2015 Depositphotos/opicobello.

Fig. 13.11: Copyright © 2020 Depositphotos/elenabs.

Fig. 13.13: Adapted from Anne Hewitt, et al, "Aligning Community Hospitals with Local Public Health Departments: Collaborative Emergency Management," *Emergency Management and Disaster Response Utilizing Public-Private Partnerships*, ed. Marvine Paula Hamner, S. Shane Stovall, Doaa M. Taha, Salah C. Brahimi. Copyright © 2015 IGI Global.

Fig. 13.14: Copyright © 2014 Depositphotos/ra2studio.

Fig. 13.15: Copyright © 2019 Depositphotos/260philip1.

Fig. 13.16: Source: https://whatfix.com/blog/kubler-ross-change-curve/.

Fig. 13.17: Adapted from Stephen L. Wagner, Patrick D. Shay, and Edward J. Schumacher, "Leadership for the Future Sector: Transformation, Innovation, and Change for Population Health Managers," *Population Health Management: Strategies, Tools, Applications and Outcomes*, ed. Anne M. Hewitt, Julie L. Mascari, and Stephen L. Wagner, p. 242. Copyright © 2022 by Springer Publishing Company.

Appendix A: Case Study: The Role of Community Health Needs Assessments for Population Health

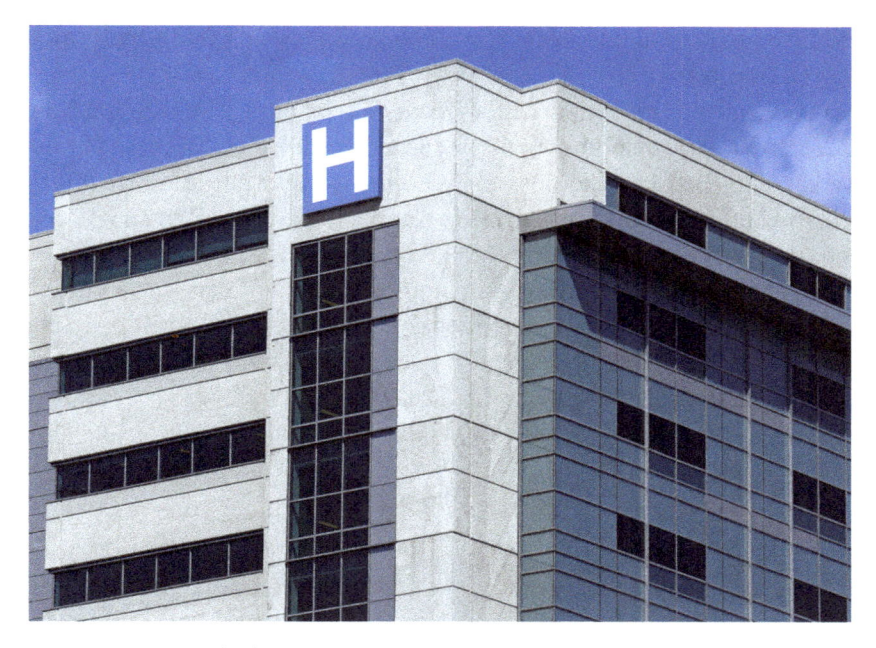

FIGURE A.1   Hospital

Introduction: Community Indicators as a Source of Population Health Data

Population health uses available data from both public and community organizations, hospitals and health systems. In 1969, the Internal Revenue Service (IRS) established a community benefit standard (James, 2016). **Community benefit** focuses on ensuring that nonprofit hospitals and health care systems serve the needs of their community to be eligible for tax-exempt status and operate as a 301(c) organization (Community Benefit Connect, 2020). Each year, hospitals and health systems submit documentation to prove their efforts meet the standards and criteria as a "public trust" initiative. What are community benefits?

They are clinical or nonclinical programs or activities providing treatment and/or promoting health and healing that are responsive to identified community needs, not provided for marketing purposes" (James, 2016). Common examples are health fairs with disease screening, mobile health vans, and community gardens, which are all sponsored by the health system or hospital. Each year hospitals collect data on the number of services they provide without charge to the community. These data supply valuable information about the needs of the local population. For example, if 200 people participate in the community garden and another 100 receive weekly food baskets, this may be an indication of food insecurity or a food desert (i.e., a location lacking fresh fruits and vegetables) in the community.

Note that community benefit differs from **charity care**. The IRS (2022) defines *hospital charity care*, also known as *financial assistance*, as "free or discounted health services provided to persons who meet the organization's eligibility criteria for financial assistance and are unable to pay for all or a portion of the services (IRS, 2022). Evidence shows that a considerable number of immigrants are recipients of charity care, which suggests a lack of care for a vulnerable population. A recent report estimated that hospitals spent $28 billion in charity care costs in fiscal year (FY) 2019, the majority of which ($22 billion) was for uninsured individuals (Levinson et al., 2022).

Community Benefits are clinical or non-clinical programs or activities providing treatment and/or promoting health and healing that are responsive to identified community needs, not provided for marketing purposes (James 2016).

Charity Care is free or discounted health services provided to persons who meet the organization's eligibility criteria for financial assistance and are unable to pay for all or a portion of the services (IRS, 2022).

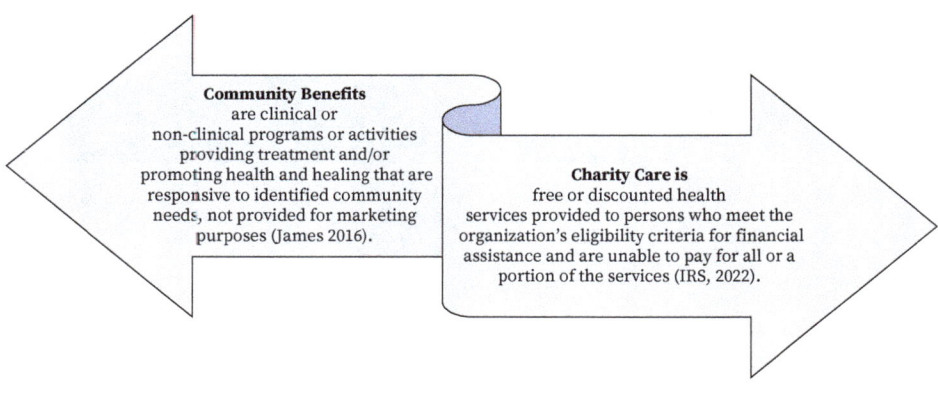

FIGURE A.2   Community Benefit and Charity Care Definitions

Since 2008, tax-exempt hospitals have been required to report their community benefit and other information related to tax-exemption on IRS Form 990 Schedule H (Catholic Hospital Association, n.d). Together, community benefit and charity care costs provide additional information for population health interventions.

Practical Skill: Essex County Community Health Needs Assessment (CHNA) 2022

Local health departments also complete mandated assessments of their constituents based on geographic location, as directed by state and federal guidelines. Public health initially referred to these evaluations as community health assessments (PHAB, 2011). Note the terms CHNA (community health needs assessment) and CHA (community health assessments) are often used interchangeably today. Many large counties, located across the country, partner with local universities that have expertise in assessment and evaluation of health conditions and population status. This example highlights a large New Jersey County which collaborated with a state university to complete their 2022 CHNA report (EC-OHPM-NJ & SPAA-Rutgers Newark, 2022). Although this report is over 170 pages in length, take the time to read the executive summary.

Access the report at: https://tinyurl.com/ea2zvtjt

1. What did you discover?
2. What are the health needs for this large metropolitan county?
3. List the top three recommendations to improve the quality of health.

Community Health Needs Assessment: A New Tool for Population Health

A new source of health data became available in 2010 with the passage of the Patient Protection and Affordable Care Act (PPACA or ACA) (PPACA, 2010). Today the ACA is regarded as one of the most far-reaching policy mandates since the beginnings of Medicare and Medicaid in the 1960s (Goldstein, Shephard & Duda, 2016). Among the many initiatives outlined in this 1,200-page legislation, was the **Community Health Needs Assessments** (CHNA) hospital requirement which focuses on accessing and meeting each community's needs to maintain non-profit status. This unique policy, located under the IRS jurisdiction, also establishes protocols detailing a hospital's financial assistance and emergency medical policy, and limitations of charges and billing and collection procedures.

Why was the concept of a CHNA a requirement? Over the years, the community benefit criteria established the necessity of addressing community need, but lacked a systematic process, plan, and assessment framework directly aligned with the hospital's delivery of health services. Hospitals needed to supply relevant and timely data that they were meeting the community's health needs to maintain their non-profit status benefits. Most importantly, the ACA stipulates a financial penalty tax of $50,000 per hospital for non-compliance or the IRS could ultimately revoke a hospital's tax-exempt status.

Every three years hospitals conduct community health needs assessments (CHNAs) in partnership with additional stakeholders, such as local health departments and other nonprofit health-related community agencies. The CHNA process must (1) assess the current population's health status (CHNA) and (2) develop an appropriate community implementation plan, commonly known as a **Community Health Improvement Plan** (CHIP) (IRS, 2020).

Completion of a CHNA is a complex and detailed process, involves many hours of data collection, analysis, and interpretation, and begins usually more than a year in advance. After the CHNA is completed, the CHIP development process requires input and collaboration with diverse and representative community stakeholders. To support local community hospitals, The American Hospital Association's (AHA) sponsored the Association for Community Health Improvement's (ACHI) **Community Health Assessment Toolkit** (ACHI, 2020). This CHNA Toolkit provides a nine-step outline that reflects a community oriented and transparent process to improve community health outcomes.

The steps in the ACHI tool are cyclical in that results from each cycle of the CHNA are integrated into strategies for the following cycle. To date, the CHNA process continues to be one of the most beneficial data collection and prioritization processes and can easily be integrated into population health interventions to ensure patient centered and community appropriate goals.

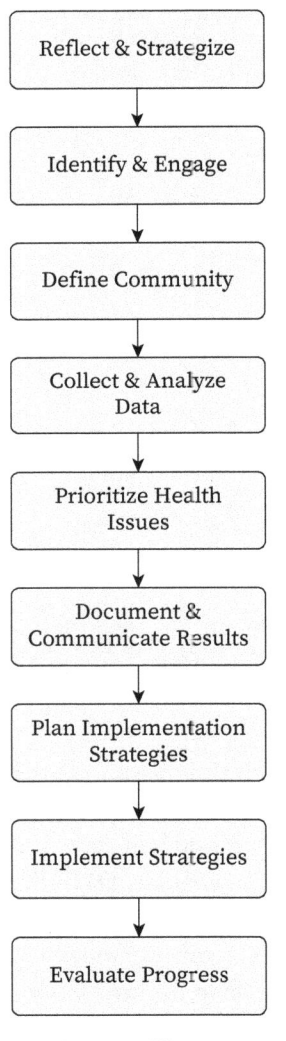

FIGURE A.3 Nine Phases of Community Health Assessment Toolkit

- Reflect & Strategize
- Identify & Engage
- Define Community
- Collect & Analyze Data
- Prioritize Health Issues
- Document & Communicate Results
- Plan Implementation Strategies
- Implement Strategies
- Evaluate Progress

County Health Rankings and Roadmap and PolicyMap Tools for Population Health

Another important community database useful for completing the CHNA is the RWJ Foundation's sponsored **County Health Rankings and Roadmap** (CHRR) (County Health Rankings and Roadmap, 2020a). This interactive platform follows the CHRR model which shows the direct relationships between three major health factors (health behaviors, clinical care, and social and economic factors) and individual and community impacts from population's activities, quality of care, and the social determinants of health.

TABLE A.1   County Health Rankings Model: Alignment of Health Factors

Health Factors		
Health Behaviors (30%)	**Clinical Care (20%)**	**Social & Economic Factors (40%)**
• Tobacco Use • Diet & Exercise • Alcohol & Drug Use • Sexual Activity	• Access to Care • Quality of Care	• Education • Employment • Income • Family & Social Support • Community Safety

Adapted from: RWJ Foundation. (2023). County Health Rankings Model. https://www.countyhealthrankings.org/explore-health-rankings/county-health-rankings-model.

The benefit of the model is the ability to create a snapshot of a specified county or municipality based on established and validated national databases. The snapshot provides valuable comparison metrics between the county and state or national data averages. The key findings are summarized year (County Health Rankings and Roadmap, 2020b).

PolicyMap is also an interactive data tool that provides diverse and expansive information from multiple databases to describe a population at a defined and specific geographic location https://www.policymap.com/maps). PolicyMap, an example of an online mapping tool or Geographical Information System (GIS), which creates a visual resource that aligns multiple determinants of health metrics that are pinpointed to a selected location (PolicyMap, 2020). Another PolicyMap benefit is the opportunity to layer personalized data or other relevant information onto a three-layer map. With this level of analysis, health planners and programmers have access to valuable visual evidence to target the most vulnerable communities.

This data mapping tool allows CHNA planners to see where vulnerable populations are located within their geographic community.

TABLE A.2 Sample County Health Ranking Snapshot

	Middlesex (MI) County	Massachusetts	United States
Health Outcomes			
Length of Life			
Premature Death	4,200	5,700	7,300
Quality of Life			
Poor or Fair Health	12%	13%	17%
Poor Physical Health Days	3.1	3.4	3.9
Poor Mental Health Days	4.0	4.2	4.5
Low Birthweight	7%	7%	8%
Additional Health Outcomes (not included in overall ranking)			
Health Factors			
Health Behaviors			
Adult Smoking	12%	12%	16%
Adult Obesity	23%	25%	32%
Food Environment Index	9.4	9.3	7.8
Physical Inactivity	22%	26%	26%
Access to Exercise Opportunities	95%	89%	80%
Excessive Drinking	23%	22%	20%
Alcohol-Impaired Driving Deaths	25%	31%	27%
Sexually Transmitted Infections	359.2	458.8	551.0
Teen Births	4	8	19
Additional Health Behaviors (not included in overall ranking)			
Clinical Care			
Uninsured	3%	4%	11%
Primary Care Physicians	780:1	960:1	1,310:1
Dentists	980:1	930:1	1,400:1
Mental Health Providers	160:1	140:1	350:1
Preventable Hospital Stays	3,836	4,202	3,767
Mammography Screening	56%	54%	43%
Flu Vaccinations	59%	56%	48%
Additional Clinical Care (not included in overall ranking)			

	Middlesex (MI) County	Massachusetts	United States
Social & Economic Factors			
High School Completion	94%	91%	89%
Some College	83%	74%	67%
Unemployment	7.3%	8.9%	8.1%
Children in Poverty	7%	11%	16%
Income Inequality	4.9	5.4	4.9
Children in Single-Parent Households	17%	24%	25%
Social Associations	9.5	9.4	9.2
Violent Crime	185	384	386
Injury Deaths	55	71	76
Physical Environment			
Air Pollution—Particulate Matter	8.0	6.3	Air Pollution—Particulate Matter
Drinking Water Violations	Yes		Drinking Water Violations
Severe Housing Problems	16%	17%	Severe Housing Problems
Driving Alone to Work	64%	68%	Driving Alone to Work
Long Commute—Driving Alone	49%	44%	Long Commute—Driving Alone
Additional Physical Environment (not included in overall ranking)			Additional Physical Environment (not included in overall ranking)

Source: County Health Rankings. Middlesex County. https://www.countyhealthrankings.org/explore-health-rankings/massachusetts/middlesex?year=2022

Summary

The Community Health Needs Assessment process systematically identifies a community's health needs and ensures that partnerships remain united to pursue community health improvement (Sachs & Skoufalos, 2021). The PPACA's increased emphasis on mandating health care system alignment with community health needs has resulted in a greater recognition of SDOH's role in the health of every American. Community and location (place-based) issues gained prominence as risk factors for positive health outcomes.

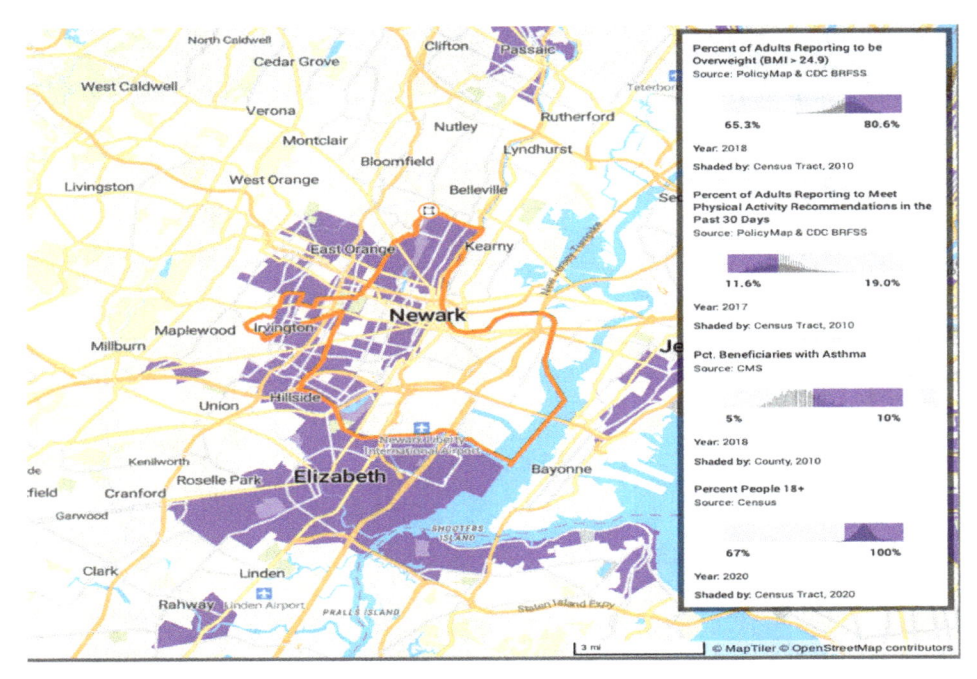

FIGURE A.4 Sample PolicyMap Risk Factors of Physical Inactivity, Asthma in Medicare Beneficiaries, and Overweight Adults

Case Study: Hunterdon Health, 2022 Community Health Needs Assessment

Hunterdon Healthcare System consists of the Hunterdon Medical Center, Hunterdon Healthcare Foundation, Hunterdon Regional Community Health, and Midjersey Health Corporation.

Hunterdon Medical Center, the flagship hospital, is acknowledged as a leader in developing comprehensive medical and health care services.

- Hunterdon Medical Center treats over 9,000 inpatients annually, with nearly 33,000 Emergency Department visits and over 570,000 outpatient visits per year. The 178-bed hospital provides a full range of preventive, diagnostic and therapeutic inpatient and outpatient hospital and community health services.
- Hunterdon Healthcare operates thirteen family practice/internal medicine offices, eighteen specialty offices and five pediatric practices. Hunterdon Healthcare has partnered with the Hunterdon Physician Practice Association to form Hunterdon Healthcare Partners LLC, an integrated delivery network dedicated to enhancing patient care.
- Hunterdon Healthcare Partners has nearly 312 providers who have come together to improve the overall quality of healthcare in the community.

Hunterdon Healthcare exists to prevent disease, illness, and injury; to seek cures; relieve pain; give comfort; and inspire a healthy way of living (AtlanticHealth, 2019).

Directions:

1. Access this CHNA report:

    Hunterdon Health. (2022). Community Health Needs Assessment: Our heart has a new look but it's still at the center of everything we do. URL: https://tinyurl.com/bddxb55m

2. Review the report and complete an analysis of the executive summary.
3. Answer the following questions:
    a. Did the CHNA include all nine components as outlined in the CHI tool? Please list.
    b. How did they define their "community"?
    c. Which stakeholder groups participated in the CHNA?
    d. What were the primary findings for lifestyle behaviors?
    e. Identify the top three findings for social determinants of health?
4. Discuss if the report presented comparisons with previous CHNAs and their conclusions.
5. How were the priority items determined, and what were they?
6. Do you feel that the report adequately addressed the community's needs as listed in the CHNA? Give an example.

References

ACHI & Community Health Improvement (2020). *Community Health Assessment Toolkit.* https://www.healthycommunities.org/resources/community-health-assessment-toolkit

AtlanticHealth. (2019, December 10). Hunterdon Healthcare and Atlantic Health System Partner to Bring Enhanced Ambulatory Services to Somerset County. https://www.atlantichealth.org/about-us/stay-connected/news/press-releases/2019/atlantic-hunterdon-partnership-bridgewater.html#:~:text=Patrick%20Gavin%2C%20President%20and%20CEO,expand%20services%20in%20Somerset%20County.%E2%80%9D

Catholic Hospital Association. (n.d.) *About community benefit.* https://www.chausa.org/communitybenefit/resources/defining-community-benefit

Community Benefit Connect. (2020). *What is community benefit?* Community Benefit Connect www.communitybenefitconnect.org/about-us/about_what-is/ https://www.communitybenefitconnect.org/about-us/about_what-is/ .

County Health Rankings & Roadmaps. (2020a). *County health rankings model.* https://www.countyhealthrankings.org/explore-health-rankings/measures-data-sources

County Health Rankings & Roadmaps. (2020b). *2020 county health rankings: State reports.* https://www.countyhealthrankings.org/

County Health Rankings & Roadmaps. (2022). *Middlesex County, MA.* https://www.countyhealthrankings.org/explore-health-rankings/massachusetts/middlesex?year=2022

Essex County Office of Public Health Management New Jersey School of Public Affairs and Administration Rutgers University Newark. (2022). *Essex County New Jersey community health needs assessment 2022.* https://essexcountynj.org/wp-content/uploads/2022/07/Essex-County-Health-Assessment-Final-Report.pdf

Hunterdon Health. (2022). Community Health Needs Assessment: Our heart has a new look but its still at the center of everything we do.:https://www.hunterdonhealth.org/sites/default/files/2022-11/2023-2025%20CHNA%20Report%20%281%29.pdf

Goldstein, F. Shephard, V. & Duda, S., (2016). Policy implications for population health: Health promotion and wellness. In *population health: Creating a culture of wellness,* Nash et al. Eds. Sudbury, MA: Jones & Bartlett Publishing.

HealthCare.gov. (2010). *Patient Protection and Affordable Care Act.* https://www.healthcare.gov/glossary/patient-protection-and-affordable-care-act/

Internal Revenue Service (IRS). (2020). Community health needs assessment for charitable hospital organizations—Section 501(r)(3). https://www.irs.gov/charities-non-profits/community-health-needs-assessment-for-charitable-hospital-organizations-section-501r3

Internal Revenue Service. (2022). Instructors for Schedule H (Form 990). Department of the Treasury. https://www.irs.gov/pub/irs-pdf/i990sh.pdf

James, J. (2016). Health policy brief: Nonprofit hospitals community benefits requirements. *Health Affairs,* February 25, 2016. https://www.healthaffairs.org/do/10.1377/hpb20160225.954803/full/

Levinson, Z., Hulver, S. & Newman, T. (2022, November 3). *Hospital charity care: How it works and why it matters.* Kaiser Family Foundation. https://www.kff.org/health-costs/issue-brief/hospital-charity-care-how-it-works-and-why-it-matters/

Patient Protection and Affordability Care Act (2010). *Read the Affordable Care Act.* https://www.healthcare.gov/where-can-i-read-the-affordable-care-act/

Public Health Accreditation Board. (2011). *Public Health Accreditation Board: Standards and measures.* https://phsharing.org/resources/public-health-accreditation-board-standards-measures/

PolicyMap (2020). 2020 PolicyMap: Online GIS maps https://www.policymap.com/maps)

Sachs, R. & Skoufalos, A. 2021. Developing the workforce to enhance population health. In A. Nash, Skoufalos, A., R. Fabius, & Oglesby, W. *Population health: Creating a culture of wellness.* Jones and Bartlett Learning.

Credits

Fig. A.1: Copyright © 2021 Depositphotos/spirope.

Fig. A.3: Source: https://www.healthycommunities.org/resources/community-health-assessment-toolkit.

Fig. A.4: Copyright © by PolicyMap. Reprinted with permission.

Glossary

Accountable care: Transitioning from fee-for-service care to value-based care.

Accountable care organization (ACO): Network of providers who come together to provide whole patient-centered care to patients, with the primary care physician (PCP) at the center of the network.

ACO Realizing Equity, Access, and Community Health (ACO REACH) Model: A model for ACOs to break down silos and deliver high-quality, coordinated care to their patients, improve health outcomes, and manage costs.

Adherence: Inference of a patient's obedience to a health professional's directives.

Advocacy: Activities that influence public opinion and attitudes that directly affect people's lives.

Agile leadership: A leadership style that emphasizes removing consumer barriers or obstacles as quickly as possible to solicit feedback and continue innovation.

Algorithm: A machine process used for solving a problem or performing a technical computation.

Alternative payment systems: A model that outlines and describes in detail a four-level continuum, with subcategories that capture clinical and financial risk for provider organizations as they move from volume to a fee-based system.

Artificial intelligence: An analysis based on sophisticated technologies that capture the complex process of human thought and intelligence.

Attack rate: A measure of disease occurrence used when a disease increases within a population over a short period.

Average life expectancy: The average remaining years an individual of a particular age can be expected to live.

Behavior economics: The incorporation of economic, cognitive, and social psychology disciplines to determine how individuals (and institutions) make economic decisions.

Big data: Extremely large data sets.

Bundled payments: Payments that include the total allowable acute and/or post-acute expenditures (target price) for a predetermined episode of care.

Case: An individual who is diagnosed with a disease or a condition.

Case fatality rate: The proportion of cases of a particular condition that are fatal within a specified time.

Centers for Disease Control and Prevention (CDC): The nation's leading science-based, data-driven, service organization that protects the public's health.

Change management: An approach and tools can be used to help people understand, accept, move forward, appreciate change, and then act.

Charity care: Free or discounted health services at a hospital provided to persons who meet the organization's eligibility criteria for financial assistance and are unable to pay for all or a portion of the service.

Chronic care model: A care coordination model designed to provide key elements for individuals who suffer from chronic disease.

Chronic disease: A disease that lasts for 3 months or more, generally cannot be prevented by vaccines or cured by medication and does not disappear.

Chronic disease self-management program: A program that features an interactive workshop for people with all types of chronic conditions and provides simple self-help education and techniques to help them self-manage their disease.

Clinical decision support systems (CDSS): A combination of computer-based programs (clinical information systems) that analyze data from electronic health records to provide reminders that assist health care providers at the point of care.

Cohort: A type of observational study in which participants are classified according to their exposure status and then followed over time to ascertain the outcome.

Collaboration: Working with others.

Collective impact: A network of community members, organizations, and institutions who advance equity by learning together, aligning, and integrating their actions to achieve population and systems-level change.

Communicable disease: Illnesses that spread from one person to another or from an animal to a person or from a surface or a food.

Community: A collective body of individuals identified by common characteristics, such as geography, interests, experiences, concerns, and values.

Community benefit: Clinical and nonclinical programs and activities providing treatment and/or promoting health and healing that are responsive to identified community needs and not provided for marketing purposes.

Community health: The health status of a defined group of people and the actions and conditions, both private and public (governmental), to promote, protect, and preserve their health.

Community health improvement plan (CHIP): A long-term, systematic effort to address public health problems based on the results of community health assessment activities and the community health improvement process.

Community health needs assessment (CHNA): A systematic process conducted by a hospital involving the community to identify and analyze community health needs and assets, prioritize those needs, and then implement a plan to address significant unmet needs.

Community health worker: Front-line public health worker who serves as a liaison between the community and needed health and social services.

Compliance: An asymmetrical relationship between the health care practitioner and the patient, in which the health care provider selects the course of treatment, and the patient is expected to follow directions.

Components of health: An individual's physical, mental, social, emotional, and spiritual well-being.

Consumer: Individual who selects who will be their health care provider and when to seek care.

Consumerism: People proactively using trustworthy, relevant information and appropriate technology to make better-informed decisions about their health care options.

Continuum of care: A pathway of care, provided over time, which includes new options for delivery of care, easier access to specialty health providers, and improved transitions through coordinated care.

Continuum of collaboration: A framework that emphasizes four relationship levels: networking, coordinating, cooperating, and collaborating.

Coordinated care: Term that implies an established health plan that ensures access to appropriate providers and health care services when needed.

Co-production of health: The idea that community organizations, clinicians, social services, government agencies, and the service recipients (i.e., patients) must be engaged and focused on the well-being of the population.

Cost-benefit analysis: A process used to measure the benefits of a decision or action minus the costs associated with taking that action.

County Health Rankings & Roadmaps (CHRR): An interactive web-based program that compares the health of nearly all counties in the United States to others within its own state and supports coalitions tackling the social, economic, and environmental factors that influence health by revealing a snapshot of how health is influenced by where we live, learn, work, and play.

Creativity: Original thought, knowledge, and imagination for generating innovative ideas.

Crude, age-specific, cause-specific, and adjusted rates: Common types of epidemiological rates where the numerator represents a condition or disease, and the denominator reflects the population size.

Cultural competence: A set of congruent behaviors, attitudes, and policies that come together in a system, agency, or among professionals that enables effective work in cross-cultural situations.

Culturally and Linguistically Appropriate Services (CLAS) standards: The National CLAS standards are a blueprint to not only eliminate health disparities and advance health equity, but also improve service quality of care.

Culture of health: Action framework combined of essential components of community, public, global, and population health approaches by establishing 10 principles that provide a foundation for four action steps.

Data justice: A proactive health sector strategy with a goal to remediate and eliminate the possibility of prejudiced or unfair data design, collection, interpretation, or use.

Decision support: Computer programming and data analysis activities that produce tailored and valuable information to make an assessment.

Design thinking: An approach to problem solving that emphasizes empathy, innovation, collaboration, and continual experimentation.

Digital assistant: A virtual assistant that provides technology designed to aid users by answering questions and processing simple tasks.

DIKW: Data, Information, Knowledge, and Wisdom.

Discrimination: Unjust or prejudicial treatment of different categories of people, especially on the grounds of ethnicity, age, sex, or disability.

Disease prevention: *Primary*, *secondary*, and *tertiary* refer to the various levels of prevention with primary focusing on the elimination of risk factors for a disease; secondary efforts focus on the early detection and treatment of disease, and tertiary activities seek to minimize disability associated with advanced disease.

Disruption: An event that interferes with the normal, whether that be a process, an activity, or a way of doing business.

Distribution and determinants of disease: Epidemiological considerations of spread (frequency and patterns), causes, and other factors of disease in a population.

Divergent thinking: Describes the process during ideation of developing multiple ideas; opposite of convergent thinking, which sifts through those ideas to explore concepts of merit and leads to iteration and experimentation.

Diversity: Encompasses acceptance and respect, meaning understanding that everyone is unique and recognizing our individual differences. Inclusion is a state of being valued, respected, and supported.

Dual eligibility: Individuals who qualify for both Medicare and Medicaid benefits.

Electronic health record (EHR [or electronic medical record (EMR)]: A universal repository of patient information.

Empathy map: Mapping that includes consumers' perceptions of what they see, hear, think, feel, say, and want in their environment.

Endemic, epidemic and pandemic: Distinguishes between the various amounts of disease within a group or location endemic being expected or constant presence; epidemic meaning more than normal expectation, and pandemic meaning worldwide distribution.

Epidemiology: Descriptive, analytical, and managerial: Refers to the various branches of epidemiology, the study of the distribution and determinants of disease in a population with analytic focusing on associations; descriptive answering questions of who, what, where, when, and why; and managerial addressing decision-making processes by applying basic epidemiological tools and principles.

Episode of care: Refers to a patient's entire treatment needed for an illness or episode.

Fee-for-Service (FFS): Refers to the payment a health care provider receives for services a patient might need; also known as *volume-based care*.

Food insecurity: The economic and social condition characterized by limited or uncertain access to adequate food.

Frequency measures of disease: Measures of the occurrence of a disease.

Global health: Collaborative transnational research and action for promoting health for all.

Grand challenge: Large, unresolved problems involving complex interactions and substantial uncertainty.

Health: A state of complete physical, mental, and social well-being and not merely the absence of disease or infirmity.

Health advocacy: Efforts to change individual behavior or a population's lifestyles or encourage development of positive health policies.

Health behavior: Actions that can directly affect health outcomes.

Health belief model (HBM): A model that suggests individuals are motivated to change their health behavior by examining three major components: expectations, threats, and cues to action.

Health data analytics: Focuses on the technologies and processes that measure, manage, and analyze health care data.

Health disparities: Preventable differences in the burden of disease, injury, violence, or opportunities to achieve optimal health that are experienced by socially disadvantaged populations.

Health education: A complex set of activities that provide diverse opportunities to acquire knowledge and the skills to make high-quality health decisions.

Health equality: A term referring to the idea that every individual has an equal opportunity to make the most of their lives and talents.

Health equity: Absence of unfair and avoidable or remediable differences in health among population groups defined socially, economically, demographically, or geographically.

Health in All Policies (HIAP): A collaborative approach that brings together policymakers and practitioners from all sectors related to the social determinants of health under the assumption that all multisectoral policies affect health outcomes.

Health informatics: A term used to describe the science of information management in health care.

Health information exchange (HIE): Access to patient data and treatment history across health care providers and organizations using a database repository of patient data that is easily accessible due to universal standards requirements.

Health information technology: Involves the processing, storage, and exchange of health information in an electronic environment.

Health Information Technology for Economic and Clinical Health (HITECH) Act: An act passed in 2009 that required health care entities to install computerized systems and demonstrate their meaningful use.

Health Insurance Portability and Accountability Act of 1996 (HIPAA): A law that established privacy and security requirements for health care providers and organizations.

Health promotion: The process of enabling people to increase control over their health and its determinants and thereby improve their health.

Health promotion program: Any type of planned combination of educational, political, environmental, regulatory, or organizational mechanisms that supports actions and conditions of living conducive to the health of individuals, groups, and communities.

Health risk assessment: Formal questionnaire used to collect data from thousands of individuals that can be aggregated to determine various disease risks across a population.

Healthscape: The situation where one is as well as the related trends in health care that accompany a particular setting that includes the entire health care environment of where one lives.

Healthy Days Measures: Four validated questions that ask each person to rate their perceived state of health.

Heuristics: Rule-of-thumb decisions based on short-cut thinking from past experiences.

High-level wellness: A desirable balance and integration between the five components of health: physical, mental, social, emotional, and spiritual.

Horizontal integration: Integration between agencies at the same level to integrate care.

Hospital-at-home: Care that integrates remote health monitoring and wearable technology strategies that enables a select group of patients to remain in the comfort of their home.

Hot spotting: A strategy of identifying those at-risk patients with multiple comorbidities who overuse emergency treatment because of a lack of coordinated care and aligning them with doctors, other caregivers, and social service providers to prevent rehospitalizations and other intensive, expensive forms of care.

Ideation: Expanding boundaries for our thoughts to propose a solution.

Implicit bias: A type of unconscious bias that occurs automatically and unintentionally and affects our judgments, decisions, and behaviors.

Incidence and prevalence: Indicators of rates of illness and disease within a population, with the incidence rate referring to the number of new cases in a population for a given time period and the prevalence rate being the total number of people having a condition at a particular time divided by the population at risk of having the condition.

Inclusion: The essential process for accepting variation and differences among a population, whether it includes American Indian/Alaska Native, Asians American, Native Hawaiian or another Pacific Islander, African American, or Hispanic.

Indicator: A measure or a value of something.

Influencer: Trusted individual who promotes an idea or a cause such as wellness and encourages populations of followers to adopt suggested preferences with the purpose of shaping behaviors.

Innovation: Execution of an idea that addresses a specific challenge and achieves value for both the company and the customer.

Integrated care delivery network (IDN): Refers to multiple options for integrating care, whether within a system, an organization, or a group of organizations.

Interoperability: The ability of various systems and organizations to work together to exchange information.

Levels of prevention: A term referring to classifying prevention intervention strategies, with *primary* meaning intervention before health effects occur, *secondary* meaning screening to identify diseases at the earliest stage, and *tertiary* meaning management of disease postdiagnosis to slow or stop the condition.

Loss aversion: When an individual has a personal preference for avoiding loss as compared to acquiring gains.

Majority: When cultural characteristics are found in more than 50% of a population.

Managed care: A type of health care delivery system organized to manage cost, utilization, and quality.

Meaningful use: A term used to describe the requirement for providers to demonstrate performance on defined metrics and measures from their electronic health record.

Medicaid: A social protection program (insurance) in which eligibility is determined by income and designed for low-income Americans.

Medical model: A model that focuses exclusively on the individual as the organizational center of the entire clinical health care delivery system with an emphasis on treatment as primary and the hospital as the center of health care.

Medicare: A federal program that provides health care coverage for individuals older than age 65, people younger than age 65 with certain disabilities, and people of all ages with end-stage renal disease.

Mental accounting: A pro-and-con system for making healthy choices.

Minority: When cultural characteristics are found in fewer than 50% of a population.

Minority health: Defined in the United States as encompassing the following groups: American Indians/Alaska Natives, Asians Americans, Native Hawaiians and other Pacific Islanders, African Americans, and Hispanics.

Mobile health applications: The use of smartphone devices and specific applications to provide health communications and increase interactions with individuals.

Mortality and morbidity: Rates that represent the presence of illness in a population (morbidity) and death (mortality).

National Center for Quality Assurance (NCQA): An organization that establishes guidelines for meeting standards and safety criteria.

Net promotor score: A rating based on a standard question asking whether consumers would recommend a health care company, product, or service to a friend or colleague.

Nontraditional competitors: New and diverse entrants into the population health sector, including drugstores, retail, venture capitalists, e-commerce businesses, third-party vendors, and Fortune 500 companies.

Nudges: A concept referring to the idea that targeted and tailored information can be used to engage consumers/patients to participate in healthy actions and activities.

Quality: A term that refers to the degree to which an object or entity (e.g., process, product, or service) satisfies a specified set of attributes or requirements; a high standard of health care services.

Pathway to Population Health: Nationally recognized document that outlines the foundational concepts to ensure hospitals and health care systems follow a successful transition to the population health model.

Patient activation: A term referring to when an individual shows they have the knowledge, skill, and confidence to manage their health care.

Patient-centered medical home (PCMH): A term referring to when multiple providers work under one organizational banner that was created with the intention of reducing costs while improving patient outcomes.

Patient empowerment: A term for what occurs when individuals are encouraged to exercise their authority and autonomy to build self-confidence.

Patient engagement: Activities or efforts to involve an individual in their own care.

Patient Engagement Capacity Model: A tool to assess patient's engagement using two sets of overlapping factors: internal capabilities and external impacts on capacity.

Patient experience: A patient's perception of the total health care interaction experience.

Patient-health care professional interaction: Refers to the interpersonal, face-to-face, and/or virtual communication between a health care practitioner and a patient.

Patient journey: A series of interactions between the individual and health care organization and personnel.

Patient Protection and Affordable Care Act (PPACA or ACA): This act provides for numerous rights and protections that make health care coverage fairer, easier to understand, and more affordable.

Patient registry: Patient information repository that stores data related to a health condition or disease.

Patient safety: A term referring to the prevention of harm to patients.

Patient satisfaction: A term referring to a patient's feelings and attitudes regarding their health expectations and outcomes.

Pay for performance: Alternative payment model that aligns performance (quality) with cost.

PDSA: Plan, Do, Study, and Act; a useful tool for documenting and piloting a change in the quality improvement process.

Performance measurement: A process used to assess the efficiency and effectiveness of projects, programs, and initiatives.

PolicyMap: A geographical information system that is an interactive, visual resource aligning multiple determinants of health metrics with pinpointed locations on a map.

Population: A term used to describe designated groups of persons that also includes the context of where they live, work, and play in their local communities.

Population health: The health outcomes of a group of individuals, including the distribution of such outcomes within the group.

Population Health Alliance Population Health Management Framework (PHA-PHMF): Developed by the industry's multistakeholder professional and trade association (Population Health Alliance); conceptualizes health care delivery systems' implementation activities for quality health outcomes.

Population health management (PHM): The organization and management of the health care delivery system in a manner that makes it more clinically effective, more cost-effective, and safer.

Post-acute care: A term referring to all health care activities following acute (treatment) care.

Preparation, Action, Sustaining Change, and Transformation (PAST) change model: A linear change model featuring four stages.

Precision medicine: A term referring to the practice of tailoring medical treatment to the individual characteristics of each patient.

Predictive modeling: The use of large databases to determine characteristics of vulnerable patients who may be at risk for infection, diseases, or other health needs.

PRO: Patient-reported outcome.

Public health: A term referring to the science and art of preventing disease, prolonging life, and promoting physical health and efficiency through organized community efforts.

Quadruple Aim: The Triple Aim with the added concept of productivity.

Quality improvement: Processes and models that help provide frameworks and guide population health through the process of improving health care outcomes.

Quality of life: An individual's perception of their position in life in the context of the culture and value systems in which they live and in relation to their goals, expectations, standards, and concerns.

Radical collaboration: Organizational strategy of working with nontraditional or unexpected organizations or entities.

Rate: A simple comparison of two numbers with different quantities or units.

Reengineering: An activity that moves reorganizing to the next level and can be the reimagination of an entire organization.

Remote home monitoring: Use of connected tools to record personal health and medical data in one location for review by a health care provider in another location at a different time.

Reorganizing: Redesigning common organizational practices that focus on configurations or structure.

Risk: The probability that an event will occur.

Risk factor: An exposure that is associated with a disease or a condition, without certainty.

Risk management: An approach to developing and implementing safe and effective patient care practices, preserving financial services, and maintaining safe working environments.

Risk segmentation: Use of current and prospective medical costs, health status, attitudes, and level of health care engagement to select individuals from a population.

Risk stratification: A systematic process for identifying and predicting patient's risk levels relating to health care needs, services, and care coordination with the goal of identifying those at highest risk and managing their care to prevent poor outcomes.

Self-efficacy: An individual's perception of their capabilities for changing a behavior.

Self-management education (SME): Programs that educate patients in ways to help manage their chronic symptoms and diseases such as asthma, arthritis, diabetes, chronic obstructive pulmonary disease, and chronic pain.

Social determinants of health (SDOH): Conditions in which people are born, grow, live, work, and age; these circumstances are shaped by the distribution of money, power, and resources at the global, national, and local levels.

Social justice: The view that everyone deserves equal economic, political, and social rights and opportunities.

Socio-ecological model: The potential scope of factors that influence health and well-being at each population level.

Specific Rates: Refers to a statistic referred to a particular sub-group of the population defined in terms of race, age, or sex.

Structural racism: Macrolevel systems, social forces, institutions, ideologies, and processes that interact with one another to generate and reinforce inequities among racial and ethnic groups.

Telehealth: A digital platform with a variety of combinations of communication options (e.g., audio, audio-video, chat-based) that also offers the capacity to store and forward options through secure communications.

Transitions of care: Linkages between primary care, acute care, and multiple options for post-acute care.

Transtheoretical (Stages of Change) Model (TTM): A model that focuses on the cycle of addictive behaviors and lifestyle behaviors needed for long-term change.

Triple Aim: An initiative that addresses simultaneously the population health issues of access, quality, and impact.

Upstream, midstream, and downstream health factors: *Upstream issues* address the social determinants of health. *Midstream issues* refer to educating individuals to improve their condition and include factors related to individual-level behavior change, such as promoting healthy eating, healthy family relationships, and exercise. *Downstream issues* include costs such as for treatment of chronic and relapsing conditions and related disease complications.

Value-based care: A term that refers to care that requires quality services, positive health outcomes, and cost reduction and that may use incentives as part of an alternative payment system.

Value equation: An equation meaning value equals outcome divided by cost.

Value over volume: Selecting value (quality) over volume (quantity).

Vertical integration: Integration between agencies on various levels (e.g., primary to secondary, secondary to tertiary); occurs when organizations at various levels of care delivery coordinate the provision of care.

Virtual care: Encompasses all opportunities for diverse digital and other interactions between a health care practitioner and a patient across the continuum of care.

Volume-to-value: A term referring to the transition from volume (quantity) to value (quality).

Wearable technology: Any type of electronic device designed to be worn on the user's body.

Well-being: A personal state of being comfortable, healthy, and happy.

Wellness: The active pursuit to understand and fulfill an individual's human needs.

Wicked problem: A major challenge with interdependent, changing, and difficult-to-define factors.

Workplace health: The alignment of meaningful work within life's balance by ensuring employees are healthy and actively engaged in wellness activities.

World Health Organization (WHO): United Nations agency that works worldwide to promote health, keep the world safe, and serve the vulnerable.

Index

A

accountability, 179–194
  cost of care, 183
  equity of care, 188–194
  impact of government health plans, 181–183
  payment models, 184–185
  quality, 188–194
  safety, 188–194
  shared financial risk, 186
  value-based payment options, 186–188
accountable care, 16
accountable care organization (ACO), 68, 211–212
ACO Realizing Equity, Access, and Community Health (ACO-REACH), 212
adherence, 225
adjusted rates, 58
advocacy, 96–97
age, 58
Agency for Healthcare Research and Quality (AHRQ), 213
agile leadership, 273–274
Alliance for Community Health Integration (ACHI), 32
alternative payment systems, 184
American Hospital Association (AHA), 9, 96, 284
American Telemedicine Association (ATA), 232
analytical epidemiology, 58–60
artificial intelligence (AI), 153, 155–156. *See also* ChatGPT
Association for Community Health Improvement (ACHI), 284
attack rate, 56–57
average life expectancy, 53

B

behavioral health, 88
behavior economics, 139–140
birth rate, 57
bundled payment, 187

C

care, 199–214
  accountable care organizations (ACOs), 211–212
  charity, 282
  chronic care coordination, 200–205
  chronic care model, 204–205
  coordinated, 207–209
  integrated, 209–211
  patient-centered medical homes (PCMHs), 212–213
  post-acute care strategies of, 208
  self-management of chronic disease, 205–206
  transition-of-care model, 206–207
Care Continuum, 95
case study
  Hunterdon Health, 288–289
  risk management, 168–173
  role of community health needs assessments, 281–289
catalysts for health care change, 14–16
Centers for Disease Control and Prevention (CDC), 14, 34, 202
challenges, 254–258. *See also* grand challenges
change, 271–273
  managing resistance to, 272–273
charity care, 282. *See also* care
ChatGPT, 156
Children's Health Insurance Program (CHIP), 181
chronic care model, 204–205
chronic conditions, 55
chronic disease in U.S. adults, 201
chronic disease, risk factors for, 131
climate change, 43–44. *See also* change
clinical decision support systems (CDSS), 204
cohort study, 59
collaborations to co-production of health, 268–271
collective impact framework, 71–72
communicable, 55
community
  benefit, 281–282
  characterization of, 29–30
  defined, 28
  indicators, 281–283
community health, 24–28
  organizations, 32–34
  population perspective, 28–34
  priorities, 31–32
Community Health Assessment Toolkit, 284
community health improvement plan (CHIP), 284
community health needs assessments (CHNA), 281–289
  community indicators, 281–283
  County Health Rankings and Roadmap (CHRR), 285–287
  tool for population health, 283–284
community health workers (CHWs), 30–31
compliance, 224
connected health, 233
consumer decision-making, 138
consumerism, 137–139. *See also* under health care

consumer/patient issues, 11–12
Continuum of Care, 98
continuum of collaboration, 70–71
co-production of health, 267–271
   initiatives, 270–271
cost of care, 183
County Health Rankings and Roadmap (CHRR), 285–287
COVID-19 vaccination, 137
creativity, 260
crude rates, 56–58
cultural competence, 120
Culture of Health model, 65, 69–70, 73, 79–80

D

data, 149–160
   challenges, 158–159
   Data, Information, Knowledge, and Wisdom (DIKW), 150–152
   health data analytics, 155–157
   health informatic tools, 152–154
   justice, 159
   role of, 150–152
   sources, 157–158
Data, Information, Knowledge, and Wisdom (DIKW), 150–152
decision support, 204
Department of Health and Human Services (DHHS), 34
descriptive epidemiology, 54–55
design thinking, 261–262
digital assistants, 243
digital front doors, 235
digital health, 244
discrimination, 114–115
disease prevention, 10, 95
disease prevention intervention, 173
disease rates calculations, 55–56
disruption, 265
disruptors, 265–266
divergent thinking, 263
diversity, 106
downstream factors, 113
dual eligibility, 182

E

efficiency, 69
electronic health record (EHR), 152–153
electronic medical record (EMR), 152, 235
emotional health, 88–89
empathy, 262–263
empathy map, 262
endemic, 55
epidemic, 55
epidemiology, 54
   analytical, 58–60
   descriptive, 54–55
   managerial, 60–61

F

fee for service, 10, 186–187
financial assistance, 282
food insecurity, 111
fragmented care patient pathway, 203
frameworks, 65–79
   collaboration, 70–72
   collective impact, 71–72
   continuum of collaboration, 70–71
   cultural of health, 69–70
   health of populations management, 66–67
   multisectoral population health initiatives, 73–79
   pathways to, 73–74
   population health alliance framework, 74–79
   population health vision for communities, 69–70
   portfolios of, 74
   Triple Aim vision, 67–69

G

gender, 58
global health, 24–28
   climate change, 43–44
   population perspective, 41–44
   sustainable development goals (SDGs), 42–43
   World Health Organization (WHO), 41–42
grand challenges, 255
gross domestic product (GDP), 12–13

H

happiness, 32
health
   advocacy, 96–97
   behavioral, 88
   components of, 89
   defined, 5, 88
   emotional, 88
   mental, 88
   physical, 88
   social, 88
   spiritual, 88
health assessments for population health, 92–94
health behaviors, 129–142
   challenges, 130–131
   decision-making and, 140–141
   defined, 132
   economics, 139–140
   frameworks, 133
   impact of consumerism, 137–139
   models, 133–137
   strategies, 131–132, 140–141
health belief model (HBM), 134–135
health care. *See also* care
   change, catalysts for, 14–16
   consumerism, 138–139
   integration, 209–210
health data analytics, 155–157
health disparities, 12, 109–110
health education, 226
health equality, 115–116
health equity, 114–120
health for all Americans, 8, 17
Health in All Policies (HIAP), 98–100
health informatics, 151
health information exchange (HIE), 154
health information systems (HIS), 151–152
Health Information Technology for Economic and Clinical Health (HITECH) Act, 152
health information technology (HIT) employees, 235
health insurance, 181

Health Insurance Portability and Accountability Act of 1996 (HIPAA), 14, 152, 235
health maintenance organization (HMO), 185
Health Maintenance Organization (HMO) Act of 1973, 185
health promotion, 10, 95–96
health promotion and wellness, 87–100
   Continuum of Care, 98
   health applications of, 95–96
   health assessments, 92–94
   Health in All Policies (HIAP), 98–100
   high-level, 89–92
   role of advocacy, 96–97
health promotion programs and activities, 95
health risk, 169
   defined, 166–167
health risk assessments (HRAs), 93–94
healthscape, 24
health silos, 12
healthy days measures, 92–93
Healthy People 2030, 37–39, 114
Herodotus, 130
heuristic, 139
horizontal integration strategies, 210–211
hospital-at-home, 240–241
hospital charity care, 282
hot spotting, 7–8

I

ideation, 263
incidence, 56
inclusion, 109
Indian Health Service, 181
influencers, 140–141
innovation, 258–264
   design thinking, 261–262
   empathy, 262–263
   framework for, 261–262
   ideate, 263
   problem, defined, 263
   prototype design, 263
   prototype test, 264
innovative management, 8, 17
Institute for Health Improvement (IHI), 67

integrated care, 209–211
integrated delivery networks (IDNs), 210
integrated delivery systems, 211
integrated health system, 210
Internal Revenue Service (IRS), 281–282
interoperability, 157

K

Kubler-Ross change curve, 272

L

Lexington Minuteman, 29
lifestyle, 55
loss aversion, 140

M

majority, 107–108
managed care, 185–186
managed care organizations (MCOs), 185
management, 8–9. *See also* risk management
   innovative, 8, 17
managerial epidemiology, 60–61
Medicaid, 181–183
medical model, 10
Medicare, 181–183
Medicare Access and CHIP Reauthorization Act of 2015 (MACRA), 14
mental health, 88–89
midstream factors, 113
minority, 108
minority health, 108
mobile health applications, 233–235
morbidity (illness), 10
mortality (death), 10
mortality rate, 57
multisectoral population health initiatives, 73–79

N

National Association of County and City Health Officials (NACCHO), 40
National Committee for Quality Assurance (NCQA), 179, 189, 212

National Culturally and Linguistically Appropriate Services (CLAS), 117–119
National Priorities Partnership (NPP), 13, 66–67
net promoter scores (NPS), 230
nudges, 140–141

P

pain points, 262
pandemic, 55
Parker, J., 29
PAST change model, 273
The Pathways to Population Health: An Invitation to Healthcare Change Agents (Saha), 73
patient activation, 228
Patient Activation Measure (PAM), 228
patient-centered medical homes (PCMHs), 212–213
patient empowerment, 221, 225–229
patient engagement, 225–229
Patient Engagement Capacity Model, 228
patient experience, 230
patient–health care professional interactions, 221–246
   mobile health applications, 233–235
   patient empowerment, 225–229
   patient engagement, 225–229
   patient experience, 230
   patient satisfaction, 229
   reframing talk, 224–225
   virtual care, 221–222, 231–245
patient journey, 229
Patient Protection and Affordable Care Act (PPACA), 14–16, 201, 283
patient-provider interactions, 224
patient registries, 154
patient-reported outcomes (PROs), 237
patient safety and equity, 189
patient satisfaction, 229

pay for performance, 11
payment models, 184–185
performance, 190–194
personalized medicine, 78
personal protective equipment (PPE), 71
PHA Population Health Management Framework (PHA-PHMF), 75–78
physical health, 89
physician hospital organizations (PHOs), 185
Plan-Do-Check-Act (PDCA) cycle, 192
point-of-service (POS) plan, 185
Policy Map, 285, 288
population-based cohort study, 59
population-focused care, 8, 17
population health, 3–17
  algorithms, 154
  alliance framework, 74–79
  as an innovation, 9–11
  catalysts for health care change, 14–16
  consumer/patient issues, 11–12
  cost of care, 183
  defined, 6
  frameworks, 65–79
  health equity, 114–120
  hot spotting, 7–8
  impact of government health plans on, 181–183
  legislation, 15
  major health systems and sector issues, 12–14
  management, 8–9, 11–16, 75
  outcomes, 114–120
  performance measures, 193–194
  portfolios of strategies, 75
  practice example, 191–192
  quality improvement, 192–193
  strategies, 23, 221–246
  to improve decision-making, 140–141
  vision for communities, 69–70
population(s), defined, 1, 5–6
precision medicine, 77–79
prediabetes, 169, 172

preferred provider organizations (PPO), 185
prevalence, 56
prevention
  levels of, 95–96
primary care physician (PCP), 168
primary care provider (PCP), 208
pro and con decision-making process, 139–140
problem, defined, 263
productivity, 69
Protocol for Responding to Assessing Patient Assets, Risks, and Experiences (PRAPARE), 152
public health, 24–28
  achievements, 35–36
  analytical epidemiology, 58–60
  as a safety net, 39–40
  assessment, 34
  assurance, 34
  core functions, 34
  disease rates calculations, 55–56
  essential services, 35
  exploring epidemiology, 53–55
  health status measurement, 56–58
  Healthy People 2030, 37
  managerial epidemiology, 60–61
  policy development, 34
  population perspective, 34–40
  relationships with community and other organizations, 35
  skills, 51–61
  strategies for population health, 52–53
  tools for population health, 53–56
  transitional phases of, 53

Q

Quadruple Aim model, 69
quality
  accountability, 188–194
  domains of, 190
  improvement, 190
  performance and, 190–194
  quality of life (QOL), 31–32

R

radical collaboration, 269
reengineering, 264–266
remote home health monitoring (RHM), 237
remote patient care monitoring, 240
reorganizing, 264–266
risk, 166
risk-based options, 186
risk factors, 166, 169
risk management, 165–176
  case study, 168–173
  defined, 166–168
  personalized care and, 174–175
  strategy, 169
risk score, 169–170
risk segmentation, 170–171
  cost and benefit of, 175–176
risk stratification, 171
  grid, 171

S

self-efficacy, 134, 228
self-management education (SME), 205
self-management of chronic disease, 205–206
shared financial risk, 186
single illness, 58
social determinants of health (SDOH), 92, 105–121, 151–152, 212
  American culture, 106–109
  categories, 110
  cultural competence, 120
  health equity, 114–120
  over a lifetime, 112
  overview, 109–112
  population health outcomes, 114–120
  population health strategies for, 113
  relationship with population health outcomes, 112
  upstream/downstream parable, 113
social health, 89
social justice, 120
socio-economic model, 27
socioeconomic (SEC) factors, 92
South End Healthy Boston Coalition, 26
specific rate, 57–58

spiritual health, 89
structural racism, 120
super utilizers, 8
Surveillance, Epidemiology, and End Results (SEER), 154
sustainable development goals (SDGs), 42–43

T
telehealth, 232
transformation, 267–268
transition, 267–268
transition-of-care model, 206–207
transtheoretical model (TTM), 135–137
Triple Aim vision, 67–69

U
upstream health factors, 113
U.S. Department of Agriculture's (USDA), 24–25

V
value, 183–184
value-based care, 77–79
value-based payment options, 186–188
value over volume, 183–184
vertical integration strategies, 210–211
virtual care, 221–222, 235–245
  challenges, 244–245
  decision-making strategies, 235–238
  for 'high-tech' population health outcomes, 231–233
  framework, 236
  mobile health applications, 233–235
  technology applications, 238–244
  wearable technology, 238–242
virtual storefronts, 235
volume to a value framework, 11

W
wearable technology, 238–242
WECANDOTHIS campaign, 97
well-being, 89–92
wellness, 89–92
Wellness Council of America (WELCOA), 90
wicked problems, 255
willingness, 228
workplace health, 32–34
World Happiness Report, 32
World Health Organization (WHO), 5, 41–42
world population by broad age groups, 131

Z
Zip code, 112